HEALTH CARE IN THE UNITED STATES

Organization, Management, and Policy

HOWARD P. GREENWALD

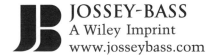
JOSSEY-BASS
A Wiley Imprint
www.josseybass.com

Published by Jossey-Bass
A Wiley Imprint
989 Market Street, San Francisco, CA 94103-1741—www.josseybass.com

Jossey-Bass books and products are available through most bookstores. To contact Jossey-Bass directly call our Customer Care Department within the U.S. at 800-956-7739, outside the U.S. at 317-572-3986, or fax 317-572-4002.

Jossey-Bass also publishes its books in a variety of electronic formats. Some content that appears in print may not be available in electronic books.

Library of Congress Cataloging-in-Publication Data has been applied for.

Printed in the United States of America
FIRST EDITION

ISBN 9780787995478
HB Printing   10 9 8 7 6 5 4 3 2 1

CONTENTS

TABLES AND FIGURES

TABLES

FIGURES

To Romalee A. Davis, MD—
Seeker, healer, teacher

PREFACE

The chapters to follow have been written as a textbook in health care management and policy. The book may serve as an introduction to problems and issues in U.S. health care for people entering related professional fields. It is also intended for use by people already experienced in a particular aspect of management or policy for attaining perspective on the system as a whole. The book will have value far beyond the classroom. Every day, large numbers of Americans become newly interested in health care management and policy for a variety of reasons. The chapters to follow constitute an introductory resource for citizens, clinicians, and officials with an emerging interest in managing or changing the system.

For no reader will the material presented here be entirely new. Without exception, everyone reading these pages will have experienced health care as a consumer. It is hoped that this book will help readers of any background see their experience as part of a large, complex, and ever-changing system. An improved view of where the reader's experience fits within this firmament will enable him to better render direct service, manage human and material resources, influence policy, and utilize health care for his own needs.

Many observations and comments in this book are based on the U.S. health care system as it was in the twenty-first century's first decade. At the end of this decade, action by the U.S. Congress envisaged sweeping changes. But even these broad measures did not address many of the basic challenges facing managers, policymakers, and clinicians. Earlier innovations hailed as system-changing in fact have had limited overall impact. The U.S. health care system has long been and remains predominantly private, decentralized, and employer-financed. These as well as certain essential characteristics of health care that prevail worldwide suggest that problems already encountered will prevail well into the future.

Present-day challenges will persist, no matter what role government plays in the U.S. health care system in the years to come or how much uniformity and regularization will be introduced into health care financing and professional practice. Throughout the world, health care is highly personal in nature, depended on for survival by many, widely viewed as a "right," and steadily increasing in cost. These basic features of health care ensure continuing controversy over access to care, quality of services, responsibility for payment, and reliability of outcomes.

For generations, critics have characterized issues facing health care in the United States as unique. Yet similar challenges occur in many other countries. The wealthy democracies of Western Europe, which all have national health plans of some kind, experience socioeconomic disparities in health and life expectancy akin those observed in the United States. Sweden, a country as strongly committed to the welfare state as any on the globe, still reports overcrowding and delay in its hospital emergency facilities, just as we see in the United States. The health care system in Canada, to which Americans have looked for generations as a model for the United States, today faces severe challenges due to increasing health care costs and deteriorating facilities and services. The problems and issues covered in this book, then, are likely to remain important in the United States for many generations.

This book is intended to help readers see their own specialized area of the health care system in the perspective of the whole. It covers a broad spectrum of health care–related subject matter, including such diverse areas as epidemiology, health behavior, the health care labor force, hospitals and ambulatory care organizations, and health care finance. The chapters to follow may not necessarily provide information that is new to specialists in the relevant area. But even for experts in a particular dimension of health care, the book will contribute to a comprehensive understanding of the system and its issues.

Within practical limits, this book attempts to be definitive and comprehensive—and to be definitive in this case requires a highly factual approach to each area addressed. Many unsupported assertions characterize management thinking and policy debate. The field of health services research, however, has produced a tremendous volume of relevant, high-quality studies. This book makes extensive use of such research.

The text attempts to be comprehensive in addressing the essential tasks of the health care system, the features of each system component, and issues relevant to the future. Truly comprehensive treatment of the U.S. health care system, however, would require many more pages than those in this volume. The more closely one examines any dimension of health care, the more complex and multifaceted it reveals itself to be.

Rather than attempting to be exhaustive, the book concentrates on matters with the broadest implications for the delivery of health services. Consistent with this approach, hospitals receive more attention than long-term care organizations or public health departments. The social and economic issues arising in long-term care are by no means unimportant. But services delivered in hospitals predominate as drivers of health care costs. Similarly, the labor supply and geographic distribution of physicians receive more attention than the supply and distribution of nurses. None would dispute the importance of the nursing profession. Physicians, however, exercise more control over the delivery process, and their decisions crucially affect health care utilization and costs.

This book is divided into three parts. Part One, The System and Its Tasks, provides an overview of the U.S. health care system's components and challenges. Chapter One addresses the characteristics and dilemmas of health care as experienced by human beings everywhere and across historical eras. The chapter points out that although health care in the United States is poorly integrated and decentralized, it is indeed a system, each of whose components is interdependent with several others. Chapter Two identifies characteristics of the U.S. health care system that distinguish it from other countries, explains why these features exist, and raises questions about the type and degree of change acceptable to U.S. citizens. Chapter Three presents a very brief summary of the field of epidemiology and the health issues that lead Americans to utilize health services. Chapter Four identifies patterns of human behavior, including individual acceptance of risks to health, that help determine both need for and utilization of health care.

Part Two addresses actual operations of the system. Chapter Five highlights the importance of formal organizations—such as ambulatory care practices, hospitals, and managed care firms—as the system's actual operating components. Chapter Six addresses the supply, demand, distribution, and management of health professionals, placing special emphasis on physicians, nurses, and health care administrators. Chapter Seven covers the ways in which Americans pay for their health care and the implications of insurance for consumer behavior and costs. Chapter Eight treats research as a sector of the health care industry with special implications for the future of health care. This chapter covers basic questions regarding the validity, usefulness, and potential misuse of research in the health field. It highlights the challenge of making decisions that are crucial for health care efficacy and cost on the basis of research findings.

Part Three examines approaches Americans have taken to improving the system, its output, and the means that will be required to put innovations into effect. Chapter Nine covers the effects of key innovations that have occurred in U.S. health care delivery over the past generation and assesses the impact of these measures. Chapter Ten addresses the contributions that prevention can make to the well-being of Americans and the control of health care costs. Chapter Eleven concentrates on government and the political process as potential agents of progress or, when misused, causes of stagnation and backsliding.

Finally, Chapter Twelve examines alternative routes that Americans have considered toward an improved health care system. This chapter pays special attention to the legislation passed by Congress at the end of the 21st century's first decade. The reader is encouraged to recall that past innovations in the U.S. health care system have neither proven uniformly successful nor provided comprehensive solutions to the system's problems. Chapter 12 concludes by highlighting past controversies that are likely to continue into the future and new ones that will almost certainly arise.

Each chapter ends with a series of discussion questions. These questions focus not on review of principles or facts appearing in the chapters, but as means of encouraging the reader to develop her own synthesis of the facts and principles. The questions are intended to serve as the basis for personal reflection and group discussion.

TO THE STUDENT

Everyone using this textbook should consider it as one of many resources that can promote an understanding the U.S. health care system. Students especially should note that any observer of this system, its operations, and its components will inevitably apply his individual experience and point of view. For this reason, students should feel encouraged to challenge material they encounter in these pages. Everyone has ample opportunity to find updated facts and competing points of view in the many specialized journals concerning health care available today and from high-quality mass media sources. Most important, students should form their own opinions and outlooks in conversation with peers.

TO THE INSTRUCTOR

Several resources will be available to instructors as companions to this textbook. These include, first, an Instructor's Manual, containing PowerPoint slides, lecture outlines, and suggested topics for class discussion. Instructors are encouraged to select materials in the Instructor's Manual that best support their own outlook on the health care field and the topics that they believe deserve the greatest emphasis.

No textbook can anticipate the character and impact of major changes at the policy level. This textbook addresses challenges and choices regarding the U.S. health care system likely to remain important far into the future. Unanticipated developments, however, are sure to occur, driven either by policy or technology.

THE AUTHOR

Howard P. Greenwald is professor of management and policy at the University of Southern California School of Policy, Planning, and Development and clinical professor at the University of Washington School of Public Health. He is a specialist in program evaluation, organizational performance, health services research, and chronic disease epidemiology. He holds a PhD in sociology from the University of California at Berkeley. He has served as a faculty member at the University of Chicago Graduate School of Business, research scientist at Battelle Memorial Institute, chairman of the Network for Healthcare Management, director of the Health Services Administration Program at the University of Southern California, and commissioner on the Accrediting Commission for Education in Health Services Administration. His current research activities include studies of innovation and effectiveness in formal organizations, the political process of policy making, long-term quality of life among cancer survivors, and outcomes of multisite interventions designed to improve the quality of life in communities. In addition to *Health Care in the United States: Organization, Management, and Policy*, he has written four other books, the most recent of which are *Organizations: Management Without Control* (Sage, 2008) and *Health For All: Making Community Collaboration Work* (Health Administration Press, 2002), with William L. Beery. He is author alone or in collaboration of approximately fifty peer-reviewed articles in journals such as the *American Journal of Evaluation*, *Journal of Clinical Epidemiology*, *American Journal of Public Health*, *Journal of Women's Health*, and *Milbank Quarterly*. His opinion pieces have appeared in the *New York Times*, the *Wall Street Journal*, and the *Sacramento Bee*.

ACKNOWLEDGMENTS

A large number of individuals have contributed directly or indirectly to the production of this book. Of the direct contributors, Martin G. Gellen and Deborah A. Dickstein deserve special thanks for reviewing draft material. Heidi Merrifield produced many of the graphic appearing in the text.

Several people deserve thanks for indirectly but materially contributing to my understanding of the health field. I wish to acknowledge the core faculty of the University of Chicago Center for Health Administration Studies, which, beginning in the mid-1970s, introduced me to the field of health administration and policy. From outstanding figures in this field, including Ronald Andersen, Odin Anderson, Theodore R. Marmor, and Selwyn W. Becker, I was privileged to receive an incredible volume of facts and an understanding of the discipline. Emory B. ("Soap") Dowell, a preeminent member of the Sacramento policy community, deserves my gratitude for many conversations regarding the politics of health care legislation. William Richardson and Doug Conrad alerted me to the importance of health insurance and finance through their writings, lectures, and informal comments. Louis P. Garrison and Suresh Malhotra helped acquaint me with the world of health economics and the sometimes tortuous methods employed by its practitioners.

Many individuals directly involved in managing systems and caring for patients have contributed to this book by talking with me about their work and allowing me to observe at their offices and clinics. I am indebted to many at the Group Health Cooperative of Puget Sound for providing direct contact with the health care industry. Bill Beery, director of Group Health Cooperative's Center for Community Health and Evaluation, has been an outstanding and forthcoming colleague. Through the Health Service Administration Program at the University of Southern California I have enjoyed the privilege of learning from highly knowledgeable students, of whom Dr. Richard Ikeda and Chris Van Gorder are only two among many. I appreciate the time taken by working epidemiologists Drs. Dennis J. Bregman and David Dassy to acquaint me with their field. Dr. Ruth McCorkle of the Yale School of Nursing has encouraged my interest and acquainted me with issues regarding chronic disease.

Jossey-Bass editors Seth Schwartz, Andy Pasternack, and Kelsey McGee have been invaluable in helping bring this project to fruition, as have the anonymous individuals from whom they obtained reviews.

Finally, I must thank the members of my family—Romalee, Phoebe, and Jared—for their patience with the writing of this book and with my other incessant preoccupations.

PART

THE SYSTEM AND ITS TASKS

Health care serves a basic human need and for this reason is one of the oldest specialized human functions. Perhaps even before the recording of history, specialized personnel in the human group acquired some degree of healing art. Imperfect understanding, and perhaps even magic and mystery, characterize healing from the layperson's point of view. Still today, the layperson views health care with varying degrees of awe, uncertainty, and suspicion. As experienced by many in the modern world, the outcomes of health care are uncertain, the cost unjustifiable, and the practitioners aloof.

The U.S. health care system shares many of the essential characteristics of health care throughout history and across the globe. But the U.S. system is unusual in the degree to which it is privately owned and operated and lacking in direction by a central authority or agency. Values central to the American mind such as belief in the private sector have helped maintain these characteristics. A belief among Americans in the right to choice and maximization of the things life has to offer also helps maintain the system as it is.

The health care system's basic tasks are to prevent and remedy illness and injury. Chronic disease represents today's principal threat to health. Diseases of this nature tend to have multiple causes, both behavioral and environmental. They require close collaboration between clinician and client for control. Because of the need for repeated treatment, such diseases tend to be expensive to care for. Recently, infectious diseases were relegated to historical accounts of epidemics and plagues. But the rise of serious pandemics such as human immunodeficiency virus (HIV) and H1N1 influenza have given infectious disease renewed currency.

Utilization of health services, and to some extent health itself, is an outcome of human behavior. Individual human beings vary significantly in the taking of health risks. Similarly, people differ in their perceptions and acceptance of illness. Demographic factors strongly influence the tendency of people to seek health care even when they perceive the need. The health care system's tasks include development of cultural competence and health literacy as means of providing quality care.

CHAPTER

1

UNDERSTANDING HEALTH CARE

LEARNING OBJECTIVES

- To obtain an overview of health care as a concern in the U.S. and worldwide
- To appreciate the challenges experienced by health care consumers and providers
- To identify objectives and goals for heath care
- To highlight the importance of public trust and professional ethics
- To frame health care issues within three perspectives: a systems approach, critical thinking, and the public interest

HEALTH CARE AS A NATIONAL CONCERN

Health and health care are subjects in which everyone has an interest. When young mothers get together, talk soon turns to the health of their children. In search of health, men and women of all ages work out at the gym. Among elders, conversation inevitably involves aches, pains, and the merits and shortcomings of their physicians. Health and health care periodically become major election issues. But acute concern for health, health care, and associated costs are only a step away from each individual, who, if he has no direct concerns, almost always has a friend, relative, or neighbor in need of care.

Health care in the United States is arguably the best in the world, and much evidence suggests that the health of Americans is today the best it has ever been. Only a few examples can convince most people that this is true. Children with leukemia, whose illness amounted to a death sentence only a generation ago, now often survive to live normal lives. Elders who at one time would have been confined to wheelchairs and nursing homes now live active, independent lives thanks to procedures such as cataract surgery and hip transplants. Effective drugs and widely available surgery are chipping away at heart disease, for generations America's leading cause of death. AIDS is now often controllable, whereas at a time still well remembered it invariably led to a miserable death. Life expectancy in the United States has steadily increased, from 69.6 years in 1955 to 75.8 years in 1995, and to 77.9 years in 2005.[1]

Health care, however, has become a major source of dissatisfaction and controversy in the United States. A challenge affecting the United States as a whole, and Americans as individuals, is that of cost. As Figure 1.1 indicates, the cost of health care increased markedly during the late twentieth and early twenty-first centuries. Despite public policy aimed at controlling costs, the upward trend appeared to be accelerating as the twenty-first century began.

Figure 1.1 takes on added significance when viewed alongside changes in the health insurance available to the American public. Most of the dollars paid for health care come from health insurance of some kind. As recently as the late 1970s, large numbers of Americans paid nothing out of pocket for their health care. Hardly anyone today enjoys such generosity. Now, both private and public insurers continuously seek ways to reduce insurance coverage for individuals. Not only are health care costs higher today, but Americans are more likely to have to pay them out of pocket.

The cost of health care has raised significant concern on many levels. Employers complain that high employee health care costs have strangled international competitiveness. Recipients of health care feel increasingly uncomfortable about increases in out-of-pocket expenses. Some researchers have reported that health care costs contribute to a majority of personal bankruptcies in the United States.[2] Programs that provide health care to the elderly and poor consumed a percentage of the federal budget far in excess of defense. Because of their responsibility to provide health care to the poor under Medicaid, individual states have experienced severe fiscal stress, forcing some to cut infrastructure maintenance and education to meet their health care obligations.[3]

FIGURE 1.1   *Growth in the cost of health care in the United States, 1960–2005*

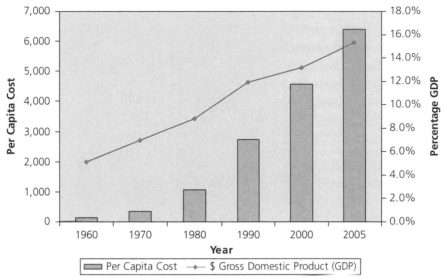

Source: National Center for Health Statistics. 2009. *Health, United States, 2008.* Table 123. Hyattsville, MD: National Center for Health Statistics.

Often, the text to follow uses the term *consumer* in preference to *patient*, the traditional designation of a seeker or user of health services. The term **consumer** recognize the health care user as someone capable of making free choices and exercising economic power. Traditionally, the term **patient** has signified a suffering, dependent individual.

The economic downturns of the early twenty-first century sharpened the issue of health care costs for many individual Americans. At that time, a majority of Americans received health insurance through their employers or those of their parents or spouses. But by 2009 it was estimated that 3.7 million working-age Americans had lost their health care coverage as a result of unemployment.[4] Millions more, though still employed, worried that they might lose their health insurance if the economy continued to slide.

Despite the resources allocated to health care in the United States, observers have expressed doubts regarding the value Americans get in return. Although the United States ranks highest in the world in per capita expenditures, it has an infant mortality rate higher than most other wealthy industrialized countries. Singapore, the top-ranked country in preventing infant mortality, recorded two infant deaths per 1,000 live births in 2004; the United States recorded 6.8.[5] In 2003, the United States ranked sixteenth in life expectancy worldwide.[6]

Concern over the quality of services received by the public is growing. A great deal of attention has focused on patient safety. A highly influential 1999 report by the Institute of Medicine estimated that between 44,000 and 98,000 Americans die each year due to preventable medical error. According to the report, more people die from such error than from motor vehicle accidents, breast cancer, or AIDS. The authors estimated total national costs (lost income, lost household production, disability, and health care costs) of preventable adverse events (medical errors resulting in injury) to be between $17 billion and $29 billion. The expense of additional health care required by the victims of medical error accounted for over half the total. In the opinion of the report's authors, health care is a decade or more behind other high-risk industries (such as aviation) in its attention to ensuring basic safety. Medication errors alone are estimated to account for over seven thousand deaths annually.[7]

The quality debate has also addressed the basic efficacy of medical procedures.[8] Strong scientific substantiation is lacking for many interventions widely used in medicine today. Consequently, patients do not always receive the most effective treatments available and may receive treatments that are ineffective or whose adverse side effects outweigh beneficial ones. Awareness of this problem has led to a movement called *evidence-based medicine,* whose goal is to develop standards of care validated through both new research and synthesis of existing studies.

Great variability has been reported in both the cost and content of medical care across geographical areas, suggesting the absence of accepted standards of care. As recently as the late 1990s researchers reported that appropriate application of scientific evidence in practice occurred only 54 percent of the time.[9] According to one observer, "most clinicians' practices do not reflect the principles of evidence-based medicine but rather . . . tradition, their most recent experience, what they learned years ago in medical school or what they have heard from their friends."[10]

Recently, health care in the United States has come under increasing criticism owing to issues of social justice. The health care system serves the nation unevenly. Inequality prevails among racial groups and economic strata in use of health services, health status, and life expectancy. People who earn high incomes, have advanced education, and are nonminorities tend to use more services, have better health status, and live longer than their less advantaged counterparts.

Table 1.1 provides an illustration of this disparity. Male African Americans have a higher mortality rate than men of any race. Women in all racial groups have lower death rates than men. But within both gender categories, people who have not graduated from high school (less than twelve years of education) have death rates roughly three times that of people with one or more years of college (thirteen or more years of education).

The differences in death rates apparent in Table 1.1 are mirrored by other indicators of well-being (or lack thereof). Similar disparities are apparent in infant mortality, likelihood of death in diseases such as cancer, and disability due to illness. Although researchers and social critics have increased their attention to these facts, public programs in the United States have long made major commitments to care for the disadvantaged. The disparities evident in Table 1.1 suggest that the billions of government and private dollars allocated to care for the poor have not yet produced the desired results.

TABLE 1.1   **Age-adjusted deaths per 100,000 U.S. residents, by gender, race, and education**

	Gender		
	Male	Female	Both
All	994.3	706.2	832.7
Race			
African American	1,319.1	885.6	1,065.9
Caucasian[a]	984.0	702.1	826.1
Asian	562.7	392.7	465.7
Latino or Hispanic	748.1	515.8	621.2
Native American	797.0	592.1	685.0
Years of education			
Less than 12	826.8	496.8	669.9
12	650.9	349.4	490.9
13 or more	252.5	171.0	211.7

[a]Excluding Latino or Hispanic.

Source: National Center for Health Statistics. 2006. *Health, United States, 2005.* Tables 29, 34, and 35. Hyattsville, MD: National Center for Health Statistics.

The issues raised here merit the serious concern of Americans. The paradox of abundant resources alongside unmet needs in the United States is striking. Basic problems in health care do not result simply from conditions that prevail in the United States. Many challenges and dilemmas regarding the objectives and delivery of health care are universal and timeless. Although many of these challenges may never be resolved, effective management and policy can do much to ensure greater benefit from health care for individuals and society as a whole.

HEALTH CARE OBJECTIVES AND GOALS

An understanding of health care requires examination of both objectives and goals. **Objectives** are short-term, measurable, and often individual in scope. **Goals** represent broad aspirations for the future, reflecting the well-being of an entire nation or society. Recognizable goals are necessary for assessing performance of any system as a whole.

Most objectives sought by consumers of health care are obvious. These include prevention of illness, relief of symptoms, restoration of function, and extension of life. Beyond these basics, though, people today seek a wide variety of health care objectives that are relatively new. Many who are biologically normal, for example, desire to improve how they look, feel, and relate to others, and look to health care for solutions. The popularity of cosmetic surgery and lifestyle-enhancing medication illustrates this development.

Objectives proposed for health care include some that are far beyond the traditional concerns of doctors and healers. Physicians today are legally required to report evidence of child, spouse, or elder abuse. Doctors crusade against youth violence in the name of protecting individuals' health. On a global scale, physician organizations have taken stands to reduce the threat of nuclear war, characterizing such action as "the ultimate form of preventive medicine."[11]

Goals of health care depend on fulfillment of a multitude of objectives, but go beyond any of those specified above. A goal of extreme breadth is implicit in the conception of health adopted by the World Health Organization (WHO), a unit of the United Nations. According to this conception, health is characterized as "a state of complete physical, mental and social well-being, not merely the absence of disease or infirmity."[12] Although this conception was formulated in 1947, it is still widely cited today.

An equally ambitious, though more concrete, goal of health care is the *rectangularization of survival.*[13] This concept refers to concentration of deaths in a population within a particular age range, presumably one approaching the natural limitation of the human lifespan. Under such a scenario, nearly everyone might live to a particular age (perhaps eighty, ninety, or one hundred years) and die rapidly thereafter.

Figure 1.2 illustrates a trend toward rectangularization of survival among U.S. women between 1900 and 1995. This graph indicates a decreasing probability of survival with every passing year in 1900, but a steady rate of survival until about age sixty in 1995. Thus, the 1995 survival curve begins to look like a rectangle. Were the trend to continue over the following century, the 2100 curve, it might be speculated, would fall off even more sharply at some natural limit. In a variation on the rectangularization concept, the goal of a health care system might be maintenance of a "wellness span," to a point where nearly everyone remained fully functional until a particular and very old age.

Both the WHO-inspired goal for health care and the rectangularization of survival present practical difficulties. Neither lends itself to straightforward measurement of progress. Documentation of "complete physical, mental, and social well-being" would require assessment of numerous features of the lives of a multitude of individuals. Though more readily expressed as numbers, rectangularization of survival is no less

FIGURE 1.2 *Survival curves by age for U.S. women in 1900 and 1995*

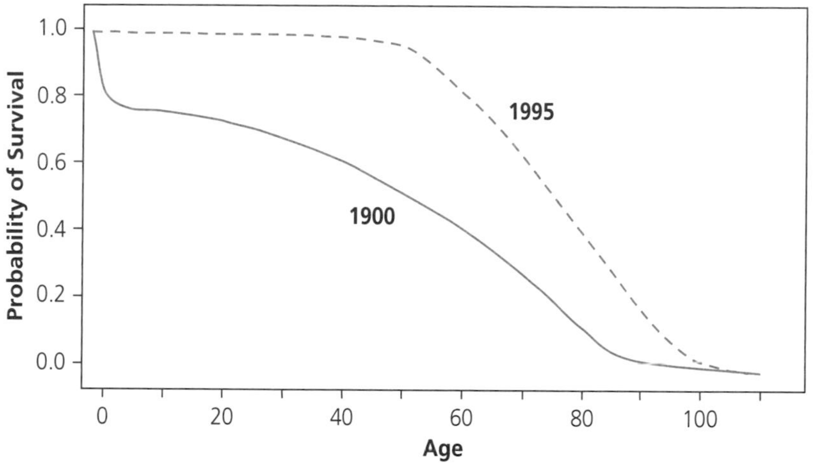

Source: Wilmoth JR, Horiuchi S. Rectangularization revisited: variability of age at death within human populations. *Demography.* 1999;36(4):475–495. Table 1.c.

definitively measured. Scientists do not agree that there is a natural limit to human life. According to some, there is little evidence that achievable human life expectancy, having increased steadily over the past century, is reaching a limit.[14]

Though important for assessing progress, widely acceptable goals are difficult to both formulate and measure. In addition, pursuit of individual objectives may undermine achievement of overarching goals. Effective treatment of chronic, heritable diseases—diabetes and certain kidney ailments, for example—increases the presence of people with such conditions in today's population and in generations to come. Antibiotics may provide prompt relief of pain from minor infections, but limit the remedies available to the seriously injured due to development of antibiotic-resistant pathogens. The goal of health care cost containment is widely endorsed in the United States. But denial of potentially useful services for reasons of cost is strongly resisted by those whose individual service needs are affected.

ESSENTIAL CHALLENGES IN HEALTH CARE

As suggested earlier, health care involves features that create challenges and dilemmas wherever it is practiced. Health care directly involves the client's body; she cannot walk away from the health care provider as readily as from a provider of other goods and services. Health care addresses the most profound of human experiences, including pain, suffering, life, and death. Across national boundaries and through the ages, healers have held special but not entirely honored status in society. As consumers, the sick seldom seem entirely satisfied. On several dimensions, tension and dissatisfaction may be universal.

Negative Demand

It is safe to say that few, if any, individuals *desire* health care in the normal sense. Except possibly for hypochondriacs, no one *wants* to see a physician or be admitted to a hospital. Even when people get sick, most would prefer to treat themselves or hope the illness would resolve on its own. People seek care—however negatively they may view it—when they feel they have no choice. In this respect, obtaining health care resembles the purchase of a casket for a deceased loved one or coughing up tuition for the feared finance or accounting course required for a management degree.

In consequence, consumers are often predisposed to viewing their encounters with health care providers and organizations negatively. The wait time at a doctor's office is experienced as more onerous than a similar delay for a table at a fine restaurant. Reasonable fees may be viewed as exorbitant. Paradoxically, some consumers seem to enjoy complaining about their health care. These individuals thus obtain some emotionally positive returns from what they perceive as a negative encounter with the system.

Uncertain Costs

Traditionally, charges to consumers are more variable in health care than they are in other areas of trade. For centuries physicians have accepted payment on a sliding scale dependent on the consumer's resources. In nineteenth-century literature, the husband of Madame Bovary, a physician, receives payment in gold from a wealthy patient, but forgets to collect the meager debts owed him by the common people. In the mid-twentieth century, physicians in the United States expected that a goodly proportion of their bills would never be paid. Traditionally, hospital administrators have referred to their receivables as *spongy*—never fully solid in terms of eventual collectability. Well into the late twentieth century, health care managers practiced various forms of *cost shifting,* in which higher charges to well-insured patients were used to subsidize lower receipts from the poorly insured, uninsured, and indigent.

It is no accident, then, that payment for health care is viewed by the public as less obligatory than payment for nonhealth goods and services. Many consumers feel a sense of entitlement to health care. A bill is seldom paid entirely out of pocket. Few patients ask a doctor how much a procedure will cost or shop for the lowest-priced practitioner. An unpaid medical bill represents less liability to the consumer than a neglected car payment—repossession of items such as pacemakers and prostheses takes place rarely if at all.

Unpredictable Outcomes

An essential unpredictability prevails in much of health care. Many standard interventions, preventive or curative, are available for a wide range of frequently encountered diseases. But the human organism is variable, and many factors—both internal and external to the individual—contribute to resistance versus expression of disease. In some cases, diagnosis is complex and inconclusive, adding to uncertainty of cure. In instances where diagnosis is evasive, physicians may treat a suspected disease in hopes that diagnosis and treatment will be accomplished in the same step.

Uncertainty of success accompanies many treatments for cancer and other chronic diseases. Standard chemotherapy and radiation protocols cure some patients and not others. Trials of new interventions are, from the patient perspective, instances of chance taking. A physician can honestly tell his patient that there are no guarantees.

Whether associated with mild or life-threatening illness, uncertainty differentiates health care from other goods and services. On the patient level, uncertainty may raise issues of trust in the provider's capability. Uncertainty may be humbling for the provider. But acknowledgment of uncertainty underscores an essential element of clinical practice. No two cases are identical. Good medicine cannot be practiced cookbook-fashion.

An Evasive Diagnosis

Baffling even the most experienced physicians at a university medical center, the case of a nine-year-old girl illustrates the evasiveness of clinical success. For six months, the patient had been chronically nauseated, vomiting, unable to eat, and losing weight. Extensive blood work and imaging failed to detect intestinal obstruction, lactose intolerance, and the autoimmune syndrome Crohn's disease. Thinking they had ruled out gastroenterological causes, doctors considered the possibility of a brain tumor and ordered an MRI.

The evening before the scheduled MRI, a family practice intern examined the girl. He examined the girl's hands—eating disorders are often revealed by calluses caused by chronic self-induced vomiting—and, finding no calluses, ruled out an eating disorder. Although there were no calluses, the intern noticed a darkening of the skin. Darkened skin can be a clue for Addison's disease, an adrenal gland disorder. Measures were taken of sodium, potassium, glucose, and cortisol, which, abnormally low, confirmed Addison's disease as the correct diagnosis.

Low levels of sodium, potassium, and glucose had been detected earlier. But other features of the girl's illness seemed to explain the low concentration of these blood chemicals, and the possibility of Addison's disease was not pursued. A simple observation of darkened skin led a physician still in training to make a diagnosis that had stumped others for months. Within hours of starting treatment for Addison's disease, the patient began to recover.[15]

Emotional Involvement

Health care is often given and received in an atmosphere inflamed by human emotion. Anxiety and fear follow hard upon injury, illness, and the possibility of death. Medical uncertainty—along with the ever-present possibility of failure—fosters disappointment, frustration, and anger at health professionals and institutions. The role of patient is the most powerless that many people ever experience. A story is told by a distinguished obstetrician about President John F. Kennedy watching as doctors struggled to successfully deliver his son. Even the most powerful man in the world could do nothing but watch in this situation.

In few, if any, societies, then, do people live in complete comfort alongside those who treat their illnesses. The uncertainty of success, unpredictability of cost, aloofness of providers, and emotional overlay—along with the fact that few, if any, individuals desire to be patients—inevitably promote fault finding. An essential discomfort with medicine throughout the ages is evident in mythology and literature as early as ancient Greece. Century after century, storytellers and commentators have connected health care with excessive expense, inexcusable error, calculated self-interest, and potential injury.[16]

Aloof Providers

In contrast to the emotional involvement of patients is a seeming aloofness of medical professionals. Many patients perceive emotional detachment on the part of their providers, particularly physicians. Researchers report that low-income and minority patients are most likely to sense absence of a caring attitude on the part of their providers.[17] A vast gulf in income, education, and privilege is evident between physicians and most patients.

Some aloofness, however, may be necessary for clinical practice. Even a practitioner who is skilled at communicating and emotionally secure requires a degree of detachment from the challenges facing her patients. According to one physician, factors conducive to detachment include fear of adverse outcomes and consequent criticism, and "an instinct to separate oneself from another's suffering."[18] Training and mutual support within a closed community of peers helps the practitioner accommodate the emotional challenges encountered in practice.

Health professionals of all types receive privileges and responsibilities allocated to few others. Practitioners are allowed to see patients naked, ask personal questions, pierce flesh with needles, and insert hands into bodies through surgical openings. The symbolism and ritual of medicine, still represented today by the snakes and staff of the caduceus, help maintain the provider's paradoxical combination of presence and absence.

Challenges on the Front Lines

Like consumers, people in the health care industry experience confusion, frustration, anger, and feelings of powerlessness. Those at the front lines most directly experience the impact of increasing demands, limitations on resources, and challenges raised by advances in biomedical science. Following are some examples:

Reacting to a reduction of compensation under the federal Medicare program, a Brooklyn physician commented, "My expenses go up and up and up every year. For the government to lower what it pays me when my expenses are rising—that doesn't make sense. It's an insult."

Also commenting on Medicare compensation changes, a doctor in Texas asserted, "I have a hard-and-fast rule. I don't take any new Medicare patients. In fact, I don't take any new patients over the age of sixty because they will be on Medicare in the next five years."[19]

Rationing, or withholding potentially useful services because of resource constraints, is a reality today. Clinicians and managers at the University of Texas Medical Branch (UTMB) must choose which indigent patients may receive potentially lifesaving care for cancer. UTMB uses a detailed playbook to help determine who gets treated and who doesn't.[20] Following are more examples in a similar vein:

Despite a federal law prohibiting patient dumping, a Chattanooga hospital dispatcher told an ambulance crew not to bring in an unconscious man found in a poor neighborhood to the hospital because, he said, the administrator "would kill us if we took another indigent."[21]

A change in federal policy regarding lung transplantation brought grievous reactions from patients moved from high to low priority. "We tried our best to educate and communicate, but many felt they had been cheated," recalls the director of a university transplantation program.[22]

PUBLIC TRUST AND PROFESSIONAL ETHICS

As suggested earlier in this chapter, health care everywhere involves elements of detachment and mystique. Consistent with the uncertainty of diagnosis and cure is an essential independence of health care providers, particularly physicians. This independence is justifiable on technical grounds. Because of the uniqueness of each case, only a large fund of knowledge and experience enables the provider to recognize the range of possibilities that may be involved. The variability in the ways that human illnesses manifest themselves and respond to treatment precludes development of formulas—or so physicians have long argued.

Still, good health care requires partnership between providers and the public. Trust constitutes a key element of this partnership—and trust depends on a widespread belief that principles of honest public service prevail in health care. Patients must feel confident in the trustworthiness of their providers to seek care, reveal sensitive information, submit to treatment, or participate in research.[23] Trust is also crucial for the operation of health care at a societywide level. Citizens will support expenditures for programs such as research and indigent care only if they believe that human beings will benefit and funds will be used appropriately.

Means of ensuring trustworthiness in the health care industry include government oversight and professional ethics. From the point of view of many in the industry, codes of ethics established by peers are a preferred means. **Ethics** may be thought of as obligations of an individual to act toward others in a manner consistent with socially reinforced values. Widely accepted principles of health care ethics include duties to help all patients in need, maintain the confidentiality of any information obtained, obtain informed consent for procedures used, avoid conflicts of interest, and apply medical skills and technology only in a competent and appropriate manner.[24]

As with other matters addressed in this chapter, resolution of issues in health care ethics is often not straightforward. Deliberately or consciously unethical behavior is rare in health care. But clinicians and managers often encounter issues that cannot be resolved via formula and whose resolution, whatever it may be, is subject to criticism. Refusal of care, examples of which were cited earlier (see box titled Challenges on the Front Lines), may be seen as unethical; however, such refusal may be necessary to preserve the operation of a health care unit. The principle of confidentiality would seem inviolate. But the need to protect the public from harm via disclosure of hazards represented by a patient's positive HIV status or homicidal intent may contradict the confidentiality mandate.

The lack of certainty in medicine itself creates ethical challenges, as the following example illustrates:

> A physician believes a course of chemotherapy using a newly licensed agent may benefit a desperately ill cancer patient. Other doctors of equal competence may consider such treatment to be of marginal value to patients with this malignancy and presumably so close to death. The physician orders the chemotherapy; the patient experiences discomfort due to the treatment and dies soon thereafter. The doctor submits a bill and receives payment.

Multiple ethical issues may be seen in this episode. Treatment with the new chemotherapeutic agent might be viewed as misapplication of medicine because it caused discomfort and ultimately failed to extend life. Some might charge that the physician's ordering of a newly developed treatment was inappropriate. The indications for newly licensed pharmaceuticals are often revised as experience is accumulated. Yet the patient and her family may have requested aggressive intervention. Since the physician will ultimately receive payment, conflict of interest may be suspected. Multiple motivations and trade-offs are made in situations such as the one described here. As in other domains of life, it may be impossible to determine whether or not an ethical transgression has occurred.

THREE PERSPECTIVES ON MANAGEMENT AND POLICY

The issues raised in this chapter are likely to appear wherever health care is practiced. Some will likely remain important in the United States, even if the mechanisms of financing and delivery fundamentally change. Practitioners involved in the delivery of health services will continue to deal with intractable dilemmas and irresolvable public debates. Within these limits, the United States can achieve maximum benefit from its investment in health care through effective management and policy. Both high-quality management and policy require a broad and accurate understanding of health care as an industry and its relationship to the society it serves. Three perspectives are presented next as tools for achieving such understanding.

A Systems Approach

A systems approach views the situation of an individual—whether a consumer, a manager, or a policy maker—in terms of his connection to the multiple and interrelated components involved in health services delivery today. Health care delivered to a single individual is the joint product of numerous individuals, organizations, and institutions. Administration of a single dose of medication, for example, is made possible only by the participation of numerous entities and individuals: the medical school at which the basic science needed to produce the drug was developed, the private foundation or government agency that funded the medical school's research, the pharmaceutical firm that produces the drug, the physician who prescribes the medication, and the technician who administers the dose.

The systems approach involves realities outside the medical field itself. Consumers must be motivated to spend money on health care. A favorable political and economic environment is required for health-related goods and services to be provided. Congressional action (often spurred by interest groups and lobbyists) may be needed to fund research agencies. Capital markets have to be sufficiently generous to enable the pharmaceutical firm to develop and test a drug. A climate of public opinion sympathetic to science is needed to permit research to take place involving human beings, animals, or cell lines of human origin. For the patient to ultimately thrive, a safe and healthful physical and social environment is essential.

The importance of a systems approach for understanding health care issues increased in the last decades of the twentieth century. In earlier generations, participants in the health care system could work in substantial isolation. Today, however, a physician ordering blood must take the blood bank's costs and safety assurances into consideration. A nursing supervisor must understand telemetry and the structuring of liability insurance. A hospital administrator must understand capital markets.

According to some observers, the United States does not have an actual health care *system*. These observers have argued that many parts of the system work at cross-purposes. Hospitals and insurance companies, for example, are viewed as adversaries, at best communicating inefficiently with each other. Acknowledging the absence of a tightly run system, this text interchangeably uses the terms *health care system* and *health care industry.*

However, it makes sense to think of health care in the United States as a *poorly integrated system.* Patients do move from community physicians to specialists, though often with delay. Physicians do receive insurance payments, although hassles may occur along the way. Newly trained health professionals do receive an education that enables them to help patients, although the relevance of some of their educational requirements may be difficult to establish. Figure 1.3 illustrates an array of organizations, institutions, and individuals whose actions ultimately produce what is needed in health care, but connection, communication, and coordination among the units are far from perfect.

Critical Thinking

Critical thinking reflects the perspective under which people question assertions made by others—peers, "experts," or administrative and political superiors. A perspective of this kind is particularly important in health care for a number of reasons. As closely as health care is tied to emotional and economic interests, ill-conceived and self-interested recommendations are likely to abound. A consultant with a new system for managing information in a hospital gains financially from adoption of that plan, just as does a physician advocating for a procedure in which she excels or a pharmaceutical

FIGURE 1.3   *U.S. health care (greatly simplified): an imperfectly integrated system*

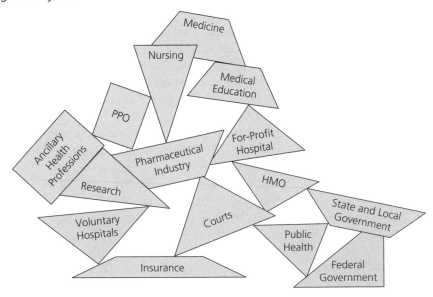

company promoting a new medication. An organization lobbying for increased research funding for a specific disease claims that the entire public is at risk, directly or indirectly, from its consequences.

The history of health policy in the United States illustrates the importance of critical thinking. **Policy** can be thought of as an approach taken by government in response to a public concern. Many vigorously promoted policies and innovations regarding health care have been adopted, only to be found less effective than first hoped or abandoned when the political climate changed. Examples of concepts whose popularity has come and gone (or at least dropped from the policy discussion) include regional health planning and public support for health maintenance organizations. It is important for leaders in health care management and policy not to let themselves get swept up in the passions of the moment.

The Public Interest

A third perspective important for today's health care leadership is that of the public interest. This term refers to the relevance of health care far beyond those directly involved as provider and recipient. Because it affects the quality of the labor force and thus the performance of the overall economy, health itself has implications for society as a whole. The general quality of life in a society is marked by the health of its members. The truth of this statement is easy to grasp by the experience of an individual from a rich country traveling in a poor one. The traveler, for perhaps the first time in his life, is likely to regularly observe people with missing teeth, clouded eyes, club feet, and open lesions.

Health care should be recognized as a *public good.* No individual, profession, or agency can claim "ownership" of health care. Medical education enjoys large public subsidies in the form of tax mitigation for universities and hospitals, as well as direct aid through guaranteed loans to students and grants to faculty. Much biomedical research is supported by government or foundations, which in turn receive direct or indirect support by the public. Service by patients as teaching cases or experimental subjects also constitutes a contribution to the health care enterprise.

Everyone is ultimately a consumer of health care. Thus, everyone has an interest in availability, quality, and affordability of health care. No matter what system a society uses to allocate health care, it more closely resembles publicly recognized necessities such as drinking water and police services than discretionary items such as automobiles, clothing, or ice cream.

KEY TERMS

Objectives	Patient
Goals	Ethics
Consumer	Policy

SUMMARY

This chapter provides a basic framework for understanding health care and taking action toward its improvement.

Health care is an issue of concern for people everywhere, particularly in the United States. U.S. health professionals are arguably the world's best trained, and U.S. health care technology is the world's most advanced. Health care in the United States is also the world's most expensive, said to bankrupt American households and hamper America's economic competitiveness. Health care is difficult to obtain or prohibitively expensive for millions. For many, the health care system seems inaccessible, culturally hostile, and emotionally cold. Many solutions have been proposed and several important ones implemented. However, none has proven sufficient.

This chapter emphasizes several themes to promote a broad-based and accurate understanding of health care. As advanced by statespersons and scientists, the goals of health care reflect large-scale social aspirations. But objectives of actual services focus on individual and immediate needs. Health care requires a balance between independence of providers and their acceptance of social obligations as manifested in public expectations and professional ethics.

This book aims at promoting effective action in developing and operating a health care system that serves Americans well. Three principles are proposed for achieving this goal: (1) seeing individual roles, interactions, and institutions in health care as parts of a broader *system;* (2) taking *a critical approach* to widely shared views among policy makers and the public; and (3) viewing health care as linked inextricably with the *public interest.*

DISCUSSION QUESTIONS

1. Making your best guess, would you say that health care today seems less "mystical" to the average consumer than it did in the Neolithic world? In medieval times? One hundred years ago?

2. How much more predictable are the outcomes of health care likely to become in the future than they are today?

3. African American men have an age-adjusted death rate over four times that of Asian American females. How much of this disparity can be explained by differences in the health care the two groups receive?

4. Should control of costs be adopted as the principal goal of the U.S. health care system at this time? Explain why or why not.

5. How widespread do you believe ethical transgressions in health care are today? In which segment of the industry are they most likely to occur?

CHAPTER

2

THE U.S. HEALTH CARE SYSTEM

Features, Development, and Controversies

LEARNING OBJECTIVES

- To understand the basic features of the U.S. health care system and its development
- To emphasize how the U.S. health care system differs from systems elsewhere
- To learn how the health care system in the United States fits with and has been influenced by the country's values and traditions
- To appreciate the system's level of acceptance among Americans
- To specify major issues facing Americans regarding health care

THE U.S. HEALTH CARE SYSTEM'S MAGNITUDE

The most striking feature of the U.S. health care industry is its size. By 2007, total expenditures for health care in the United States exceeded $7,000 per person and topped 16 percent of gross domestic product (GDP). The total national outlay for health services in the United States approximated $2.2 trillion.[1] This figure exceeded the entire GDP of every country in the world except China, Japan, India, and Germany.[2] The United States spent more for health care than the value of all goods and services produced in such countries as the United Kingdom (U.K.), Russia, and France.

Health care constitutes a major source of employment in the United States. By the twenty-first century's first decade, health care employed nearly 15 million individuals—over 10 percent of the U.S. labor force. Included in this total during 2006 were about 2.4 million registered nurses; 1.4 million nursing aides, orderlies, and attendants; 921,000 physicians; 720,000 licensed practical nurses and licensed vocational nurses; and 240,000 pharmacists.[3] Health care personnel saw patients in physician office settings 964 million times and made 34.9 million admissions to hospitals. U.S. pharmacists filled 2.4 billion drug prescriptions or medication orders.[4]

UNIQUENESS OF THE SYSTEM

Chapter One emphasized the potentially universal features of health care. But the health care industry in the United States is distinct from those in the rest of the industrialized world in several respects. The distinguishing features of the U.S. health care system may become less prominent in the years to come. For the immediate future, however, they represent the reality with which management and policy must deal. The private sector is more important to health care in the United States than it is elsewhere. In comparison with most systems, health care in the United States is less centralized and integrated. The U.S. health care system is newer in some respects than Europe's systems, and it continues to evolve.

Dominance of the Private Sector

Newcomers to the United States are often surprised that the U.S. health care system is predominantly *private*. Unlike most other countries, hospitals are privately owned. Of 5,747 hospitals operating in the United States in 2006, 3,808 were private, either nonprofit or for-profit.[5] In the United States, most physicians work as members of private partnerships or corporations or as independent professionals. Even those who work for hospitals or managed care plans do so predominantly as contractors, rather than employees. The majority of dollars charged for health care are remitted by private insurance companies or collected directly from the pockets of individual consumers. In 2006, 54.7 percent of all health care dollars were paid by private insurance, out of pocket by consumers, or other private dollars.[6]

The private sector in the United States conducts a great deal of health-related activity beyond direct provision of health services. Health insurance used by employed individuals is purchased by their employers from private firms. Government programs themselves are operated in part by the private sector. Private firms known as *fiscal intermediaries* provide interface between public health care programs and the hospitals and doctors receiving payment under them. Like other potential private contractors, firms compete with each other to be selected as fiscal intermediaries. Firms such as Mutual of Omaha, Blue Cross, and Blue Shield process claims on behalf of the Centers for Medicare and Medicaid Services (CMS), the federal agency responsible for Medicare and Medicaid.

Other examples of the private sector's dominance include organizations concerned with maintaining professional standards and quality in the health care industry. These include most prominently **The Joint Commission**, formerly the Joint Commission on Accreditation of Healthcare Organizations, or JCAHO. CMS recognizes Joint Commission accreditation as a requirement for hospitals' participation in the Medicare and Medicaid programs, a crucial line of business for most. Joint Commission policy is made with the participation of five corporate members representing hospital-oriented interests in the health care industry. These include the American College of Physicians, the American College of Surgeons, the American Dental Association, the American Hospital Association, and the American Medical Association, all private-sector organizations. In addition to hospitals, The Joint Commission evaluates and accredits home health agencies, hospices, nursing homes, rehabilitation centers, and independent laboratories.

Another private agency involved in quality assurance on behalf of health care purchasers and the public is the National Committee for Quality Assurance (NCQA). A private, nonprofit organization, NCQA reviews, accredits, and certifies managed care organizations, utilization review organizations, and several additional types of health care organizations. In making accreditation and certification decisions, NCQA applies capacity-related criteria, such as physician credentialing review, and outcome measures, such as health risk reduction and patient satisfaction. NCQA maintains the Healthcare Effectiveness Data and Information Set (HEDIS), widely used in industry to assess the quality of care in employee health plans. HEDIS measures address areas such as asthma medication, hypertension control, antidepressant medication, and smoking cessation. As with The Joint Commission, NCQA offers a range of commercial products to help health plans prepare for accreditation procedures. On a proprietary basis, NCQA offers health plan reports on peer health care organizations. Through a process known as *benchmarking*, the recipient organizations are expected to work toward performance at the level of the highest-scoring plans.

Yet another instance of the private sector's importance is visible in biomedical research. For 2009, officials of the National Institutes of Health (NIH) asked Congress for a budget allocation of $29.5 billion, a figure supplemented later by funds from the 2009 Recovery Act. Most of these funds were spent to support research outside NIH, under what is known as the *extramural research program.* NIH distributes approximately 85 percent of its budget to outside organizations in the form of grants, contracts, cooperative agreements, and training support. The majority of NIH's extramural support goes to colleges and universities, many of which are private nonprofit organizations. In 2005, two of the three universities that had received the most funding, Johns

Hopkins and the University of Pennsylvania, were private. Johns Hopkins received over $449,000,000 and the University of Pennsylvania over $399,000,000.[7]

Multiple Subsystems

No single financing arrangement or means of providing care dominates in the United States. A variety of subsystems provide care for different segments of the population. Division into these subsystems reflects the imperfect integration that characterizes health care in the United States. Potential segregation of consumers within individual subsystems raise questions about adequacy of services provided by each.

Subsystems and Populations Served. Table 2.1 summarizes basic characteristics of each subsystem and the primary population it serves. Two of the subsystems utilize privately owned facilities, are privately operated and staffed, and are funded primarily from private sources. These subsystems, which serve a majority of Americans, include private *fee-for-service* and private *managed care.*

Unrestricted fee-for-service care provides consumers with the most choice. Individuals receiving private fee-for-service care are free to obtain services from the professional or facility of their choice. Payment is made according to charges for each encounter between consumer and provider. Evidence suggests that relatively older, wealthier, and Caucasian consumers are drawn to such plans despite their higher costs.[8]

Private managed care plans today serve a majority of Americans. Much will be said about managed care in later chapters. For now, it is sufficient to understand **managed care** as an arrangement under which *an administrative structure is placed between provider and consumer to regulate expenditure of resources.* Although individuals may pay for fee-for-service care out of pocket, managed care is always linked to a health insurance plan for which an individual or his employer has prepaid. Traditionally, managed care plans have paid only for services provided by health professionals employed by or contracting with the managed care organization (MCO). More recent managed care innovations have covered services provided by larger panels of providers and offered partial coverage for services by providers outside these panels.

A variety of public programs serve specific segments of the U.S. population. **Medicare** finances health care for the elderly and some others, paying primarily private providers to deliver actual services. The Department of Veterans Affairs (VA), which operates hundreds of facilities throughout the United States, serves veterans with service-connected disorders and in some instances other complaints. An agency known as *Tricare* serves military dependents and civilian employees of the armed services. The Indian Health Service (IHS) provides care to Native Americans and Alaska Natives. **Medicaid**, a federal program designed for poor people, pays for care at public and private facilities for individuals such as public welfare clients and indigent elderly in nursing homes. Historically, many poor people have not been eligible for Medicaid. These individuals have obtained care from public and charity-funded clinics, medical practices, county hospitals, and hospital emergency departments. Specialized units in prisons, military installations, and universities provide care for individuals with restricted access to services in the community.

TABLE 2.1 **Population-specific health care subsystems in the United States**

Subsystem	Description	Primary Population Served
Private fee-for-service	Consumer choice from among all qualified providers	Employed individuals and dependents able to pay high coinsurance
Private managed care	Consumer choice from restricted groups of providers	Employed individuals seeking convenient, economical care (or fee-for-service option is not offered)
Medicare	Federal program to fund care for elders; managed care options available	Virtually everyone age 65 and over
Tricare	Department of Defense provides choice of plans and some direct service	Civilian employees of military services, dependents of active duty military
Veterans Administration	Federally operated hospitals and clinics	Disadvantaged veterans
Indian Health Service	Clinics and referral to contract providers	Primarily reservation-based and rural Indians
Medicaid	Health insurance provided under joint federal-state funding; increasingly from designated managed care providers	Historically, members of welfare families
Local clinic system	Emergency rooms, low-fee and free clinics, county health facilities, charity care	Working uninsured, undocumented immigrants

Segregation of Subsystems. No one is absolutely confined to a single health care subsystem, and subsystems overlap, providing services to each other's populations. Most veterans, for example, do not regularly use the VA system, opting to receive care under other plans to which they may have access. Research suggests that veterans most likely to use the VA are younger, have service-connected health problems, are African American, and live in cities. Those in need of services related to mental health and alcohol and drug use often turn to the VA.[9] People in private managed care plans have the option of paying out of pocket for outside, fee-for-service care. Many managed care plans today offer *point-of-service* (POS) options that provide some insurance coverage for care obtained by providers outside the plan.

Access across subsystems is more difficult among disadvantaged consumers. A trend toward establishment of MCOs primarily or exclusively treating Medicaid beneficiaries was clear as early as the 1990s.[10] At least one study has found that requiring Medicaid beneficiaries to obtain care only from designated MCOs reduces utilization and increases unmet needs.[11] Referral of poor people treated at public and charity clinics to outside specialists is particularly difficult, since these specialists are often unsure of how (or how much) payment will be made.[12] Many private physicians do not accept Medicaid patients or accept only a limited number into their practice.

Operation of the IHS illustrates the difficulties that result from division of U.S. health care into subsystems. This agency both delivers and finances care to members of federally recognized Native American and Alaska Native tribes and bands. Historically, the agency has concentrated its resources on reservation-based clinics that provide direct care. The scope of clinic capabilities tends to be routine care, requiring consumers with nonroutine issues to seek care from contracted health service providers outside the IHS.

Critics comment that it is in fact difficult for IHS beneficiaries to obtain care from outside providers. The story of a fourteen-year-old girl in Arizona provides an illustration. When the girl hurt her foot in gym class, her mother took her to an IHS clinic, where it was recommended that the girl have magnetic resonance imaging (MRI) and possibly surgery—services not available through IHS. The girl was referred to an outside contract service provider. However, the IHS would not pay for the service. The mother was told to apply for Medicaid, which took more than forty-five days to grant approval while her daughter "limped through school on crutches." Even after receiving approval from Medicaid, the private doctor to whom they had been referred refused to perform the MRI because the daughter had Medicaid coverage.[13]

An Evolving System

Recent development of key components and continuous change help distinguish the U.S. health care industry from systems elsewhere. Despite its size and importance, the U.S. health care industry is new when viewed in broad historical context. Some of the system's most basic features developed within living memory. Since the end of World War II, moreover, the U.S. health care system has undergone a continuous process of dynamic evolution. This process has resulted in a system with whose features no manager or policy maker has complete familiarity or expertise. The newest of innovations may still be under development as health care managers put them into use.

Table 2.2 presents selected milestones in the system's development and the decades in which they were achieved. These milestones represent developments in the organization, delivery, regulation, and financing of care. All can be said to reflect scientific, demographic, epidemiological, economic, ideological, and political developments in both health care and the broader society.

TABLE 2.2 **Some milestones in the development of the U.S. health care system**

Milestone	Decade
Medical licensure	1900s
Hospitals serving the mainstream public	1920s
Private health insurance	1940s
Proof of efficacy required for licencing pharmaceuticals	1960s
Hospital accreditation	1950s
Managed care	1970s
Selective contracting	1980s
Corporate health care	1990s
Major government programs	
Research	1930s
Training of health professionals	1960s
Health insurance for elderly and poor	1960s
Health insurance for children	1990s
Insurance exchanges, subsidies for insurance purchases, Medicaid expansion	2000s

Health Care Institutions and Professions. Health care systems outside the United States are also relatively new in the scheme of world history. But they are typically older, better established, and less subject to change than the U.S. system. Founded in 1150, the University of Bologna provided medical education to an international clientele.[14] In 1523, an act of Parliament gave the Royal College of Physicians the power to license physicians throughout England.[15] It should be noted that the licensure act did not prevent certain nonphysicians, such as surgeons and apothecaries, from practicing medicine. As early as 1883, German Chancellor Otto von Bismarck established a state-mandated, payroll tax–funded national health insurance system.[16]

Events in the history of U.S. health care are, of course, much more recent. It is difficult to imagine that it was ever legal to practice medicine without a license in the United States. New York City was the first American jurisdiction to enact a medical licensure law, which it did in 1760. However, the requirement of a license to practice medicine did not become law in every state of the union until 1901. The first American medical school began operation as part of the University of Pennsylvania in 1765. The United States has yet to equal Bismarck's achievement in national health insurance.

Hospitals and Health Insurance. Hospitals achieved a central position in U.S. health care only in the 1920s. The precursors of modern hospitals had begun in America as early as the eighteenth century as charitable or government-supported facilities. These institutions resembled modern hospitals only slightly. They functioned first as custodial facilities for people without family resources for their care, admitting individuals with a wide range of physical and mental dysfunctions. They also functioned as quarantine quarters for people with contagious diseases. Only with the development of professional nursing and reliable, antiseptic surgery did hospitals emerge as organizations focused primarily on treatment of illness. With this added capacity, hospitals began supporting themselves through billing of middle-class users for services such as birthing and surgery.

Health insurance, a fundamental feature of today's health care system, became widespread only in the 1940s. It is likely that some form of health insurance always existed in America, as communities and benevolent societies passed the hat for the ill or injured. Historians often look to the establishment of a hospitalization plan by Baylor University Hospital for Dallas teachers in 1929 as the first formal health insurance product in the United States. Under the plan, each subscriber paid $6 per year in return for which they were entitled to twenty-one days in the hospital. This concept was developed as the Blue Cross plans, nonprofit organizations with statewide territories under the auspices of the American Hospital Association. By 1940, Blue Cross plans had enrolled six million members; for-profit insurance companies that had trailed Blue Cross into the hospital insurance business had enrolled an additional 3.7 million by that year.[17] Health insurance received a boost as an employee benefit during World War II and became a standard element of employee compensation thereafter.

Government Participation. Today the U.S. health care industry would be unthinkable without the strong participation of government, because it would lack professional licensure and health insurance. U.S. government agencies have been involved in health and health care since 1798, when Congress established the U.S. Marine Hospital Service—the predecessor of today's Public Health Service (PHS)—to provide health care to sick and injured merchant seamen. State and local governments established health departments and boards of health throughout the latter half of the nineteenth century.

A trend toward massive government involvement in health care began as biomedical research. The signing of the National Cancer Institute Act by President Franklin D. Roosevelt in 1937 created the National Cancer Institute within the National Institute of Health, a PHS subunit. Funding was quite modest, with the entire PHS research budget under $3 million in 1938. By the end of the 1940s, several new institutes had been added, each at the behest of groups interested in specific categories of disease. During the remainder of the twentieth century, a number of additional institutes and centers were created within NIH, with a proposed funding level for 2008 of $28.8 billion.

Though significantly expanded during the latter half of the twentieth century, federal support for biomedical research pales before outlays in other areas. The federal government began providing funds for health professions training in the 1960s. By the mid-1990s, Titles VII and VIII of the Public Health Services Act were receiving annual appropriations in the $300 million range. These titles aim at adding to the number of health care professionals, placing these professionals in underserved areas, and training more minority health professionals. Mechanisms for accomplishing these objectives include direct student assistance such as loans and grants to institutions for expansion or maintenance of health professions education and training.[18]

Most notable in government's participation in health care is the funding of Medicare and Medicaid, programs that became operative in 1966. Requested appropriations in the president's 2008 budget for these programs totaled roughly $600 billion. In that year, the president also requested $6.6 billion for the State Children's Health Insurance Program (SCHIP), begun in 1997.[19] As a new program, SCHIP was a rarity in the late twentieth century. The program provided low-cost health insurance to children in low-income homes. Eligibility was more liberal than that of Medicaid, in that children whose parents had limited income but weren't technically poor could be beneficiaries. In California, children whose family incomes were 300 percent of poverty level could still enroll. California officials contemplated expanding eligibility to the parents of qualifying children, but abandoned the prospect when the state encountered an unexpected fiscal shortfall.

Accreditation, Managed Care, and Competition. The Joint Commission, identified earlier in this chapter as a key institution in U.S. health care, began operation in the early 1950s. The organization began operation in its current form in 1951 as the Joint Commission on Accreditation of Hospitals and began offering accreditation in

1953. A more expansive name, the Joint Commission on Accreditation of Healthcare Organizations (JCAHO), was adopted to include a broader range of organizations. The Joint Commission today accredits over ten thousand hospitals, laboratories, and other health care outlets.

Managed care, another ubiquitous feature of health care today, became prominent in the United States in the 1970s. This form of health care delivery, initially provided on the health maintenance organization (HMO) model, existed in the United States from at least the 1940s, but it occupied a limited niche in the health care market. Organizations such as the Health Insurance Plan of Greater New York, Group Health Cooperative of Puget Sound, and Kaiser Permanente began during and just after World War II and served restricted populations of voluntary subscribers for the decades to follow. In 1973, the federal HMO Act made incentives available for offering managed care products to a much broader market.

Like managed care, *selective contracting* is a fundamental part of health care today. Private preferred provider organizations (PPOs) and contracting for state Medicaid programs would be impossible without legal enablement of selective and competitive contracting. Prior to the 1980s, insurance companies and government insurance programs were required by law to pay "any willing provider" for serving their enrollees. After a California law enabling selective contracting passed in 1983, financing entities could select the providers they were willing to pay, thus directing their enrollees to specific health professionals and facilities. This legislation, eventually reproduced in other states, made a competitive market possible in health plans of all kinds.

Corporatization of Health Care. The "corporatization" of health care became apparent in the 1980s and 1990s, as profit-seeking business organizations acquired hospitals and bundled them into national networks. Corporations such as National Medical Enterprises (later Tenet) and Humana raised capital by the sale of stock to make acquisitions. In 1975, for-profit hospitals operated 5.0 percent of the hospital beds in the United States. By 2003, the percentage had more than doubled, to 11.4. By 2005, Columbia/HCA became the world's largest for-profit hospital chain. The corporation was established in a merger of the Columbia and HCA systems, both of which had aggressively bought smaller health care businesses during the 1980s and 1990s. By 1995, the new company operated some 180 hospitals and nearly 100 surgery centers, with annual revenues of roughly $25 billion.[20]

Strictly speaking, the 1980s and 1990s did not introduce corporate management into health care. Many conventional health care operations are legally corporations and utilize familiar corporate management techniques. Late twentieth-century corporatization, though, saw strong involvement of Wall Street, large profit margins, and eventual scandals among industry leaders Tenet and Columbia/HCA.

Pharmaceutical Regulation. Several important changes occurred in the regulation of pharmaceuticals in the period covered by Table 2.2. Signed by President Theodore Roosevelt in 1906, the original Food and Drug Act focused on enforcing the purity of foods and medicines sold to the public. Although the measure was also intended to prohibit unproven claims of pharmaceutical efficacy, court rulings precluded enforcement. Successor legislation in 1938, the Pure Food, Drug, and Cosmetic Act, emphasized detection and control of toxic components in medications. Only in the 1962, through an amendment of the 1938 act, did federal legislation actually require proof of efficacy as a requirement for release of a new drug onto the market.

Beginning in 1992, the Prescription Drug User Fee Act allowed the Food and Drug Administration to collect fees from drug manufacturers to cover part of the cost of regulation. Resources generated in this fashion have enabled the agency to accelerate the drug approval process, long criticized as a bottleneck to innovation. Critics of the charges, however, have objected that dependence on user fees may compromise the FDA's independence.

Attempts at System Change. The period covered in Table 2.2 saw major initiatives toward health care reform led by four presidents of the United States: Truman in the 1940s, Nixon in the 1970s, Clinton in the 1990s, and Obama in the 2000s.

Changes initiated by Presidents Ronald Reagan and Barack Obama were the most far-reaching. Characterized by a free-market orientation, the Reagan administration promoted the use of *prospective payment* mechanisms on health care organizations and individual providers. These mechanisms, which include diagnostic-related groups and capitated contracts, designated fixed payments to providers for each patient encounter or illness episode—a marked departure from traditional cost-plus payments that assured providers of a profit. The Obama Administration looked to more direct government action. On President Obama's initiative, both houses of Congress passed different versions of a measure known as the Patient Protection and Affordable Care Act in 2009. This measure aimed at making publicly-funded and subsidized health insurance available to millions of previously uninsured Americans and expanding regulation of the health insurance industry.

AMERICAN VALUES AND HEALTH CARE

It is not difficult to identify drawbacks in U.S. health care. The system is unquestionably high cost and serves different members of the public unequally. Some critics have conceived of the system as one involuntarily imposed on the public by special interests intent on maintaining their privileges and income. This may explain some features of the industry. But a powerful set of values widely shared among Americans does much to hold the system in place. These have strong historical grounding and appear likely to endure well into the future.

Table 2.3 presents examples of these values. In the table, they are characterized as two types: social values and political culture. **Social values** concern the manner in which people are expected to behave and what they have a right to expect from others. **Political culture** addresses how public decisions should be made, how government should treat the citizen, and the claims that the public sector may make on the individual.

TABLE 2.3   **The impact of social values and political culture on U.S. health care**

Value	Impact
Social Values	
Private property and the free market	Keeps health care within the private sector; has historically restricted involvement of government to programs for the poor, disadvantaged, and senior citizens
Meritocracy	Prevents generous funding of programs for the poor and disadvantaged; protects employee benefits and non-means-tested public programs
Maximization	Encourages obtaining and utilizing resources to increase personal benefit
Personal choice	Restricts growth of closed-panel managed care plans and centralization of health care delivery
Political Culture	
Equality	Supports maintaining opportunity for all; discourages special privilege
Pluralism	Restrains any tendency for central direction or financing of health care
Incrementalism	Discourages rapid, large-scale changes in the system

Social Values

Private Property and the Free Market. The right to private property is taken as fundamental in the United States. It receives emphasis in such iconic documents as the Declaration of Independence and the Constitution and is ramified throughout public law. Closely associated with the holding of private property is the right to exchange goods and services in a free market—one facilitated rather than restrained by government and protected from monopolies and unfair competition.

Business values are lionized in America. Socialist movements have crossed the political stage but have never achieved national predominance or had electoral success beyond state and local government. Class rhetoric in the United States has typically been restrained, and proposals for redistribution of wealth from the well-off to the disadvantaged have been unpopular.

In keeping with this value, Americans are suspicious of "big government." Economists such as Milton Friedman who support the free market gain national prominence. Simple-sounding concepts have captured an important element of the public spirit, such as that attributed to President Calvin Coolidge: "The business of America is business."

America's reliance on the private sector for health services, then, would appear to be no accident. Many Americans believe that business can do the job better than government. In addition, business is often perceived as less dangerous to personal liberty and well-being than government.

Meritocracy. **Meritocracy** is the belief that those who work and achieve should receive the highest rewards. Like private property, the value of meritocracy is readily observed in the United States. Its reflection is visible in practices such as pay for performance, bonus giving, promotion examinations in bureaucracies, and standardized tests for admission to college and graduate school. Meritocracy can be thought of as the opposite of a human being's worth *qua* human being or the equality of all men and women before God.

The idea of meritocracy contradicts that of the *welfare state.* The welfare state, which exists to some extent in most of the wealthy countries of the world, provides an economic floor below which no citizen is permitted to fall. Countries such as Sweden, Germany, and the U.K. have strong welfare states. A strong sense of community prevails in these countries, and health care is provided to all with a strong measure of equality. Americans generally believe that the poor should receive basic health services. But they may not believe that the disadvantaged should receive health care in the same facilities or with the same amenities as the middle class.

Maximization. A concept reflecting the desire of individuals to achieve the best possible results of any effort, *maximization* captures a desire widespread among Americans not to settle for "just good enough." Americans have high expectations. They believe in progress and intergenerational advancement up the social and economic ladder. They want the best products and services.

It cannot be expected, then, that many Americans willingly refrain from demanding the best that health care has to offer. Few, it seems, would forgo a new medication, surgery, or device only because it would save money for the government or an insurance company. Americans would have great difficulty accepting the style of health services offered in countries such as Canada or the U.K. These nationally financed systems operate at considerably lower expense than does the United States and cover a higher proportion of their citizens. Due to stretched resources, however, they skimp on maintenance and place patients on long waiting lists for services readily available in the United States.

Personal Choice. The value to Americans of personal choice has an enduring quality evocative of the words "life, liberty, and pursuit of happiness." Throughout the republic's history, U.S. citizens have enjoyed more choice in their lives than their counterparts elsewhere. Religious freedom was a fundamental guarantee. As late as the nineteenth century, some Europeans needed government permits to move from city to city. Americans could head west on a whim.

The issue of personal choice had great visibility during the early 1990s, when comprehensive health care reform was first under serious discussion. Because health care is a highly personal service, perceived limitation of choice catalyzes resistance in America. Opponents of reforms proposed by President Clinton and others emphasized the possibility that they might compel people to join government-supervised plans or to purchase health insurance.

The rise and fall of the HMO as a model for the future illustrates the degree to which Americans reject perceived limitation of personal choice. From the 1970s on, federal policy encouraged the formation of HMOs. Enrollment of consumers in HMOs grew rapidly at first. But their popularity was soon outstripped by managed care plans that offered greater choice of providers. By 2002, more than half of Americans enrolled in private health plans received their care from PPOs, plans offering a wide choice of health professionals and facilities.[21]

Political Culture

Equality. The value Americans place on equality would at first seem to contradict that of meritocracy. The focus of this value in America is equality of opportunity to participate in public life. Key beliefs of this nature include visibility in government operations and the principle of "one person, one vote."

Rejection of elites, particularly when they are secretive or hereditary, is an important manifestation of this value. The Constitution explicitly states that no citizen of the United States shall accept a title of nobility. Thus, the cornerstone of elite life in Europe was banned from the earliest days of the republic. Modern Americans may no longer fear domination by a titled nobility, but they tend to be suspicious of experts, particularly when these experts meet behind closed doors to discuss public issues. Public enthusiasm for the reforms proposed in the early 1990s diminished as elites in Washington, D.C., secretively deliberated over details.

America's longstanding valuation of equality and its suspicion of elites helps explain a long delay establishing licensure as a requirement to practice medicine in the United States. As noted above, the first U.S. jurisdictions to enact the licensure requirement did so in the mid- to late 1700s. States in the newly independent nation enacted new licensure laws into the early years of the nineteenth century. However, most, if not all, of these laws had been rescinded by 1852.

Pluralism. A second value closely tied to U.S. political culture that in turn affects health care is **pluralism**—the belief that society should encompass many distinct repositories of power, centers of decision making, financial structures, and educational systems. Pluralism is most visible in America's religious history, in which no one denomination has ever dominated.

Pluralism is a definite feature of health services in the United States. There is no central institute or bureau mandating the elements of care or procedures that must be used to diagnose and treat specific conditions. Physicians are free to prescribe any licensed drug for any condition they believe appropriate. Physicians who graduate from one residency program are likely to differ somewhat in their practice of medicine from physicians trained in another residency program. Hospitals tend to offer the same treatment at different prices and, depending on the resources possessed by the hospital, deal with different presenting conditions differently. At bottom, Americans oppose overriding, all-powerful authorities, be these King George III of England in 1776 or a "health care czar," as has been proposed under some reform plans.

Incrementalism. Incrementalism is a longstanding feature of the Anglo-American tradition. In addition to being a value in itself, incrementalism represents a method of bringing about social change. **Incrementalism** involves pursuing change in a patiently applied series of small steps. Incrementalism is the opposite of political sectarianism. Ideally, an incrementalist tries to coalesce support around measures that have limited impact but no clearly obnoxious contents. Thus, supported by successive coalitions backing small-scale proposals, a piecemeal process of progress toward a broader goal may take place.

Incrementalism militates against rapid and fundamental change. Historically, Americans have preferred that change occur in small increments. This value may have contributed to the failure of the Clinton health care plan proposed in the early 1990s, which would have revolutionized the financing and delivery of health care in the United States. In contrast, little opposition arose to the SCHIP program, which later expanded in scope.

How Satisfied Are Americans with the System?

The U.S. health care system appears compatible with some key values in American society. But how well do Americans actually like the system? How much confidence do they have in it? To what degree, and in what direction, would they like to see the system change? Answers to these questions have important implications for the likelihood of basic change in the foreseeable future.

Three recent studies address these questions from slightly differing perspectives. All are based on high-quality surveys.

The first study, supported by the Commonwealth Fund, compared findings from surveys in Australia, Canada, New Zealand, the United Kingdom, United States, and Germany.[22] This study was particularly valuable because it reported results obtained from people who were sicker than the population average, and hence more sensitive to health care issues.

(Continued)

(Continued)

This study found that only 23 percent of U.S. respondents thought that the system worked well, and only minor changes might be needed. However, the percentages of individuals reporting satisfaction according to this definition were lower for Canada (21 percent) and Germany (16 percent). The United Kingdom and New Zealand were higher (30 and 27 percent, respectively).

The second study reported data from the Employee Benefit Research Institute's Health Confidence Survey (HCS), an annual survey conducted on a random sample of one thousand Americans over the age of twenty-one.[23] Conducted annually, the HCS makes it possible to track changes in the thinking of Americans over time.

Following are some of the findings:

- A majority (53 percent) of respondents surveyed in 2006 felt extremely confident or very confident about their ability to get needed treatments, compared with 55 percent in 2002.

- Only a minority (29 percent) of those surveyed in 2006 felt extremely or very confident about their ability to afford health care without financial hardship, down from 35 percent in 2002.

- Only 39 percent of those surveyed in 2006 rated the U.S. health care system as good, very good, or excellent; 31 percent rated the system as poor, up from 15 percent in 1998.

- A majority of 2006 survey respondents (54 percent) said that they were extremely satisfied or very satisfied with their current health plan, up from 52 percent in 1998.

The third study,[24] combining information from over one hundred public opinion polls conducted between 1945 and 2000, found the following:

- In 1991, at the start of an era of intense national concern over health care, 42 percent of Americans believed that the U.S. health care system needed to be completely rebuilt; by 2000, only 29 percent continued to hold this view.

- Over twenty years of surveys have indicated basic satisfaction among Americans with their health care; in 2000, 84 percent of respondents said they were satisfied with their last visit to a doctor (compared with 88 percent in 1978); 72 percent thought that hospitals were doing a good job.

- A majority of Americans (67 percent) surveyed in 2000 felt confident that they had enough money to pay for a serious illness; in 1978 the figure had been 50 percent.

The authors conclude that most of the U.S. public has never been completely satisfied with the system. Still, no consensus regarding solutions is apparent. In 2000, when asked in general about national health insurance financed by taxes, 56 percent of respondents said they were in favor. But when a clause was added specifying that all Americans would get their health insurance from a single government plan, support fell to 38 percent of registered voters. To underscore this finding, only 21 percent of survey respondents in 2000 indicated that they trusted the federal government, down from 77 percent in 1958.

Finally, a survey just preceding the U.S. presidential election of 2008 found that only 24 percent of likely voters believed "there is so much wrong with our health care system that it needs to be completely overhauled."[25]

CONTROVERSIES IN U.S. HEALTH CARE

Key values of Americans appear consistent with distinguishing features of the U.S. health care system, and there is a high level of satisfaction with the health care Americans receive. Yet concern about rising costs and insecurity about health care coverage has troubled many. Although they espouse values such as private property and meritocracy, Americans do not lack compassion. According to a 2005 study, a majority of Americans favored government insurance for all, even if a tax increase was required.[26] The interplay of concerns, values, and ever-advancing technology and costs has given rise to four fundamental controversies. Many day-to-day challenges facing managers, policy makers, and citizens boil down to these basic questions, none of which can be readily resolved. These four controversies are (1) what care should be allocated and to whom; (2) what should be done for the disadvantaged; (3) what are the appropriate roles in health care for government and the market; and (4) who should pay for the care of people who cannot pay for themselves?

How Much and What Kind of Health Care Should Be Provided?

The volume and type of health services delivered to any given individual has become a continuing issue in U.S. health care. The issue has arisen in part because the marginal benefit of a unit of care is often quite small. An initial operation for breast cancer, for example, will often bring added years of life for the patient, at relatively low cost. However, intensive radiation and chemotherapy for advanced disease may extend survival only a few weeks, at great expense. The phenomenon of declining marginal utility of health service is illustrated by Figure 2.1, from health economist Henry Aaron's influential book *Serious and Unstable Condition*.[27]

The presence of health insurance encourages the use of interventions of marginal benefit. This is because the patient pays only a small part of her costs. Thus, additional treatments may be quite expensive for the insurance plan, but insignificant for the patient. This is particularly true for desperately ill individuals. For many patients and their families, extreme remedies (of uncertain benefit) are worth the cost; the

FIGURE 2.1 *Declining benefits from units of health care*

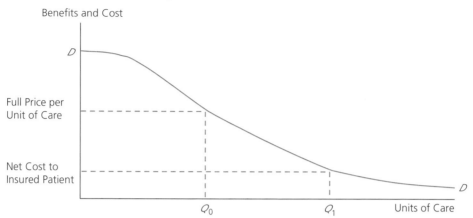

alternative is reconciling to the certainty of death. Trained to do the maximum for their patients, physicians tend to try any potential remedy, unless restrained by the mechanisms of managed care.

Out of this dilemma comes the question of who should decide when an element of care should be delivered. Should such decisions be based on science? If so, how should the science be interpreted, and by whom? Should the decision be based on economics? In such cases, there would need to be widely acceptable estimates of the value of the individual's health, function, or survival. Should the quandary be resolved by experts on the relative value of an individual's contributions to society? What role should the patient's position in the community or the socioeconomic ladder be allowed to play?

What Should We Do for the Disadvantaged?

The United States made substantial commitments to the disadvantaged during the 1960s. These commitments have slowed but have continued on a substantial level in the 1990s and 2000s. The problems with health care in the United States are still greatest among the disadvantaged. A sense of justice, it would appear, would require that the disadvantaged receive some measure of equality.

However, the mechanism and generosity of health care for the disadvantaged is a matter of contention. Criteria for eligibility are an example. It may be argued, for instance, that undocumented aliens should be denied coverage. But millions of such individuals live in the United States today. Should the SCHIP program be expanded to include entire families? What level of income should be the eligibility cutoff? Should recipients of such benefits enjoy choice of health care providers, or should they be restricted to contracted entities?

Another fundamental dilemma concerns whether U.S. health policy should be driven by concern for the disadvantaged. An argument in this direction might say that if the system were run more economically, sufficient resources could be saved so that the disadvantaged would be covered *without* new taxes on working people. Such a reconfiguration of the health care system, though, might require a diminution in the choice and quality of care available to those who today enjoy private insurance coverage.

What Are the Appropriate Roles for the Market and Government?

At present, goods and services related to health care are distributed by a combination of market forces and government mandates. Americans today face a dilemma regarding the proper balance of these mechanisms of distribution.

A complete free market in health care may make sense when viewed in the abstract. Under such as system, the consumer can choose what he thinks best. Health insurance rates would reflect the degree of choice the consumer wished to enjoy.

On the other hand, the market does not always lead to the best long-term choices. Of course, reliance on market forces would leave some disadvantaged Americans without needed services. In addition, free choice over the use of one's health care dollars might lead to significant waste. An example of such waste is expenditure of large sums on services and medications that are close to useless.

Who Shall Pay?

Perhaps the ultimate controversy in U.S. health care concerns wherewithal. Resources will be required to implement any decisions that are made and to empower whoever is asked to carry them out. Like all goods and services, the items in the health care package are ultimately scarce. Decisions must be made about whether limited resources are allocated to health or other purposes. Sources of funds will need to be designated. Some consumers will rely on others for resources. The disadvantaged need to be subsidized, as do people temporarily without resources and at the end of life.

Financial responsibility for health care has shifted among potential payers over the past half-century. Health insurers and ultimately employers took on the burden in the 1950s. Government agencies and ultimately taxpayers started playing a major role in the 1960s. In the last decades of the twentieth century, consumers had begun to assume an increasing share of health care costs.

Over the years, paying for health care began to resemble a shell game, with different sectors of the industry seeking ways to make other segments pay. Hospitals, becoming the predominant recipient of health care dollars in the mid-twentieth century, developed invisible mechanisms for subsidizing uninsured patients, shifting their costs onto the bills of the well-insured. Government agencies and private insurers countered by adopting prospective payment schemes. Employers increased the worker's share of company health insurance premiums and offered plans with increased cost sharing. Government ratcheted down payments to providers through selective contracting with hospitals and reduced compensation to physicians and other health professionals. Although polls suggest willingness by the public to increase taxes so that all will have access to health care, resistance to increased taxation for any purpose may be anticipated.

As illustrated in Figure 2.2, U.S. health care today seems like a kind of tug-of-war. Insurance companies try to shift costs to doctors and hospitals. Employers increasingly

FIGURE 2.2 *Contradictory concerns in the U.S. health care system*

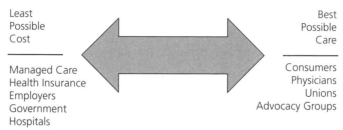

Least Possible Cost		Best Possible Care
Managed Care Health Insurance Employers Government Hospitals		Consumers Physicians Unions Advocacy Groups

attempt to shift costs to individual employees. The federal government tries to shift costs to the states, which in turn look to local governments to make up the shortfalls. At every level consumers assert their right to the best possible care. Pressure groups of many kinds agitate for higher quality and more advanced care without increased financial responsibility. Examples include unions, health professionals, and advocates for poor people or victims of specific diseases. A more equitable and secure health care system in the United States will require development of a mutually agreed-upon set of expectations regarding division of financial responsibility.

It is noteworthy that the Patient Protection and Affordable Care Act referenced earlier had insufficient power to resolve these controversies. The measure did not address the system's essential features. Health care in the United States remains privately delivered and pluralistically financed. Concerns about costs and who will ultimately pay them remain prominent. Public beliefs regarding incrementalism and the limited role of government keep reform limited.

KEY TERMS

Managed care

Medicare

Medicaid

Social values

Political culture

Meritocracy

Pluralism

The Joint Commission

Incrementalism

SUMMARY

This chapter summarizes basic features of the U.S. health care system and the issues it faces. The U.S. health care system is different from its counterparts in most of the world. Ownership and financing of health care in the United States are primarily private. It is pluralistic, with distinct subsystems serving specific segments of the population. By historical standards, most features of the system have developed only recently. The values that prevail in the United States have done much to shape the current system and have helped prevent fundamental change.

Americans express dissatisfaction with certain aspects of the health care system, but reject the idea of a government-run plan. The cost of insurance and personal health care appears to be the most prevalent cause of discontent. Support of coverage for the uninsured at taxpayer expense is widespread.

Within America's unusual system and the values that support it, the public and policy makers continually grapple with several core issues. These include (1) what care should be allocated and to whom; (2) what should be done for the disadvantaged; (3) what are the appropriate roles in health care for government and the market; and (4) who should pay for the care of people who cannot pay for themselves? Pressure by payers to restrict expenditures versus desire by consumers for readily accessible and high-quality services constitutes the master controversy in U.S. health care.

DISCUSSION QUESTIONS

1. The U.S. political culture and the values associated with it have helped keep the health care system from fundamental change. In general, have these values helped or hurt the quality of care available to most Americans?

2. Programs such as SCHIP and the Patient Protection and Affordable Care Act have mandated subsidies for purchase of insurance by families earning incomes well above the federal poverty line. What are the pros and cons of such subsidies.

3. The U.S. health care system depends heavily on private conduct of functions that are allocated to public agencies in other countries. What are the advantages and drawbacks of this American practice?

4. Do you see the pluralistic feature of the U.S. health care system as a positive or negative?

5. Following are a number of assertions regarding health care in the United States which, though widely made, might be disputed by critical thinking. Consider each, and explain why you believe it to be true or false:

   a. The United States spends too much on health services.

   b. The poor lack health care.

   c. Systems in other countries are better.

   d. The U.S. health care system today is in crisis.

   e. Health care is a right.

CHAPTER

3

MAJOR HEALTH PROBLEMS IN MODERN SOCIETY

LEARNING OBJECTIVES

- To understand health and illness as basic challenges to the health care system
- To learn about the causes of illness and injury
- To become familiar with the basic concerns, concepts, resources, and applications of epidemiology
- To appreciate the relative importance of specific threats to health and longevity in the United States
- To recognize the implications of demographics and epidemiology for health care management
- To see how epidemiology can be applied in management and policy

CONCEPTIONS OF HEALTH AND DISEASE

The health care industry's manifest task is to maintain and improve the biological functioning of Americans despite the ever-present threat of illness and injury. This chapter provides an overview of the diseases and other biological challenges to health that create the need for health care. This material provides the reader with concrete information about the job of the health care system. It also presents controversies about how that job is actually defined. Definitions, conceptions, and expectations regarding health and illness play a crucial role in the decisions made by consumers, managers, and policy makers.

Conceptions of health and illness vary by frame of reference. The purely biological frame of reference sees health and illness in terms of observable and measurable parameters. These include microscopic, metabolic, or clinical variables. Evidence of disease can be pathological, as in the examination of tissue; cytological, as in the examination of cells; chemical, as in levels of cholesterol, prostate-specific antigen, or blood sugar. Ultimately, though, objectively measurable data are less important than human perceptions about health within the context of individual expectations and social surroundings.

Medical Criteria and Classifications

Traditionally, medicine has relied on signs and symptoms as signals of the presence of disease. *Signs* refer to objective *physical findings* detected by an examiner. *Symptoms* are subjective evidence of disease as perceived by the patient.

Sometimes a single sign may suffice for diagnosis. A low hematocrit is a marker for anemia. A throat culture giving rise to colonies of streptococci is diagnostic in a straightforward manner. Jaundice imparts a characteristic skin color. Microscopic inspection of tissue can identify cancer cells.

Diagnosis of disease usually requires more than a single sign or symptom. Specific combinations and sequences of observations are more often required to make a diagnosis. Some diseases are never specifically diagnosed. Systemic lupus erythematosus (or simply lupus) is such a disease, designated by convention as present when four or more symptoms or signs on a list of eleven are observed. In some instances, diagnosis is made through treatment, as when a physician gives an antibiotic for a disease that she believes is bacterial and the possibility is substantiated when signs and symptoms disappear.

Despite the uncertainty that sometimes attends diagnosis, the health care industry today uses an extensive set of metrics to indicate the presence of disease and its severity. Two of the most widely used systems for disease classification are the *International Classification of Diseases* (ICD)[1] and the *Diagnostic and Statistical Manual of Mental Disorders* (DSM).[2]

The ICD, currently published by the World Health Organization, has appeared in successively updated editions since 1900. The ICD provides codes that classify diseases and a wide variety of signs, symptoms, abnormal findings, complaints, social circumstances, and external causes of injury or disease. Every health condition receives a unique code and is often placed in a category of clinically related and similarly numbered diseases. The ICD is used worldwide for morbidity and mortality statistics and insurance payment.

Table 3.1 presents the major categories of disease included in the tenth major revision of the ICD, or the ICD-10. These classifications correspond roughly to disease categories successively considered by health professionals in the processes of history taking and diagnosis. Some of the categories are linked with specific tissues, organs, or organ systems. Other disease categories are defined in terms of their **etiology**—the causes of and factors leading to the disease.

TABLE 3.1   Major ICD categories and codes

Code Range	Title
A00-B99	Certain infectious and parasitic diseases
C00-D48	Neoplasms
D50-D89	Diseases of the blood and blood-forming organs and certain disorders involving the immune mechanism
E00-E90	Endocrine, nutritional, and metabolic diseases
F00-F99	Mental and behavioral disorders
G00-G99	Diseases of the nervous system
H00-H59	Diseases of the eye and adnexa
H60-H95	Diseases of the ear and mastoid process
I00-I99	Diseases of the circulatory system
J00-J99	Diseases of the respiratory system
K00-K93	Diseases of the digestive system
L00-L99	Diseases of the skin and subcutaneous tissue
M00-M99	Diseases of the musculoskeletal system and connective tissue

(Continued)

TABLE 3.1   *(Continued)*

Code Range	Title
N00-N99	Diseases of the genitourinary system
O00-O99	Pregnancy, childbirth, and the puerperium
P00-P96	Certain conditions originating in the perinatal period
Q00-Q99	Congenital malformations, deformations, and chromosomal abnormalities
R00-R99	Symptoms, signs, and abnormal clinical and laboratory findings not elsewhere classified
S00-T98	Injury, poisoning, and certain other consequences of external causes
V01-Y98	External causes of morbidity and mortality

The *Diagnostic and Statistical Manual of Mental Disorders* is the primary diagnostic system for psychiatric and psychological disorders in the United States and elsewhere. Like the ICD, it is used for both statistical and insurance purposes. The DSM contains five dimensions or *axes* according to which clinicians make diagnoses. This multiaxial approach enables diagnoses to capture multiple dimensions of the patient's complaint, reflecting the complexity of many psychiatric diagnoses. For example, an individual may have an Axis I diagnosis of major depression, an Axis III diagnosis of arthritis (presumably contributing to depression), and an Axis IV diagnosis of severe stress due to a job situation.

In addition to classifications of disease, the health care industry has developed an elaborate set of standard measures of the severity of individual diseases and their impact. Perhaps most familiar is cancer stage, with people in late stage having more disseminated disease and shorter life expectancy than those in early stage. A staging methodology for chronic kidney disease divides this condition into five categories (mild kidney damage through kidney failure), according to the kidneys' filtration rate.[3] Forced expiratory volume is an index of severity of asthma and other diseases of the lung.

Physical or mental dysfunction has been widely adopted as a criterion for illness or as a measure of its severity. Examples of widely used metrics include counts of impairment of specific activities of daily life or general level of dysfunction (Karnofsky scale);[4] pain (McGill Pain Questionnaire and visual analogue scales);[5] mood (Profile of Mood States);[6] and multidimensional questionnaires that include both mental and physical dimensions (RAND MOS-36).[7]

Health service researchers have also developed quantitative measures relevant to specific diseases or individual disease dimensions. Researchers, for example, have formulated scales to assess the severity of gastrointestinal involvement in scleroderma (an autoimmune disease), sexual function in cervical cancer, and incontinence following prostate cancer surgery. Later chapters in this volume will address measurement of disease severity and impact in greater detail.

Despite the objectivity with which twenty-first-century medicine approaches health and illness, it is difficult to define disease without an element of subjective interpretation. Some commentators define *illness* in terms of the individual's perception and *disease* as a biological condition. This distinction is especially useful for so-called mental illness. An individual's behavior may appear bizarre, yet he cannot be considered "ill" if there is no sense of personal distress or dysfunction.

Social, Cultural, and Political Interpretations

Culture, politics, and other social forces help determine how individuals interpret signs of illness and what society will accept as a disease. In this sense, biological factors are only one dimension of illness. A society's conception of disease determines what will be treated as disease rather than normal variation among individuals, divine intervention, or criminality. Society's conception in turn determines the public's consumption of medical care, release of the sick from social and work responsibilities, and support for biomedical research.

Ethnicity and Disease. A person's ethnic background can strongly influence how he recognizes disease and explains its development. A classic study of disadvantaged U.S. African Americans in the mid-twentieth century provides an illustration. People interviewed in this study identified "high blood" as an illness not to be confused with high blood *pressure*. High blood was thought to concern the amount of blood in the body or a shift in its location, resulting from improper diet or emotional shock. An interview subject described the condition as "too much blood, the blood goin' to your heart, to your brain or somethin'," and its cause as "eatin' too much and gettin' too fat, [as a result of which] the blood goes up to your head too fast."[8]

Members of other ethnic groups have identified diseases unrecognized by mainstream medicine. Examples from Latino communities include *mollera caida* and *empacho,* linked with gastroenteritis in infants and children.[9] Mollera caida refers to the fallen fontanelle (soft spot) on an infant's head. It is believed to be caused by a fall or by sudden withdrawal of the breast during breastfeeding. Empacho is a gastrointestinal disorder believed to be caused by an obstruction in the stomach or intestines. Empacho is often associated with eating too much, eating the wrong type of food, eating poorly prepared food, or eating at the wrong time. Treatments for empacho include massages; ingestion of teas, oils, and purgatives; dietary restrictions; mercury; and lead.

A classic study of pain addressed ethnically conditioned interpretation of a symptom rather than the presence versus absence of disease.[10] Around 1950, Zbrowski interviewed members of New York City's then-prominent ethnic communities regarding their interpretations of pain due to serious illness. Comparison of old ethnic stock (predominantly Irish), Italian Americans, and Jews revealed significant differences. Descendants of old ethnic stock tended to be stoic, either minimizing the importance of their pain or denying it altogether. Italian Americans freely expressed their pain and felt satisfaction when it was reduced via medication. Jewish patients also freely expressed their pain, but, concerned with its implications for their underlying medical condition, were less satisfied even when their pain was effectively controlled.

In a broader sense, society and community determine the individual's perception of a normal and desirable condition versus a disease or illness. Psychiatric conditions provide good illustrations. A culture encouraging stoicism and reserve, for example, would be less likely to identify depression as an illness than a culture encouraging exuberance and emotional display. Modern Japan provides an illustration. Producer Kenichiro Takiguchi, who worked for Japan's biggest television broadcaster, read Peter Kramer's *Listening to Prozac*,[11] a book that had helped popularize selective serotonin reuptake inhibitors (SSRIs) in the United States. As the *Wall Street Journal* described subsequent events,

> *Takiguchi persuaded his bosses to air a fifty-minute prime-time special presenting depression as a treatable disease rather than a character flaw. Millions watched and more than 2,000 viewers called in afterward to thank the network.*
>
> *It was the beginning of an extraordinary transformation in Japan. Once, says Mr. Takiguchi, "no one would say, 'I have a psychiatric illness.' . . . It was really a shameful disease."*
>
> *Japan's attitude toward mental illness . . . offers an insight into the country's culture. As the nation plunged into deep economic slump in the late 1990s, widespread bankruptcies and layoffs contributed to an increasing divorce rate and a suicide rate that is now double that of the U.S. Yet . . . Japanese psychiatrists continued to focus almost exclusively on psychosis and depression severe enough to require hospitalization.*
>
> *Hiroko Mizushima, who was a medical student specializing in psychiatry at prestigious Keio University in the early 1990s, says, "We weren't taught anything about how depression is increasing or how it's the disease of the modern age." Instead, the traditional Japanese view prevailed, that depression was just a figment of the imagination that could be solved with konjo, or willpower.*[12]

Politicization of Disease. In addition to ethnicity and social climate, politics often influences what is considered disease and the actions considered appropriate in response. *Politics* in this sense is a process by which a person or group attempts to influence collective thinking or action. Groups and individuals use politics to accomplish a deliberate purpose—for example, to preserve or challenge prevailing expectations and practice. Individuals and groups use politics to mobilize collective resources to their benefit or that of their allies. Politics is a competitive process. In politics, people promote the thinking or action they desire over the preferences of others.

Agitation over chronic fatigue syndrome (CFS) illustrates the interrelationships that sometimes develop between politics and disease. The health care industry recognized CFS as a disease in the 1980s, with criteria for diagnosis including "debilitating fatigue . . . present for at least six months, some functional impairment, and . . . this fatigue and impairment have not been caused by any other identifiable clinical condition."[13] Other characteristics sometimes cited include flulike symptoms, chemical sensitivities, balance impairments, and cognitive difficulties. The vagueness of the condition still leads some to question its legitimacy as a disease. It seems doubtful that CFS would have been recognized and research on the condition funded without public advocacy.

Individuals to whom the disease description applies and at least one national organization have advocated vocally for people with CFS. Much of this agitation has focused on public resources. CFS advocates have argued for more research funding, commenting that current funding levels are consistent with a policy of neglecting women's health (a majority of people with CFS are female). Advocates have also demanded antidiscrimination legislation for CFS, a single-payer health care system ensuring choice of physicians, and a "toxic-free environment."

Other conditions await potentially successful advocacy. Multiple chemical sensitivity provides an interesting example. This condition is alleged to predispose those affected to react adversely to a wide range of scented products, ranging from perfume to laundry detergent. Despite lack of scientific evidence, the condition seems to be gaining recognition. The San Francisco mayor's disability coordinator has commented that "ten years from now it will be politically incorrect to wear perfumes in public." An organization known as the Human Ecology Action League has announced that "perfume is going to be the tobacco smoke of tomorrow."[14]

Medicalization of Deviance. Sociologists use the term *deviance* to mean violation of cultural norms in a fashion suspect or repugnant to the broader society. Crime constitutes a prime example of deviance. Less obtrusive forms of deviance include adverse forms of behavior and lifestyle such as alcoholism or drug abuse, chronic (and voluntary) unemployment, sexual experimentation or excess, and disruptive behavior. Subsistence on welfare among the nonelderly is sometimes regarded as deviant, as are fringe lifestyles such as homelessness, sadomasochism, and bohemianism.

A seminal work of the 1980s, *Deviance and Medicalization: From Badness to Sickness,* identified several areas in which medicalization has helped transform public and official views.[15] Instances of the transformation include insanity, at one time seen as possession by evil forces, though today the clear province of psychiatry. Alcoholism constitutes another example, with severe susceptibility to alcohol abuse today widely recognized as appropriate for medical intervention. Inattentive and disruptive children who at one time were considered ill behaved are diagnosed today with ADD and treated with drugs.

Criminal behavior is sometimes viewed as a proper focus for medical intervention. A long lineage of biomedical and social scientists has attributed criminal behavior to genetic flaws or other heritable factors. Medical interventions have been developed for such crime-related predispositions as low threshold for violent reactions to stress. Repeated sexual crime has been attributed at least in part to a high testosterone level. In response, nine U.S. states have passed laws mandating interventions to reduce repeated or pedophilic offenders' circulating testosterone, either through surgical castration or drugs that drastically reduce testosterone secretion ("chemical castration").[16]

Medicalization of deviance raises the fundamental question of whether some people are actually "evil" or "bad" or whether they are violating social norms because of illness. Medicalization of nondeviant behavior raises other issues. Birth and death have been considered natural processes throughout most of human history and usually took place at home. During the twentieth century, these great passages of life moved from the home to the hospital. Movements favoring natural childbirth and death at home have arisen in reaction. Aging presents another instance of questionable medicalization. In the decades following initiation of Medicaid, people have asked whether actual medical need justifies placement of the elderly in residential long-term care facilities. Some would argue that the practice simply reflects an unwillingness of offspring to cohabit with their aged parents.

Supernormality. People are increasingly unwilling to accept limitations that were once considered normal. The term *supernormality* refers to transcendence over limitations placed on the individual by heredity, aging, or the natural features of the human body. Modern health care offers many opportunities for pursuit of supernormality.

Resources for achievement of supernormality include sports performance–enhancing drugs, human growth hormone for normal individuals, Prozac and other SSRIs for the slightly depressive, and cosmetic surgery of many kinds. Agents such as Botox and its successors have become popular for smoothing foreheads and crows' feet, filling wrinkles and creases, and reshaping noses, chins, and cheeks. Liposuction, aesthetic lip modification, and, if advertising on the Internet is to be believed, even penis enhancement are big business. For men, Viagra promises restored potency, and products offering similar benefits for women are in the pipeline.

It is tempting to view the desire for supernormality as only a manifestation of human vanity and narcissism. But creditable reasoning lies behind the desire of many to surpass traditional normality. The parent seeking human growth hormone for a son may share the widespread belief that tall men are more likely to succeed than men who are average in stature. Often rightly, the athlete believes that she cannot compete at a sport's highest level without the aid of the drugs used by her peers. Taking an SSRI to attain supernormal sociability and pep is understandable in a person who desires to live life to the full.

It is important to remember that only a few decades ago normality meant something different from its meaning today. Before the development of in vitro fertilization and SSRIs, it was considered normal for some couples to be childless and some individuals to suffer lifelong intractable depression. Some considered coronary bypass surgery, hip replacement, and laser cataract surgery for elders to be medical extravagance. It seemed normal for an elderly person to suffer regular bouts of pain, require the aid of a walking cane, and wear heavy-lensed eyeglasses.

THE CAUSES OF DISEASE

Knowledge about the causes of illness is essential to understanding issues facing the U.S. health care system. Factors leading to the occurrence of disease are of primary concern to public health, a professional field responsible for disease prevention and control. Knowledge of the causes of disease is important to the consumer, because it will likely help him avoid illness and, in the event of illness, take steps toward recovery. An understanding of the causes of disease is a crucial ingredient in public policy formulation, for example, regarding funding of biomedical research, public health interventions, health services, and disease prevention. Some causes of disease may be unavoidable. But others, such as the individual's **environment**—his biological, physical, and social surroundings—can often be made less hazardous.

Microorganisms

To the professional and the layperson alike, germs are the most familiar cause of disease. Germ theory explains disease on the basis of infection, multiplication, and adverse action by pathogenic microorganisms. The nineteenth-century pioneers of germ theory investigated diseases caused by bacteria such as anthrax, cholera, tuberculosis, and plague. But the explanation of diseases as infection by microorganisms originating outside the host applies more broadly. Larger microorganisms such as protozoa give rise to diseases such as giardiasis and malaria. Viruses, much smaller than either bacteria or protozoa, also produce disease through infection and self-replication. Pathogenic microorganisms tend to seek out and multiply in specific organs or tissues, a fact that helps explain why each disease produces characteristic signs, symptoms, and impact. In this fashion, the poliomyelitis virus infects muscle tissue, and HIV infects a specific category of T lymphocytes—white blood cells that play a key part in the body's immune response.

As is true in much of science and health care, germ theory is of relatively recent origin. The theory emerged from the work of prominent nineteenth-century scientists such as Louis Pasteur (1822–1895), Robert Koch (1843–1910), and Joseph Lister (1827–1912). Science had known of the existence of microorganisms since the 1600s, when Anton van Leeuwenhoek (1632–1723), an early experimenter in microscopy, became the first to see bacteria, yeast plants, and protozoa.

But humankind was slow to learn the connection between microorganisms and human diseases. Only in the mid-1800s did scientists demonstrate this connection, and the remainder of the nineteenth century passed before germ theory was widely accepted. Pasteur's experiments (see Chapter Eight) demonstrated that weakened bacteria could produce immunity from infection when injected into susceptible hosts. Koch's work conclusively demonstrated the causative nature of bacteria in disease. The surgeon Lister, suspecting that what was becoming known about pathogenic bacteria might explain the widespread mortality among surgical patients of his day, began applying antiseptics to surgical wounds. The marked reduction in mortality he thus achieved made possible the era of modern surgery. Similarly, the experiments of Koch and Pasteur laid the groundwork for modern pharmaceutical immunization.

In the twentieth century, germ theory achieved new relevance. Scientists found associations between viral infection and certain forms of cancer. Human papilloma virus is associated with cervical cancer[17] and hepatitis B virus with liver cancer.[18] Epstein-Barr virus has been linked to cancers of blood-forming tissues.[19]

Immune System Malfunction

Although infection by microorganisms accounts for much disease, the host's immune status plays a parallel role. Mechanisms for resisting microorganisms and larger parasites were established early in the history of organic evolution. These have been passed on and improved for the benefit of modern organisms, including humans. Weakening or disruption of the immune system predisposes any organism to disease.

HIV provides an important illustration. This virus replicates in and destroys CD4 cells, a key component of the body's immune response. With the destruction of these cells, the immune system becomes inoperative. Frequently present but usually resisted microorganisms then have a chance to proliferate and cause disease—an outcome known as *opportunistic* infection. Patients frequently die of a form of pneumonia caused by *Pneumocystis carinii.* Spores of this organism are present in the lung tissues of many, if not most, individuals. However, they do not cause disease as long as the host's immune system remains intact.

Immunosuppression results from many conditions other than HIV. A number of medical procedures either deliberately or incidentally involve immunosuppression. Tissue and organ transplantation, for example, require suppression of the patient's immune system to promote acceptance of the transplanted material. Adverse conditions that result from medical suppression of the immune system fall into the category of *iatrogenic* disease—illness resulting from an attempt at cure.

Immune suppression also occurs naturally. A number of hereditary diseases reduce the competence of the immune system, particularly in children. Poor diet may weaken immune response. Linkages have been reported between low protein intake and impairment of several components of the immune system; it has been asserted that "malnutrition is the most common cause of immunosuppression worldwide."[20]

Some evidence suggests that an environment rich in disease-causing microorganisms reduces the strength of the human immune system.[21] Reduced immune system capability may explain the devastating effect of AIDS in Africa.

Diminution in ability to fight infection is not the only way the immune system can malfunction. The immune system can also misdirect its powers against normal and healthy tissues and organs. Such conditions are known as *autoimmune* diseases. They include such widespread illnesses as systemic lupus erythematosus and rheumatoid arthritis.

Physical Environment

Along with germ theory, factors in the physical environment are broadly identified by the public as causes of disease. Environmental effects on individual health are clearest in instances of industrial exposure. Historically, coal miners, textile workers, and shipbuilders have suffered from occupational respiratory illnesses such as black lung (pneumoconiosis), brown lung (byssinosis), asbestosis, and lung cancer. The discovery among chimney sweeps of old London of a relationship between coal tar exposure and testicular cancer constituted one of the first discoveries of occupational disease.

Public concern has also focused on air pollution. Of historical significance was the so-called Killer Fog of 1952 in London. In five days during a December temperature inversion, a mixture of trapped fog and dirty fuel effluent killed as many as 12,000 Londoners. A recent field study in London focused on more normal levels of exposure to air pollution. The study demonstrated that asthmatic individuals exposed to diesel exhaust experienced small reductions in pulmonary function. Although reduction of this magnitude was not accompanied by clinically significant symptoms, the study team concluded that individuals with more severe asthma would be likely to sustain greater impact.[22] Longer-term studies have demonstrated increased risk of cardiovascular disease among individuals living in areas with high levels of particulate matter from automobile emissions.[23]

Several notorious events following the London Killer Fog have alerted the public to the health threat represented by environmental toxicity. In the United States, a housing development known as Love Canal in New York State was found to have been built on a chemical waste dump. Prior to evacuation of the site in 1978, exposure to hazardous materials appears to have caused more than half the pregnancies in the development to end in stillbirths. Radioactive products from the 1986 nuclear plant explosion in Chernobyl, Ukraine, are expected to produce four thousand excess deaths from cancer in the surrounding area. Tougher antipollution laws have made similar environmental catastrophes less likely in England and the United States. But countries undergoing rapid industrial growth today, such as China, face catastrophic health risks.

Chemical compounds in food, water, and consumer products also increase the risk of disease. A review of agents of this type identifies widely encountered substances as carcinogenic, including halogenated plastics such as polyvinyl chloride compounds (PVCs), pesticides such as hexachlorobenzene, and pharmaceutical and cosmetic products such as certain hormones and hair dyes.[24] Exposure to chemical carcinogens may occur directly or through contact with persons who have had direct contact. Thus, the families of asbestos workers have contracted asbestos-specific cancers due to residues on the workers' clothing. Unborn children and infants receive carcinogens through the placenta or the mother's milk.

Public health researchers have recently become interested in the structures and streets in which people spend their lives—the so-called *built environment.* These researchers identify lack of open space as a cause of disease. An absence of open spaces such as parks denies people the opportunity to exercise, socialize, and relax.

Streets made unsafe by excessive automobile traffic or violent criminals expose residents to risk of trauma. Buildings themselves can represent hazardous environments due to use of hazardous construction materials (such as PVCs and asbestos), toxic cleaning agents, tobacco smoke, dust mites, and molds.

Heredity

It is natural for people to look to ancestors and relatives for clues to their own health risks and life expectancy. Genetic variation does indeed play a role in individual risks for specific diseases. Well-researched examples include heart disease, certain types of cancer, asthma, Alzheimer's disease, and systemic lupus erythematosus. The appearance of diseases recurring over multiple generations in prominent families illustrates the inherited component of disease etiology. Hemophilia in the court of the nineteenth-century Russian czars constitutes a familiar historical illustration.

Some of the strongest evidence linking diseases with genetic heritage has emerged from research on so-called cancer-prone families. A prominent study of colon cancer, for example, has demonstrated that individuals with several near relatives who have had colon cancer have a 50 percent lifetime risk of contracting the disease.[25] This compares with a 2 percent risk in the general population. Similar results have been found for other cancers, most prominently cancer of the breast.

Studies of identical twins have also helped scientists understand the contribution that genetic background makes to development of disease. In one important investigation of cancer risk, scientists studied the health histories of 44,788 pairs of twins in Scandinavia. Generally, a person whose twin had a particular type of cancer experienced an elevated risk of developing that same cancer.[26]

Similar findings have been reported in mental illness. In a U.S. study of 794 pairs of female twins, the investigators compared the importance of genetic and environmental factors (particularly concerning family) in the development of conditions such as conflicted interpersonal relationships, anxious-depressive symptoms, substance use, lack of social support, and low self-esteem. Genetic effects were observed for all these dimensions; total heritabilities ranged from 16 percent to 49 percent. Genetic factors had more comprehensive effects than family environment.[27]

Despite ample evidence of genetic influence on health and illness, the relationship is not necessarily a simple one. Single genes or genetic mutations do explain the appearance of some conditions. In many instances, though, the effects of multiple genes interact with each other to produce disease. In still other cases, genetic predisposition interacts with environmental conditions to initiate or promote a disease process.[28]

Individual Behavior and Attitude

The biological and physical causes of disease discussed earlier by no means exhaust potential explanations of health and illness. A great deal of evidence suggests that lifestyle and diet cause many cases of disease. Public health authorities predict that today's overweight adolescents will become tomorrow's diabetes and heart disease patients.[29] Tobacco and alcohol are obvious factors in development of disease. People who seldom exercise are likely candidates for heart disease, stroke, and perhaps cancer. Those who engage in hazardous occupations place themselves at risk of injury or illness. People who look for good times in activities and venues ranging from drugs and sex in high-crime neighborhoods to double-diamond runs in Aspen or Switzerland risk injury. Relationships between behavior and health risk will receive detailed attention in Chapter Four.

A number of widely read commentaries have asserted that adverse emotion and personal outlook contribute directly to poor health.[30,31] Rigorous investigations have produced mixed results. A team of researchers, for example, reviewed a large number of studies on the effects of stress due to loss of a job, death of a spouse, lack of control over life, war, and natural disaster. They found that stress was associated with development of cardiovascular disease, but not cancer.[32] Attitude, outlook, and emotional state will remain important considerations even if future studies show that they do not directly affect physical health. People with positive attitudes toward life and who believe they can control their destiny seem more likely to follow doctors' orders and to exercise conscientious self-care.

Geography and Community

Occurrence of diseases and life expectancy tend to differ across geographical area. Life expectancy is longer in some parts of the United States than in others. Heterosexual HIV/AIDS, for example, occurs more frequently in the southeastern United States than on the west coast. Violent crime occurs more often in big cities than in suburbs. However, methamphetamine manufacture and use are highly prevalent in rural areas.

To some extent, individual outlook and behavior explain the influence of place on health. Mormonism, which is predominant in Utah, promotes family life, a health-preserving practice, while forbidding use of tobacco and alcohol. Nevada, on the other hand, attracts holiday-seekers oriented toward smoking, drinking, gambling, and prostitution. The relatively unstable population of Nevada makes it more difficult for people to maintain strong social ties, a personal asset that research has linked with life expectancy.[33]

In addition to individual behavior, though, public health researchers now pay serious attention to factors outside the individual that influence her thinking and actions. These include social norms, forms of behavior viewed as acceptable in a given community. Local laws regarding advertising of alcohol and tobacco as well as enforcement of building codes affect the health of residents. Availability of fresh fruits and vegetables in a neighborhood promotes healthful diets, while a predominance of fast food joints does the opposite. Together, these diverse factors define communities that are healthful versus illness-prone.

A strong body of research has developed attempting to explain these differences on the basis of the strength of communities. The frequency of contact among individuals with intimate ties to each other has been found to increase longevity.[34] This finding has been replicated in both rural and urban settings and in different regions of the United States.

The strength of social ties across the community as a whole has also been credited with promoting health and longevity. The town of Roseto, Pennsylvania, for example, has attracted the attention of researchers. In the tradition of south Italian immigrants who originally founded Roseto, residents in the mid-twentieth century consumed a lard-rich diet. They used tobacco at about the national average. However, they suffered heart attacks at about half the national rate. Researchers have attributed Roseto's surprisingly low heart attack rate to the strength of community ties. Both modest- and high-income earners in Roseto interacted regularly and participated in civic activity.[35] Reinforcing this interpretation, a national study found that communities with relatively small differences in the incomes of individuals tended to experience lower death rates than communities with large income differences.[36]

Health Risks and Local Culture

Although towns like Roseto may represent a model healthy community, other places represent just the opposite. Poverty and exposure to environmental hazards can make a neighborhood an unhealthy place. However, factors associated with local culture can also foster disease and reduce life expectancy. The city of New Orleans furnishes an example, as illustrated by observations reported in the *Wall Street Journal*:[37]

> Gluttony and excess are to New Orleans what pilgrims and prayer are to Mecca. The city's catchphrase, "Let the Good Times Roll," has become a cliché, and even the names of places and events—Bourbon Street, Desire, Fat Tuesday, the Sugar Bowl, the Big Easy—are redolent of debauchery. But living the good life, it seems, may also mean living the short life. Recent studies by the federal Centers for Disease Control and Prevention and other groups have named New Orleanians the fattest people in America, the most likely to contract lung cancer and among the shortest-lived, with an average life span roughly equal to citizens of Mauritius, North Korea, and Uzbekistan.

> The city also has held the dubious title as America's murder capital, and it has ranked in the top tier for AIDS, infant mortality, and other afflictions.

> In many cities, statistics like these would spark cries of shame, alarm, or outrage. In New Orleans, they are generally received fatalistically, or with black humor and raffish pride. Andrei Codrescu is a poet and editor of a literary journal, *Exquisite Corpse*. Told that at fifty-one he is only thirteen years short of the average age of death for males here, he gestures around the crowded bar where he sits drinking whiskey and smoking at 3 a.m.

> "You have to allow for one fact," he says. "We're awake twenty hours a day, so really we live much longer even if we drop dead at sixty-four."

NONDISEASE THREATS TO HEALTH, FUNCTION, AND SURVIVAL

In addition to disease, accidents and other adverse events in daily life must be handled by the health care system. Table 3.2 presents the most frequent nondisease causes of death in the United States in 2004. These are generally designated as *external causes* of mortality (ICD-10 codes S00-T98 and V01-Y98)—meaning external to normal or abnormal processes within the individual organism. The numbers of individuals who survive each event indicated in Table 3.2 are much larger than those who succumb. Thus, the numbers in the table are merely suggestive of the need for health services associated with accidents and injury. Numbers corresponding to a few widely known but infrequently occurring causes of death not presented in the table provide perspective. In 2004, for example, 52 Americans were killed by legal execution, 46 by lightning strikes, 22 by floods, and 6 by contact with venomous snakes and lizards.

TABLE 3.2   Nondisease causes of death in the United States, 2004

Cause of Death	Number of Deaths
Motor vehicle accidents	44,933
Intentional self-harm (suicide)	32,439
Poisoning and exposure to noxious substances (including narcotics)	20, 950
Falls	18,807
Assault (with firearms, sharp objects, and so on)	11,624
Accidental suffocation, strangulation, or obstruction of airway	5,891
Drowning	3,308
Fire and smoke exposure	3,229
Complications of surgical and medical care	2,883
Mechanical forces (such as machinery) and explosions	2,759

Source: National Safety Council. www.nsc.org/lrs/statinfo/odds.htm. Accessed February 21, 2008.

EPIDEMIOLOGY: THE SCIENCE OF THE DENOMINATOR

Personal health services aimed at curing or ameliorating threats to an individual's health, function, and survival constitute the most visible work of the health care system. **Epidemiology,** by contrast, focuses on the health of populations. In this fashion, epidemiology serves as an essential resource for management and policy making. Health services achieve results on the level of individual patients. But managers configure resources on the basis of an entire community's needs. Policy makers develop legislation, regulations, and interventions that address the health challenges ranging from local to global in scope.

The science of epidemiology provides information on risk of specific diseases observable in a city, state, or country's population. Epidemiology identifies the means through which pathogens survive in the environment to periodically spawn new outbreaks. Identification of the mechanisms and routes by which disease is transmitted within and across communities is a classic focus of epidemiological investigations. In the absence of direct biological evidence, epidemiology can help identify the causes of disease by determining common characteristics among those affected—in this manner, tobacco and asbestos were first identified as causes of lung cancer.

Epidemiology is sometimes known as the *science of the denominator.* This is because epidemiologists concern themselves primarily with rates of disease—obtained by dividing the number of people with an illness by the population at risk—rather than the ill individuals, as do clinicians. Epidemiology covers many manifestations of diseases. Often, it addresses **incidence** of diseases (the number of new cases occurring in a population within a specified time period) and **prevalence** (the number of cases that exist within a population at a given point in time). Epidemiologists study consequences of disease such as pain and disability.

An early example illustrates how characteristics of people who frequently contract a particular disease may provide clues to the disease's immediate, if not ultimate, cause. Percival Pott, the famed eighteenth-century London surgeon, noticed high rates of scrotal cancer among the city's chimney sweeps. Inferring that chimney soot was somehow responsible for the disease, Pott advised chimney sweeps to take precautions against excessive and prolonged contact with soot. It was not until the twentieth century that Japanese scientists identified the specific chemical compound in coal residue responsible for scrotal cancer. The epidemiological evidence observed by Pott had the capacity to save lives threatened by a disease whose actual cause was unknown in his time.

Early epidemiologists also made inferences based on the geographic points around which epidemic cases occurred. Such findings often pointed to *reservoirs of disease*—human groups, neighborhoods, or manmade facilities that harbor and maintain disease-producing factors, known or unknown. The British physician John Snow's discovery during a severe epidemic of cholera between 1853 and 1854 provides a classic example. Snow discovered that the residences of cholera victims tended to cluster around a water supply source known as the Broad Street Pump. The pump in fact dispensed water contaminated by cholera-bearing sewage. Snow stopped the epidemic by removing the handle of the now-infamous pump, whose tainted water comprised, quite literally, a reservoir of disease.

It is instructive that Snow never learned the actual cause of cholera. He believed it to be a water-borne poison somehow associated with sewage. Only some thirty years later did Robert Koch identify *vibrio cholerae* as the responsible bacillus. Even before the actual cause of a disease has been determined, epidemiology can serve as the basis for effective action.

The Concept of Relative Risk

Epidemiologists sometimes use the concept of relative risk to compare likelihood of morbidity or mortality in two distinct populations or population segments. Relative risk (or risk ratio) is computed by dividing the probability of an event—for contracting a disease, for example—in one group by the probability of that event in another. As a hypothetical example, consider the potential effect of exposure to a certain chemical on the likelihood of contracting cancer. An experimental situation compares 462 nonexposed individuals with 851 exposed. It is found that over an extended period of time, 154 people who were not exposed contracted cancer, while 709 of those exposed did. The risk experienced by the nonexposed people would be 33 percent (154/462); the risk of those exposed would be 83 percent (709/851). The risk ratio of individuals exposed to the chemical and those not exposed would be 2.5 (.83/.33), clearly suggesting that the chemical causes cancer.

Alternatively, epidemiologists compute odds ratios to compare the likelihood of an event's occurring between two groups. In the above example, the odds of a non-exposed individual's remaining cancer-free would be 2 to 1 (decimally expressed as 154/308 = .5). The odds of an exposed person's contracting cancer would be approximately 5 to 1 (expressed as an exact decimal of 709/142 = 4.993). The odds ratio would be 4.99/.5 = 9.99, again indicating the chemical's strong carcinogenicity.

Both statistics have advantages. Relative risk has a more intuitive meaning: in the above example, people exposed to the chemical have a risk of developing cancer 2.5 times greater than those not exposed. However, relative risk cannot be computed in all experimental designs and may overstate small differences in likelihood of an event's occurring within comparison groups.

Adapted from: Simon SD. Understanding the odds ratio and the relative risk. *Journal of Andrology.* 2001;22(4):533–536.

Traditional Epidemiology

Identifying features that many individuals with a given disease have in common remains a model for epidemiology today, as it did in the time of Edgar Snow. Both the risk groups and the routes of transmission for AIDS were determined in this fashion.

In 1983, epidemiologists at the federal Centers for Disease Control and Prevention (CDC) analyzed data on the first one thousand cases of AIDS reported to the agency.[38] All but sixty-one of the cases could be classified into one or more of the following groups: homosexual or bisexual men, intravenous drug abusers, Haitian natives, or patients with hemophilia. These findings suggested that AIDS was caused by a blood-borne pathogen and served as the basis for public health alerts to the relevant risk groups. Identification of the specific virus that caused AIDS, however, was still years away.

Identification of reservoirs of disease and routes of transmission to susceptible populations has been a source of international concern since the fourteenth century. Realizing that bubonic plague originated in Asia Minor and was disseminated along trade routes, officials in Italian port cities such as Venice instituted the practice of quarantine, prohibiting ships from the East to dock until their occupants were proven disease-free. Today international systems of influenza surveillance have been established to identify potential sources of global epidemics and to initiate measures to mitigate them.

Action against avian flu in the early twenty-first century provides an example. Localized cases of the disease were identified in Southeast Asia and Hong Kong, where domestic chickens apparently transmitted the virus from wild birds to humans. Chickens in huge numbers were killed and burned in an effort to prevent global exposure.

The following examples illustrate the contemporary importance of epidemiological detective work:

- An epidemic of diarrhea in Rome, New York, during the mid-1970s also illustrates the techniques and continuing relevance of traditional epidemiology. The epidemic was traced to a species of protozoa known as *Giardia lamblia.* This microorganism causes diarrhea of explosive intensity, along with cramps and fever, and is occasionally fatal. Over 10 percent of the residents of the city of Rome became infected with *G Lamblia,* the largest epidemic of its kind in U.S. history. The epidemic was traced to the city water supply.[39] A combination of antiquated chlorination and filtration systems, plus an increase in human habitation in the watershed, appear to have produced the infestation.

- A well-known epidemiological investigation in the 1990s traced a Florida woman's HIV infection to her dentist.[40] An absence of typical risk factors (such as intravenous drug use or sexual contact with potentially infected men) alerted public health officials to the possibility of a new source of infection. The woman identified her dentist as a possible source, and he indeed was suffering from AIDS and had ceased to practice. Examination of additional former patients identified several others with HIV infection. Retrospectively tracing the source of infection to a specific individual or reservoir is sometimes called *look-back procedure.*

- An outbreak of syphilis in San Francisco during the late 1990s was traced to a gay Internet chatroom. Users made contact with a single infected individual, or *index case,* through the chatroom. They contracted syphilis upon subsequent physical contact with this individual and went on to infect others.[41] Although syphilis bacilli do not literally travel through cyberspace, a series of social contacts initiated through the Internet promoted spread of the disease. The chatroom may be thought of as a virtual reservoir of disease.

■ In an instance of food-borne illness, a case control study was used to identify the source of an outbreak of *salmonella saphra* in southern California.[42] Although only a few cases of this infection normally occurred each year, public health officials were notified of fifteen cases occurring within a period of three weeks. The officials performed a *case-control* study, in which salmonella patients, designated as *cases,* were compared with *controls,* individuals unaffected by the organism. Both cases and controls were intensively interviewed regarding the foods they had eaten recently. Patients were more likely than controls to have consumed cantaloupe (88 percent versus 45 percent). Through interviewers with grocery store managers and distributors, the officials identified the source of the epidemic as a particular growing region in Mexico. The investigation pointed up health risks from food importation and the importance of washing produce.

The Florida HIV outbreak and the Rome diarrhea epidemic illustrate concerns and controversies in epidemiology. Both examples illustrate the importance of unusual occurrences to epidemiologists. In themselves, AIDS and giardiasis are widely encountered. However, AIDS occurs largely within recognized risk groups such as gay men and injection drug users (IDUs). The disease is said to be *endemic* in these populations—continuously present and neither markedly increasing nor declining in prevalence. Similarly, infection by *G. lamblia* occurs regularly among backpackers and travelers returning from countries with faulty infrastructure. An AIDS diagnosis would be very serious, and giardiasis troubling for any individual. But AIDS in an IDU or giardiasis in an adventure tourist would spark no extraordinary concern purely for epidemiology.

The Florida HIV case also illustrates challenges for epidemiology. Epidemiological techniques can provide strong clues about the origin and spread of disease. But they can seldom provide conclusive proof. Critics, for example, have argued that the HIV victims in Florida may have contracted the disease from sources other than the dentist. These critics also raise the possibility that some of the individuals may have lied about their sexual history or orientation.

The Epidemic Cycle

Scientists have repeatedly demonstrated that epidemics occur in cycles. Plotted against time elapsed from a zero point, incidence of an epidemic disease approximates a normal distribution. Figure 3.1, for example, illustrates the increase followed by the decline in incidence of an atypical strain of influenza in Mexico during April 2009. This influenza strain, the H1N1 or swine flu virus, later gave rise to widespread disease in the United States and elsewhere. But its incidence rose and fell in its venue of origin, a sequence ultimately expectable worldwide.

FIGURE 3.1 *Epidemiological curve of swine-origin influenza A (H1N1) virus infection: Mexico, April 2009*

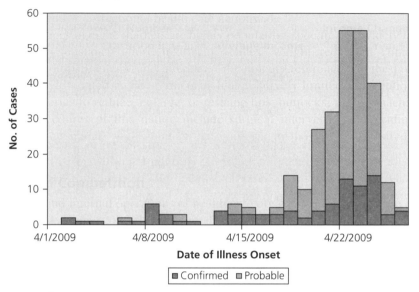

Source: Centers for Disease Control and Prevention. Outbreak of swine-origin influenza A (H1N1) virus infection: Mexico, April 2009. *Morbidity and Mortality Weekly Report.* 2009;58(17):467–470.

Epidemics since ancient times seem to have arisen and declined in similar fashion. A classic formulation known as *Farr's law* offers an explanation.[43] Accordingly, a virulent microorganism eventually runs out of new individuals to infect. All individuals are not equally susceptible, nor are they equally exposed. As the availability of susceptible but as yet unaffected individuals declines, the chain of transmission is broken. Thus, even the most fearsome epidemics have burned themselves out.

Modern Applications

Like traditional epidemiology, today's investigators monitor and analyze the occurrence of disease (morbidity) and death (mortality). But epidemiology can also address derivative phenomena such as pain, disability, avoidable hospitalization, and survivorship. Related studies go beyond observations of which clinicians themselves are capable. Thus, studies of pain in the general population alert health professionals to potential undertreatment of pain in doctor's offices and hospitals. Epidemiological studies of disability have demonstrated that resources such as flexibility in working hours can help keep people with physical dysfunction in the mainstream.[44] Research on hospitalization for conditions potentially treatable in community settings—so-called *ambulatory care–sensitive disease* such as asthma and congestive heart failure—point up the need for more community medical resources.[45] Studies of cancer survival have identified the consumer's access to care and ability to navigate the health care system as factors capable of extending life expectancy.[46]

An Epidemiology of Violence

The city of Los Angeles is sometimes viewed as a place where gang violence flourishes. News reports of drive-by shootings make people elsewhere think that gunplay is rampant among citizens driven mad by road rage.

Using a database on gangs maintained by the Los Angeles Police Department, researchers conducted an epidemiological study of drive-by shootings that occurred in a single year.[47] The researchers found that 429 individuals had been killed or wounded.

Of this total, 303 (71 percent) were gang members. The majority of shootings occurred in areas plagued by violent street gangs, typically economically deprived African American and Hispanic neighborhoods. Most shootings result from gang rivalry and largely affect gang members.

The researchers concluded that "drive-by shootings are not random events," but a phenomenon particular to the inner city.

Traditional epidemiology focused on acute disease and physical routes of transmission. Today epidemiologists must also concentrate on what may be termed *modern diseases,* whose development is often obscure, complex, and slow. Applications of epidemiological principles today, whether focused on acute or chronic conditions, extend to social, economic, and environmental factors. Diseases that are caused by human efforts to *prevent* disease are also concerns of the modern epidemiologist. Generally, such diseases are known as *iatrogenic.* The creation of drug-resistant bacteria through overuse of antibiotics illustrates the iatrogenic process. Infections that occur in hospitals, known as *nosocomial* infections, constitute a special case of iatrogenesis.

Today's epidemiologists are concerned with the rapid development and worldwide transmission of new strains of disease and perhaps even new diseases. The potential exists for pathogenic microorganisms to mutate into new forms with greater capacity to harm human populations. Thus, bacteria in time become resistant to antibiotics and cancer cells become immune to chemotherapeutic agents. Viruses that breed in animals acquire the ability to infect human hosts. An exchange process taking place within the intestines of pigs on farms of mainland China has worldwide implications.

In this process, viruses in the pigs' guts exchange DNA fragments with human DNA that the pigs have ingested via household waste. It is feared that the process may give rise to contagious and lethal forms of influenza, readily spread worldwide by migrating birds and the global transportation network.[48]

Outbreaks of diseases heretofore confined to isolated outposts of humanity have begun to spark international concern. Ebola and Marburg, two viral diseases, produce extreme morbidity in the form of massive hemorrhaging. Originally, these diseases occurred in isolated African jungle locales. Transmitted only by contact with body fluids, they have devastated individual villages, but did not readily spread to neighboring settlements. However, acquisition by the Ebola or Marburg virus through mutation of a capacity for aerosol transmission (via coughs and sneezes) could create a disease with the potential of becoming widespread.

Managerial Epidemiology

Today epidemiology contributes directly to the work of managers and policy makers. Contributions of this nature are sometimes grouped under the label of *managerial epidemiology*. Management of many types of health services benefits from epidemiological methodology. A good example may be found in the planning and pricing strategy of health plans offering prospective payment contracts to consumers (typically employee groups). Under such contracts, the plan is required to provide or pay for care required by the insured group at a fixed price. Epidemiology provides an understanding of the likely disease burden of the insured group, allowing the health plan to price its services appropriately. Planning and locating health facilities constitutes another application. Health care entities contemplating where to establish new facilities may wish to place them in areas where the complaints in which they specialize are most frequent.

HEALTH AND ILLNESS IN THE TWENTY-FIRST CENTURY

Compilations of figures by state and federal agencies help define the task of the U.S. health care system. Table 3.3 indicates the most frequent causes of death in the United States. Heart diseases, cancer, and strokes are now the predominant causes of death, both in the United States and other economically advanced countries.

Morbidity and Mortality

The twentieth century saw striking changes in the predominant causes of death in the United States. Early in the century, infectious diseases accounted for a much higher proportion of deaths. The three most frequent causes of mortality were influenza, pneumonia, and tuberculosis, which together accounted for almost a quarter of all deaths. Food-borne and water-borne diseases such as cholera, diarrhea, and intestinal ulceration constituted another frequent cause of mortality, accounting for 8 percent of all deaths. The public health systems and antimicrobial drugs deployed in the

TABLE 3.3   The most frequent causes of mortality in the United States, 2005

Cause	Number of Deaths (Thousands)	Percentage of Deaths
All causes	**2,448**	
Diseases of heart	652	26.6
Malignant neoplasms	559	22.8
Cerebrovascular diseases	143	5.8
Chronic lower respiratory diseases	131	5.4
Unintentional injuries	118	4.8
Diabetes mellitus	75	3.1
Alzheimer's disease	72	2.9
Influenza and pneumonia	62	2.8
Nephritis, nephritic syndrome, nephrosis	44	1.8
Septicemia	34	1.4

Source: National Center for Health Statistics. 2009. *Health, United States, 2008.* Table 30. Hyattsville, MD: National Center for Health Statistics.

twentieth century brought infectious diseases under control. However, it is important to remember that the causes of these diseases are still prevalent in the environment and may not have been controlled permanently.

Notable differences in the most frequent causes of death are found across age and racial groups. Among men, suicide was the eighth leading cause of death in 2005. Among African Americans, human immunodeficiency virus (HIV) disease was the ninth leading cause. Among individuals twenty-five to forty-four years of age, unintentional injury was the leading cause of death, accounting for 24.4 percent of deaths in this age group. Suicide, homicide, and HIV accounted for 9.1, 6.1, and 4.5 percent of deaths respectively among Americans ages twenty-five to forty-four.

Like the differences observable over the past hundred years, more recent changes in prevalence of mortality causes are important. Although heart disease is still the most frequent killer of Americans, its frequency as a cause of death has declined significantly since the mid-twentieth century. The proportion of cancer deaths, however, has increased over time. Effective medical and surgical treatments for heart diseases and underlying circulatory pathology have come into widespread use. These include drugs for prevention of sclerotic plaque and cardiac arrhythmia, as well as coronary artery bypass surgery. But progress in treatment for some of the most lethal cancers, such as lung and pancreas, has, despite well-funded efforts, been frustratingly slow.

Although the diseases named in Table 3.3 represent the immediate causes of death, many public health scientists would seek the root causes of mortality beyond these figures. These observers point to smoking as the actual cause of many cancer deaths, overweight and sedentary lifestyle as the cause of much heart and vascular diseases, and poverty and racial discrimination as the cause of many deaths from other immediate causes.

Tables 3.4 and 3.5 provide other perspectives on the tasks facing the U.S. health care system. These tables indicate the reasons people have sought care in doctors' offices and hospitals.

TABLE 3.4 The most frequent reasons for office visits in the United States, 2006

Reason for Visit	Number of Visits (Millions)	Percentage of Visits
All visits	**902.0**	
General medical exam	66.4	7.4
Progress visit, not otherwise specified	51.3	5.7
Cough	26.7	3.0
Postoperative visit	23.4	2.6
Prenatal exam	21.7	2.4

TABLE 3.4

Reason for Visit	Number of Visits (Millions)	Percentage of Visits
Gynecological exam	19.4	2.1
Medication	19.0	2.1
Stomach pain or cramps	16.0	1.8
Knee symptoms	15.0	1.7
Well-baby exam	13.6	1.5
Back symptoms	13.3	1.5
Symptoms referable to throat	13.3	1.5
Test results, not otherwise specified	13.1	1.4
Visual dysfunctions	12.2	1.4
Fever	12.2	1.3
Hypertension	11.6	1.3
Earache or ear infection	11.4	1.3
Headache or pain in head	10.2	1.1
Skin rash	10.1	1.1
Nasal congestion	9.4	1.0
All other reasons	512.7	56.8

Source: Cherry DK, Hing E, Woodwell DA, et al. National Ambulatory Medical Care Survey: 2006 summary. *National Health Statistics Reports.* Table 8. August 8, 2008 (No. 3).

TABLE 3.5 Leading discharge diagnoses from U.S. short-stay hospitals, 2004

Category of First-Listed Diagnosis	Number of Discharges (Millions)	Percentage of Discharges
All conditions and diseases	34.9	
Heart, stroke, or circulatory system	4.4	12.6
Females with deliveries	4.1	11.7
Psychoses	1.6	4.6
Pneumonia	1.3	3.7
Cancer	1.2	3.5
Fractures	1.0	2.9
Cerebrovascular disease	.9	2.6
Complications of surgical or medical care	.9	2.6
Osteoarthritis and related	.7	2.0
Diabetes	.6	1.7
Cellulitis and abscesses	.6	1.7
Dehydration	.5	1.4
Asthma	.5	1.4
Chronic bronchitis	.5	1.4
Urinary tract infection	.4	1.1

Source: Kozak LJ, DeFrances CJ, Hall MJ. National Hospital Discharge Survey: 2004 annual summary with detailed diagnosis and procedure data. *Vital Health Statistics.* 2006;13(162):1–209.

Table 3.4 presents the most frequent reasons identified by physicians for visits by their patients. People most often visit the doctor for a general medical examination, a "progress visit" to follow up on an intervention such as medication, or postoperative care. Of general patient-perceived symptoms, coughs appear most frequent, followed by stomach, knee, and back problems.

Table 3.5 presents data on the most frequent reasons for treatment in the hospital. Diagnosis charted at discharge, or *discharge diagnosis,* is commonly used as the basis for statistics on reasons for hospitalization because a diagnosis may not be readily available at admission. Heart and circulatory disease, including strokes, are the most frequent reasons for hospitalizations. Women giving birth account for the second most frequent category. Emergent conditions such as fractures are included among the leading discharge diagnoses. Surprisingly, serious mental disorders (psychoses) account for more instances of hospitalization than cancers.

The Concept of Modern Disease

It is useful to think of the diseases that cause the most deaths in the contemporary United States—and also account for many doctor visits and hospital stays—as *modern* diseases. These include cancer, heart disease, stroke, diabetes, and chronic obstructive pulmonary disease. These diseases existed in earlier times as well. However, with the control of infectious disease, they have become more prominent as causes of mortality.

Modern diseases involve a cluster of the following distinguishing characteristics:

■ *Chronicity.* Modern diseases are *chronic* in nature; that is, they are often never fully cured, but remain part of the patient's life, to be lived with and managed. Cancer and AIDS are examples. Like other chronic diseases, cancer and AIDS are distinguished from diseases that posed the greatest problems in yesteryear, which were *acute* and *self-limiting.* Diseases of this kind would rapidly reach a crisis, at which time the patient would die or survive, retaining a measure of immunity from further infection. Measles and smallpox are examples.

■ *Multifactorial in etiology.* Early life scientists such as Koch and Pasteur thought of diseases as being caused by a single, identifiable agent. Modern diseases, however, usually arise from a combination of factors. Biologically, a person may be predisposed to contracting a cancer or heart condition due to genetic heritage. The environment, including one rich in damaging radiation or lacking healthy nutrition, may potentiate the biological predisposition. The individual's social surroundings, which promote or deter healthy behavior, may affect risk of the disease.

■ *Expensive to treat.* Modern diseases are more expensive to treat than acute, self-limiting ones. This is because the individual requires continuing treatment for a number of years, until he succumbs to the diseases or is done in by a competing cause of mortality. Episodes of treatment are also more expensive than a single episode of a familiar, infectious disease.

■ *Require physician-patient collaboration.* Unlike the case of many acute, self-limiting diseases, patients need to be participants in their care. Many modern diseases require behavior changes and dietary revisions. For most such diseases, the patient bears responsibility for collaborating with the medical regimen.

Although so-called modern diseases today account for most mortality and morbidity in the industrialized world, diseases of the contagious, acute, and self-limiting variety are still present in the human environment. Modern diseases, moreover, may ultimately decline in importance, as scientists chip away at the threats represented by heart disease, cancer, AIDS, and similar conditions. A new class of challenges to health and survival may emerge, perhaps fitting the label *postmodern diseases.* Postmodern threats to health and survival arise from a combination of social, economic, and environmental factors. Although colon cancer is often cured, for example, mortality may result from a combination of factors including an absence of practical assistance in the subject's neighborhood, inadequate opportunity for screening and treatment, poor nutritional resources, and lack of skills in self-care.

FUTURE THREATS TO HEALTH

Conditions in the world today expose populations to new health threats. Disease can migrate from an isolated African cave to the heart of Western Europe in a matter of hours. Modern medicine enables individuals with heritable diseases to survive long enough to pass dysfunctions on to succeeding generations, increasing the prevalence of heritable diseases. Economic abundance itself has pathogenic effects. As leisure time and inexpensive carbohydrates become more widely available, pathological consequences such as obesity and diabetes become more prevalent. Other emerging and potential health hazards are illustrated below.

Drug-Resistant Microorganisms

As humankind has fought disease with antibiotics, it has helped create strains of pathogenic organisms that are resistant to these drugs. Thus, a new generation of "superbugs" has begun to emerge. Methicillin-resistant *Staphylococcus aureus,* or MRSA, has become a major problem in U.S. hospitals. New drug-resistant strains can be expected to emerge in the coming years.

Broadly speaking, the emergence of drug-resistant microorganisms may be considered an iatrogenic phenomenon. Use of antibiotics for conditions in which they are unnecessary or ineffective has stimulated mutation to immunity by microbes. Reducing such use of antibiotics in the community, however, has proven difficult. Consumers demand treatment for diseases such as ear infections that, though painful, are likely to spontaneously resolve themselves in time. Antibiotics are used to prevent disease in some settings. Livestock are fed such drugs to enable them to survive in crowded pens. Prostitutes in some cities take antibiotics to prevent infection by clients, promoting the development of drug-resistant strains within their bodies.

These drug-resistant microorganisms are then spread worldwide by sailors, sex tourists, and others global transients.

Species-Threatening Epidemics

In addition to the perspective on epidemics as self-limiting presented above, it is important to note that unique events in organic evolution may occur in the future as they undoubtedly have in the past. *Homo sapiens* have evolved some immunity to most pathogens in their environment. Thus, infectious microorganisms seem to eventually run out of hosts. However, an alternative scenario underscores the importance of both surveillance and the capacity of civilization to rapidly develop and deploy remedies to unexpected threats.

> *Begin with a thought experiment: What might it take to produce a virus with the potential to eliminate* Homo sapiens*? For a start, it should be one that we are unfamiliar with; our physical naiveté ensures only perfunctory resistance to virulent infection. To preserve the element of surprise, the virus must cross to humans from another species. Airborne transmission would encourage such a leap—a cough or simply sharing a breath, especially if only a tiny amount of virus were needed to establish a human foothold. Once inside us, the virus must multiply with extraordinary rapidity, producing catastrophic and irreversible damage to all major organs: liver, heart, lungs, brain, kidneys, and gut. During this phase of fertile proliferation, subtle but significant changes to its structure (mutation) would enable the virus to evade any rear-guard attempt by our immune system to reestablish control. To give the virus the ultimate upper hand, we should possess neither drug nor vaccine to challenge the infection. Finally, we should be denied the means to restrain viral spread, an easy condition to fulfill if one is ignorant of where it normally (and peacefully) resides.*[49]

KEY TERMS

Etiology
Environment
Epidemiology

Incidence
Prevalence

SUMMARY

This chapter identifies the illnesses and injuries that are most often encountered by health care providers today, illustrates the most important health risks presently facing the public, and describes new threats to health that are possible in the future.

The health care industry aims at maintaining normal biological functioning among Americans despite the challenges posed by illness and injury. Defining the health care system's proper domain, however, is more difficult now than in the past. Social, cultural, and political factors affect conceptions of health and illness. Definitions of normality themselves are subject to change. The causes of illness, moreover, are not fully understood.

The science of epidemiology contributes to understanding of health and illness by identifying sources of disease and the means by which risk of illness is distributed within a population. Unlike other branches of the health care industry, epidemiology concerns itself with health of a society, jurisdiction, or neighborhood. Information of this kind has wide implications for policy, planning, and marketing. In this connection, the term *managerial epidemiology* has come into use.

Pain, depression, allergies, respiratory diseases, high cholesterol, hypertension, and peptic disorders comprise the most frequently encountered health problems in the United States. Cancer, ischemic heart disease, and stroke, followed by unintentional injuries, chronic obstructive pulmonary disease, pneumonia or influenza, diabetes, and chronic liver disease are the most frequent causes of death. Subjective perception and intercultural differences help determine whether an individual considers himself in need of health care.

The diseases that represent the greatest threats to health and longevity in the United States today are chronic in nature and of multifactorial etiology. They are caused by combinations of environmental, hereditary, and behavioral factors. Their treatment and control often require multiple interventions, which raise issues for the health care system. Once thought to have become unimportant, infectious diseases today represent an increasing concern.

DISCUSSION QUESTIONS

1. Health risks and causes of death vary among people of different genders, age groups, and races. What issues does this observation raise for American society?

2. Of human concerns today that are considered normal, are any likely to become legitimate targets of medical intervention in the future?

3. Since the mid-twentieth century, decline in tobacco use has contributed markedly to the health of Americans. Can you identify any public health or policy interventions capable of contributing similarly to public health in the years to come?

4. The causes of death in the United States today are different from those of a hundred years ago. What will be the most frequent causes of death a hundred years hence?

5. How likely do you consider the occurrence of a species-threatening epidemic in the next twenty years?

CHAPTER

4

HUMAN BEHAVIOR, HEALTH, AND HEALTH CARE

LEARNING OBJECTIVES

- To learn about individual perceptions of illness
- To understand why people accept some health risks but not others
- To see how social, economic, and cultural factors affect the seeking of health care and demand for health services
- To become familiar with steps intended to promote appropriate utilization of health care and favorable outcomes
- To appreciate key consumer preferences in health care

THE BEHAVIORAL DIMENSION

This chapter focuses on the thinking and the behavior of health care consumers. As discussed in the preceding chapter, human behavior can promote or reduce risk of disease. This chapter takes a closer look at human behavior related to health and health care. It addresses not only behavior but the reasons why it takes place, including the individual's thinking and forces outside the individual. The availability to an individual of medical facilities and effective treatments does not ensure that she will benefit from them. Even people who make use of available medical resources may not do so appropriately. Social factors as well as individual experience affect utilization. Acceptability of risk plays a part not only in exposure to disease but utilization of health care. In a feedback cycle of major importance, the behavior of health professionals and organizations can affect the thinking and actions of consumers in a positive or negative fashion.

THE CONCEPT OF THE SICK ROLE

A classic concept in medical sociology known as the **sick role**[1] helps make sense of the differences in how individuals respond to symptoms. The concept provides insight into how illness may change an individual's relationships with those around him or her and society as a whole. It also provides a framework for characterizing individual patients and anticipating how they might respond to the offerings or instructions of health professionals.

Dimensions of the sick role concept include self-conception and social relations considered appropriate in the event of illness. The term *role* in this context reflects the characteristics and behavior that society expects of a sick person. Expectations of this kind include both privileges and responsibilities. The sick role, for example, grants the individual release from work and social obligations. But it requires the individual to seek care, adopt lifestyle modifications required for recovery, and avoid exposing others to infection.

Differing tendencies prevail among individuals with regard to acceptance of the sick role. Some individuals readily accept the role. Gross symptoms contribute to acceptance of illness. Social pressure to accept the sick role may come into play, as, for example, when someone with a bad cold is urged by colleagues at the workplace to go home. Other social influences may discourage an individual from accepting the sick role. Many people keep working despite obvious disease or take drugs to mask the appearance of illness in order to recreate or socialize.

Psychological and personality factors frequently impel individuals to reject the sick role. People are often reluctant to admit to themselves that they have a life-threatening disease. Rejection of the sick role in such instances has been characterized as *denial.* Denial may occur in less severe instances. Some people, for example, think of themselves as "never getting sick." Others place so high a value on self-sufficiency that they cannot accept the privileges of help from others or release from work.

People do not adopt the sick role, then, simply because they develop symptoms of disease. Adoption of the sick role also depends on the individual's values, personality, and social background. Women, for example, seem to adopt the sick role more readily then men.[2] Stress can motivate people to embrace the sick role, or to reinforce the sick role in motivating people to seek medical care.[3] The need to justify nonachievement of personal objectives or unfavorable social status can induce people to adopt the sick role. According to one study, public welfare recipients unable to become self-supporting looked to illness as an acceptable explanation.[4]

Despite its potential for abuse, the sick role should not be confused with malingering or fraudulent claim of illness. When adopting the sick role, an individual makes a positive contribution to the society around him. The individual's adoption of the sick role invokes compatible responses from the holders of other roles (by substituting at work or caretaking, for example). By going home or staying away, the person adopting the sick role protects others from contagion.

HEALTH RISK BEHAVIOR

Along with acceptance versus rejection of the sick role, an individual's choices regarding risk help determine her health status and utilization of services. Chapter Three addressed risks over which an individual may have little or no control, such as heredity, environment, or exposure to microorganisms. Individuals, however, may exercise substantial choice over other risks. To varying degrees, individuals are free to choose their lifestyles, occupations, neighborhoods, and exposure to substances. Choices such as these in turn affect the individual's health.

Personal Acceptance of Risk

Lifestyle. Many Americans pursue lifestyles and use substances that place their health in jeopardy. Despite increased understanding, acceptance of personal health risks in these areas remains widespread. Table 4.1 indicates that over one-third (37.6 percent) of Americans are physically inactive. A large majority of Americans are overweight (65.1 percent), and 21.5 percent now smoke tobacco. The percentage of U.S. adults who smoke fell considerably during the late twentieth century, declining by 50 percent during the century's closing decades. Still, over one in five continue this highly lethal practice.

Table 4.1 also illustrates differences in the degree of risk across major demographic categories. Females, for example, are less likely to smoke than males, but more likely to be physically inactive. Higher levels of education correspond to lower levels of inactivity and smoking. Latinos and Asian Americans are less likely to smoke than Caucasians or African Americans. Not shown in the table is a growing tendency among Americans to become overweight. During the period 1960 to 1962, 44.8 percent of Americans were overweight, compared with 65.2 percent during the period 1999 to 2002. Overweight occurs most frequently today among African American women (77.1 percent) and Mexican American men (73.2). While rates of smoking and inactivity are higher among the disadvantaged, the tendency to be overweight is shared by all socioeconomic categories.

TABLE 4.1   **Major health risks by demographic characteristics**

	Health Risk (%)		
	Inactive	Overweight[b]	Current Smoker[c]
All	**37.6**	**65.1**	**21.5**
Gender			
Male	35.4	68.8	23.7
Female	39.5	61.7	19.4
Race			
African American	48.5	70.1	18.1
Caucasian[a]	33.4	69.4	22.7
Asian	35.9	n.a.	6.3
Latino or Hispanic	51.9	72.7	10.9
Native American	54.7	n.a.	31.3
Years of education			
Less than 12	61.2	65.2	29.7
12	45.5	68.8	27.8
13–15	28.1	64.9	21.1
College graduate			10.2

[a]Excluding Latino or Hispanic.

[b]Race percentages for overweight are approximate (average male and female); "years of education" in this column are "poor, near poor, and nonpoor."

[c]Adults over 18.

Source: National Center for Health Statistics. 2006. *Health, United States, 2005.* Tables 63, 64, 65, 72, 73. Hyattsville, MD: National Center for Health Statistics.

Table 4.1 underscores the fact that lifestyle and consumption choices are not independent of people's social conditions and background. The personal health risks addressed in the table are concentrated among the socially disadvantaged. Data on some of the most acutely lethal health risks reinforce this impression. Deaths due to illicit drug overdose, for example, are most likely to occur among racial minorities.[5] A majority of habitual users of illicit drugs overdose from time to time, though not always with fatal results. However, overdose is a major cause of death in large American cities, constituting, for example, the ninth leading cause of death in 2000 in the city of New York. In 1998, male rates of fatal overdose were 21.3 per 100,000 for African Americans, 18.9 for Latinos, and 15.2 for Caucasians.

Relatively advantaged people engage in behavior that, while neither socially frowned upon nor illicit, nevertheless places them at risk of ill health and mortality. Many, in fact, consider such activity to be healthful, wholesome sport. An estimated 425,900 Americans aged six though seventeen were treated at U.S. hospitals for gymnastics-related injuries between 1990 and 2005.[6] About 200 million people worldwide ski Alpine-style. Among these individuals, risk of anterior cruciate ligament injury is comparable to that of college football players.[7] Sports that place their participants at risk of spinal cord injury and paralysis include diving, horseback riding, trampolining, and air sports such as hang gliding. A total of 14.5 percent of paralyzed patients brought to a trauma rehabilitation facility had been injured in sports, a majority of these in diving.[8]

The influence of an individual's subculture on acceptance of health risks may be strong. It has been observed, for example, that few teenage skateboard enthusiasts consistently wear helmets, wrist guards, or kneepads.[9] A culture of youthful bravado and invulnerability discourages visible risk avoidance. The writer of an article in *Skateboarder* magazine comments, for example, that "pads make you look like a dork" and that "elbow pads, kneepads, and wrist guards are equally dorky-looking."[10] Similarly, networks, neighborhood, and affinity-group cultures seem likely to affect willingness of individuals to take a broad range of risks.

Drugs favored by poor people and minorities, as well as daring maneuvers by skateboarders, may be seen as risks engaged in by the backward or immature. But the thinking of educated, presumably progressive-minded people may also give rise to increased risk. The gender-equality movement, for example, appears to have increased the average young woman's risk of traumatic injury. In comparison with years past, many more women today participate in competitive sports such as soccer and basketball. Women are considerably more likely to sustain serious injuries in soccer, basketball, and other sports than are men.[11]

Across the globe, other forms of risk taking with roots in culture and tradition may be observed. One such risk is consanguineous union, or marriage ranging from cousin-cousin to more distant relatedness. Prevalence is highest in Arab countries, followed by India, Japan, Brazil, and Israel. Within the United States, pockets of consanguineous union prevalence exist within religious communities such as Utah Mormons and Pennsylvania Old Order Amish. In Saudi Arabia, where consanguineous union is common, offspring are at elevated risk of juvenile rheumatic disease[12] and retinoblastoma,

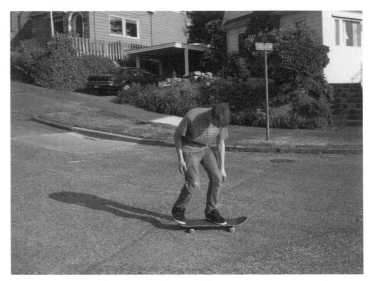

A teenager practices skateboarding. Note absence of protective gear strongly recommended by public health authorities such as helmet, kneepads, and wrist guards. Culture, whether defined by ethnic or age group, significantly affects the risks an individual will accept.

an eye cancer that usually occurs among young children.[13] Both Utah Mormons and Old Order Amish experience high rates of mortality among the young men in their communities.[14,15]

Medical Risk. The choices an individual makes regarding health care may itself involve risk. Some medications have side effects that for selected individuals outweigh their benefits. Physicians and pharmacists today take pains to inform patients of risks associated with prescription drugs. Surgery for conditions such as spinal disk disorders and certain cancers may or may not help the patient, but involve risk to both function and survival.

A study of individuals with cystic fibrosis (CF), a progressive, disabling, and ultimately fatal lung disease, illustrates the trade-offs patients must consider at the extreme. Today many CF patients are offered the option of lung transplantation. A successful lung transplant can allow previously compromised individuals an essentially normal life. However, most lung transplants are not successful. The procedure fails perhaps 75 percent of the time. Those who receive the failed transplants suffer greatly, with lower quality of life and often shorter life expectancy than they would have had if they had not undergone the procedure. In a study of people faced with this choice, Maynard comments:

> *Many patients, if they are willing to accept a more circumscribed life with less function, will live a longer life without transplant. If patients are unwilling to live a more circumscribed life, then transplant may be a gamble they wish to pursue, a gamble that poses a sequelae of risks and benefits for them to consider. Does transplant*

represent a beacon of light and hope or a series of half measures by which life has the possibility of being extended just a little bit more? Does transplant represent a form of cure or the acquisition of another disease haunted by its own series of declines and disabilities? Is transplant a last desperate measure or a calculated gamble for a "normal" life with fully functional lungs?[16]

As in other instances, the decisions an individual makes regarding risky medical interventions are influenced by peers and the surrounding culture. According to Maynard, values such as being able-bodied and strong and fighting illness through heroic means are fundamental elements of American culture. Indeed, the sick role emphasizes an obligation to achieve wellness through whatever means may be available.

Health Risks: Measurement and Intervention

Government, business, and the public health profession consider personal health risk taking of vital importance. The willingness of individuals to accept risk increases demands on public agencies, threatens corporate profits, and diminishes the health and well-being of the population. Means for understanding and changing patterns of personal health risk include the Behavioral Risk Factor Survey and the Health Risk Appraisal.

The Behavioral Risk Factor Survey (BRFS) is a continuous data-gathering effort spearheaded by the Centers for Disease Control and Prevention (CDC) and conducted independently by all fifty states.[17] Through telephone surveys, each state determines the prevalence of practices such as tobacco use, excessive alcohol consumption, unsafe sex, and keeping of loaded guns in the home. BRFS results have identified significant differences among states in health risks and their outcomes. In 2006, for example, nearly 10 percent of adults in Mississippi were diabetic, compared with half this percentage in Connecticut.

Because it is continuously administered, the BRFS makes it possible to detect trends in the risk behavior of Americans. An analysis of BRFS results from 1995 to 2004, for example, alerted public health authorities to the increase that was taking place in the percentage of Americans who were overweight, obese, and diabetic.[18]

The Health Risk Appraisal (HRA) is a questionnaire on health variables and practices that enables analysts to predict an individual's likelihood of death within the next ten to twenty years. Many such instruments have been developed since the 1970s. Items appearing on them typically include blood pressure, family history of disease, HDL cholesterol, seatbelt use while driving, and drinking behavior.[19] These instruments also include behavioral dimensions such as hours of sleep, social ties, involvement in violent arguments, and frequenting high-crime neighborhoods and bars.

(Continued)

(Continued)

> Survival models associated with HRA instruments enable them to provide individuals with information about the degree to which their behavior patterns place them at risk of mortality. Computerized versions of HRA instruments deliver instant feedback. Messages based on an individual's responses on an HRA instrument are often presented as "risk age"—the age a typical person has to reach to have the same mortality risk. A person whose risk age is greater than her actual age is in excessive danger of sickness and death.
>
> Health promotion efforts have utilized HRAs as tools for both assessment and motivation. Through HRAs, individuals learn that they may increase their years of healthy life by changing their habits and practices. HRAs can also help individuals formulate concrete objectives for modification of lifestyle and behavior.

Occupation. Occupational hazards comprise risks incurred as a consequence of choosing a job or career. Risks of traumatic injury in a variety of occupations in 2006 are presented in Table 4.2. Individuals involved in mining, agriculture, forestry, fishing, and construction had the highest rates of fatal injury. Workers in white-collar occupations such as finance and insurance were much safer.

Job-related mortality due to accidents represents only one type of industry-specific health risk. Risk of disability due to accidents is also important. In addition, risk of particular diseases is often associated with exposure to particle and chemical substances found in specific industries. Black lung (coal workers' pneumoconiosis), caused by breathing coal dust, is perhaps most familiar. Increased risk of chronic obstructive pulmonary disease (COPD) has been reported among workers in industries such as rubber, plastics, leather, office building services, textiles, food, trucking, health care, and armed services.[20]

Studies of relatively advantaged job holders also report occupational health risks. Law enforcement personnel have been found to experience increased health risks due to overweight, high cholesterol, stress, shift work, lack of exercise, and poor dietary habits.[21] The night-shift work required of many nurses is associated with increased intake of fat and refined carbohydrates, reduced physical activity due to fatigue, and decreased social contact outside work.[22] People who travel regularly on business face a variety of associated health risks. Extended airplane trips expose travelers to infectious diseases of fellow passengers and to blood clots from long periods of inactivity. Time away from home is conducive to family disruption and associated stress,[23] as well as to risks such as poor nutritional and sleep practices, alcohol abuse, and unsafe sex.

It is important to remember that although people choose their jobs, they often do so within a limited range of options. Individuals in many communities have limited choice regarding employment and disinclination or inability to move away. In rural areas, for example, employment is typically scarce. People may be disinclined to relocate, however, making lifestyle choices favoring proximity to family, friends, and familiar places.

TABLE 4.2 **Number and rate (per 100,000 workers) of traumatic occupational fatalities by industry, 2006**

Industry	Rate per 100,000	Number of Deaths
Agriculture, forestry, and fishing	30.0	655
Mining	28.1	192
Transportation and warehousing	16.8	860
Construction	10.9	1,239
Utilities	6.3	53
Wholesale trade	4.9	222
Professional, scientific, management, and administrative	3.2	459
Manufacturing	2.8	456
Retail trade	2.2	359
Finance, insurance, real estate, rental, and leasing	1.2	126
Total for 2006	4.0	5,840

Source: National Center for Health Statistics. 2009. *Health, United States, 2008.* Hyattsville, MD: National Center for Health Statistics.

Residence. Residence in a disadvantaged, inner-city neighborhood is associated with multiple health risks. Scientists have not yet determined the full range of neighborhood-level health hazards that may exist, but a complex of interrelated factors seems to prevail. As cited in a *New York Times* report, the following facts stand out:

■ There are three times as many bars in poor neighborhoods as in rich ones

■ There are four times as many supermarkets in white neighborhoods as in black ones

■ There are fewer parks in low-income neighborhoods than in higher income ones[24]

Although people are technically free to live where they please, actual choice is highly constrained. Racial discrimination and unequal income distribution create ghettos. Conditions in such areas further constrain individual choice. As the *New York Times* report comments, "Poor people are more likely to have unhealthy habits because fast food and cigarettes are abundant and cheap in their neighborhoods, and healthy alternatives tend to be limited."

Public Perceptions and Responses to Risk

Most people's behavior is guided not by scientific inquiry but by perceptions and beliefs. Individuals' perception of risk may not match the findings of scientists. This disparity between fact and perception has important implications. Inaccurate perception of risk can lead people to ignore serious hazards. Beyond the personal level, inaccurate perception of risk can lead to faulty public policy. Many government decisions are driven by public perceptions, rather than scientific facts. Thus, public officials may be tempted to support interventions that address health concerns other than those representing the greatest risk to the most people. Adverse decisions in areas such as lawmaking, regulation, and research funding may result.

The public suffers from many misperceptions regarding health risks. Perceptions about risk of contracting diseases illustrate this fact. Surveys in the late twentieth century found U.S. women to be far more concerned with the risk of contracting breast cancer than other cancers or heart disease. One review quotes a survey of one thousand women ages forty-five through sixty-five, 61 percent of whom said they were concerned about developing breast cancer, but only 9 percent of whom were concerned about having a heart attack. In fact, at the time the survey was conducted, a woman's chance of dying from lung cancer or heart disease was much higher than her likelihood of dying from breast cancer.[25]

Misconceptions about cancer in general are widespread in the United States. A study published in 2007 compared perceptions of the general public with those of professional epidemiologists. Over two-thirds of the general public thought that the risk of dying from cancer in the United States was increasing; over one-third thought that living in a polluted city was a greater risk for lung cancer than smoking a pack of cigarettes per day. None of the epidemiologists thought that either proposition was true. Nearly one-third of the public (29.7 percent) thought that electronic devices like cell phones could cause cancer. All the epidemiologists who were familiar with this topic expressed doubts, considering the link between electronic devices and cancer to be false, likely to be false, or difficult to evaluate.[26]

Areas of public misconception are evident in infectious disease. The scare over West Nile virus at the turn of the twenty-first century provides an example. West Nile virus is transmitted by mosquitoes that feed on infected birds and then infect humans. Public officials fretted about the spread of West Nile virus from the eastern United States to the Pacific coast states. Yet West Nile virus generally produces mild symptoms and is seldom fatal, except in the elderly.

Diseases that are much more widespread and potentially lethal arouse scant public concern. A New York state outbreak of West Nile virus in 1999, for example, made headlines. At the same time, outbreaks of *E. coli* and whooping cough aroused little public attention.[27] These diseases in fact endangered a far greater number of New Yorkers. Both *E. coli* infection and whooping cough can be life-threatening, particularly in young children. Both diseases are readily controllable through conventional means—proper food handling in the case of *E. coli,* and immunization in whooping cough. Control of West Nile virus, however, may require extensive and costly mosquito eradication programs.

A synthesis of research by psychologist Paul Slovic summarizes the nonfactual basis on which most people assess risks. According to Slovic, response to hazards is mediated by social influences transmitted by friends, family, fellow workers, and respected public officials. People may downplay the level of risk associated with behavior in which they regularly engage. Slovic adds: "Experts' judgment appears to be prone to many of the same biases as those of the general public, particularly when experts are forced to go beyond the limits of available data and rely on intuition." [28]

Generally, Americans express greater concern with health risks imposed on them than the ones they incur on their own. Unions negotiate for engineering solutions to workplace health risks rather than for solutions involving self-protection by workers. Lawsuits are launched against industrial polluters. Increasingly, municipalities and states have banned workplace smoking to protect nonsmoking workers from exposure to sidestream smoke. Research on public perception of risks associated with technology can be readily applied to health. A review of research in this field has concluded that the public will accept risks from voluntary activities (such as skiing) that are roughly one thousand times as great as risks from involuntary hazards (such as food preservatives) that provide the same level of benefits.[29]

However, Americans neglect some of the most widespread heath risks. The natural environment, for example, contains a number of carcinogens. In recent years, the public has become more familiar with risk of cancer associated with sun exposure. Risks associated with natural carcinogens in vegetables such as mushrooms and peanuts are as potent as widely feared PCBs and DDT.[30] Yet cancer risks associated with vegetable consumption have not yet attracted the public's attention.

In summary, three factors seem consistently important in determining how people perceive health risks:

■ *Newness of threat.* A newly recognized health risk is likely to draw more attention than one that has been known for many years. West Nile virus, as described above, illustrates this phenomenon. The disease was new to most Americans; hence, it created more concern than *E. coli* infection and whooping cough. Alzheimer's disease today attracts considerable public attention. Although "senile dementia," as the disease was once known, has always occurred, greater recognition of its prevalence and a renaming have transformed the condition into a seemingly new disease capable of arousing increased concern.[31]

■ *Political promotion and media exposure.* Advocacy around health issues is big business in the United States. Powerfully organized and well-funded advocacy groups have raised public consciousness about breast cancer, AIDS, Alzheimer's disease, and a number of other conditions. The process by which advocacy groups promote the importance of specific diseases is detailed in Chapter Eleven. Skilled advocates use the media as a tool in their promotion efforts, increasing the public's knowledge and perceived vulnerability to the relevant disease.

■ *Imposition of risk.* The importance of imposition versus personal acceptance of risk is crucial. Americans tend to emphasize risks for which they can blame forces outside themselves. Despite the known hazards, millions of Americans still use tobacco and ride bicycles and motorcycles without helmets. Public outcries, however, have arisen upon introduction of supposedly risky technologies such as genetically engineered crops and exposure of food products to radiation for preservation and pest control.

The Famous (or Infamous) Delaney Clause

Responding to vastly increased use of artificial chemicals in food production and distribution, Congress amended the federal Food, Drug, and Cosmetic Act to require the following:

> No additive shall be deemed to be safe if it is found to induce cancer when ingested by man or animal, or if it is found, after tests which are appropriate for the evaluation of the safety of food additives, to induce cancer in man or animal.[32]

Introduced by Representative James Delaney in 1954, the provision became known as the Delaney Amendment or the Delaney Clause. It remained unchanged for over forty years amid continual controversy. A literal interpretation of the clause (which was supported by the courts) required the Food and Drug Administration (FDA) to ban from the food supply substances that exposed consumers to even a statistically negligible (*de minimis*) risk of cancer.

For decades, food producers and pesticide manufacturers argued that the clause actually undermined the public interest by banning agriculturally important chemicals and potentially jeopardizing an adequate and economical food supply. Scientists pointed out that carcinogens naturally occurring in foods such as peanuts and grains posed greater risks to humans than many of the banned artificial additives.

Fearing a public outcry, Congress has been unwilling to repeal the Delaney Clause, although its importance was reduced in 1996 by exemption of pesticides from its jurisdiction. The decades-long endurance of the Delaney Clause is testimony to the public's sensitivity to risks that are imposed and poorly understood.

USE OF HEALTH SERVICES

Research on human behavior is particularly important in predicting utilization of health services. This chapter has already discussed the variability of utilization. People who accept the sick role are more likely to visit a health care provider than those who resist the role. As in the example of cystic fibrosis presented earlier, people weigh the risks and benefits associated with treatment and make utilization decisions accordingly. As in the case of health risks, many elements of an individual's thinking other than awareness of physical symptoms determine whether he will obtain health care.

Understanding of the differences in utilization patterns among segments of the population is of key practical importance. Managers require this information, along with associated epidemiological facts, to ensure that their facilities have appropriate professional staffing and physical capacity for the expected patient volume. Policy makers need to ensure levels of funding and revenue for the needs of clients in public programs. Both managers and policy makers require information on utilization differences to design and operate programs that encourage the populations they serve to obtain appropriate care.

Demographic Variation

Distinction along demographic lines is the most elementary step in understanding variations in health service utilization. *Demographics* refers to the distribution of age, gender, race, ethnicity, immigration status, and national origin within a population. Scientists who study demographics also concern themselves with population dynamics such as birth rates, death rates, and population changes due to excess of births over deaths ("natural increase") or migration. Beyond their traditional concerns, demographers today examine income distribution and chances for moving up the social ladder as important features of a city, regional, or national population.

Table 4.3, addressing health care and dental visits over the past year, provides an illustration of demographic variation in health service utilization. The table indicates that gender, race, and income all affect the likelihood of an individual's having received services at least once in the past twelve months. The independent effects of poverty and minority race are most visible in dental services. Only 36.7 percent of poor Latinos saw a dentist within the past twelve months. Among poor, non-Latino African Americans and Caucasians, 39.9 and 50.6 percent respectively visited a dentist.

Age, race, and gender—the three principal demographic variables—affect utilization of many forms of health care other than doctor and dentist visits. Some research findings suggest disparities potentially affecting quality. One study, for example, reports that African Americans and Latinos are less likely to utilize new medications than non-Latino Caucasians.[33] Among individuals with arthritis, utilization rates for hip and knee surgery differ by both age and race. Among older individuals (sixty-five and up) but not among younger individuals, African Americans are less likely to have hip or knee surgery than Caucasians.[34] Immigrant women are less likely to have mammograms or Pap smears than women born in the United States.[35] The differences

TABLE 4.3 **Percentage utilizing health care and dental services in past twelve months by major demographics**

	Service Utilized	
	Health Care[a]	Dental[b]
All	82.8	62.2
Gender		
Male	77.2	57.7
Female	88.2	67.1
Race		
African American	84.0	55.6
Caucasian	82.8	63.3
Asian	78.1	68.7
Latino or Hispanic	72.9	47.2
Native American	79.5	51.0
Poverty status		
Poor	79.4	44.8
Near poor	79.9	46.8
Nonpoor	85.5	69.6

[a]Includes visits to doctor's offices, emergency departments, and home visits, 2006.

[b]Includes individuals ages eighteen through sixty-four, 2006.

Source: National Center for Health Statistics. 2009. *Health, United States, 2008.* Tables 75, 84. Hyattsville, MD: National Center for Health Statistics.

between immigrant and native-born women decline when the effects of insurance coverage, having a usual source of care, and acculturation to life in the United States are taken into account.

Personal Outlook

Several dimensions of personal outlook introduced in this chapter affect individual consumption behavior. People who readily accept the sick role would appear more likely than others to utilize health services of all kinds. Individuals who acknowledge risk of illness and take personal responsibility for reducing their risks are relatively likely to utilize preventive services. Not surprisingly, for example, researchers have found that women who perceived their risk of developing cervical or colon cancer as moderate to very high were more likely to get screened for these diseases than women who considered themselves at no or very low risk.[36] Parental attitudes about the health care needs of their children, again not unexpectedly, have much to do with the health care that the children utilize.[37] The absence of a father in the household and the presence of large numbers of children reduce the likelihood that an individual asthmatic child will receive appropriate health care or that her asthma will be controlled.[38]

Clearly, many personal and social factors explain the utilization behavior of individual consumers of health care. Many factors in addition to those already cited appear important as well. Health services researchers since the 1950s have investigated and catalogued these predictors of utilization behavior.

The Behavioral Model of Health Care Utilization

The many factors shown to affect health care utilization can be summarized according to the so-called Behavioral Model of Health Care Utilization. Table 4.4 presents the basic elements of this model. According to the model, multiple interacting factors strongly influence the individual's tendency to use or not to use health services. The original model explained variations in health care utilization through three factors: need, predisposing, and enabling.[39] In later years, factors associated with the health care system itself were added to the model. Health services researchers have periodically augmented the model further.

In the version of the model summarized in Table 4.4, *need* is the most obvious factor. The individual must believe he is ill or may potentially become ill to seek health care. Need is experienced as the classic signs of illness such as fever, pain, redness or other skin manifestations, and swelling—the *calor, dolor, rubor,* and *tumor* articulated by the ancient Romans to describe inflammation. Other dimensions of need are more subjective. As discussed earlier in this chapter, acceptance of the sick role involves acknowledgment of need for health care. Denial of illness is the opposite and a quite widespread phenomenon. Awareness of personal risk and acceptance of personal responsibility for its reduction contribute to the feeling of a need for health services, particularly of the preventive variety.

TABLE 4.4   Factors in the Behavioral Model of Health Care Utilization

Population Factors			System Factors
Need	**Predisposing**	**Enabling**	**System Factors**
Perception of illness: pain, function, disability, observations of others	Belief in benefits of health care	Health insurance status	Policy
		Income or wealth	Resources
	Ethnicity or history; Culture	Ambulation	Organization
Perception of risk: exposure to illness, desire for immunization, screening	Immigration status or years in the U.S.	Ability to drive or use public transit	
	Gender	Accessibility of facility	
	Education	Availability of assistance in community	
		Language or translation services	
		Child care	
		Self-efficacy	

The relationships of basic demographics to visits to health professionals visible in Table 4.3 may reflect differences in perception of need. Women, for example, seem more comfortable with the sick role than men. Interethnic differences may arise in part because of differences in the ways Latinos (particularly immigrants) and Native Americans recognize illness in comparison with Caucasians. People with more years of education may be more sensitive to early signs of illness than those with fewer years. The more educated are relatively high utilizers. The greater tendency of the educated to use health services is particularly strong in the absence of apparent disease. People with more years of education are relatively likely to have general physicals, tests, immunizations, preventive procedures, and prenatal care (within the first three months of pregnancy) in comparison to people with fewer years of education.

Predisposing factors are associated with the feeling of potential benefit from health care and emotional comfort with the health care system. The concept of predisposition to health care utilization offers an additional explanation of the impact of demographics. Additional years of education may foster a stronger belief in the benefits of science and medicine. Immigrants often feel uncomfortable approaching mainstream institutions such as those involved in health care. This is particularly true among undocumented individuals. Whether immigrants or not, members of ethnic minority groups may have similar feelings of discomfort with mainstream U.S. institutions. Women, who often have primary responsibility for the health care received by their families, may be more sensitive to the need for such services than men.

Enabling factors constitute the ways and means associated with utilization of health services. Today insurance coverage is paramount. As a later chapter will demonstrate, the uninsured tend to consume less (and lower-quality) health services than the insured. Money, either as disposable income or accumulated wealth (such as investments or home equity), may substitute for or supplement insurance. Nonmonetary enabling factors are important as well. These include convenience, such as the geographical proximity of a health care facility, its accessibility by public transportation, and accommodation to people with disabilities. For young families, a child-friendly environment (with or without actual child care) is often important. Factors related to health care personnel include their ability to communicate in the patient's language (directly or through a translator), and, whatever language may be involved, to be good listeners. For women, particularly those from third-world cultures, the presence of female providers may be important.

Specific dimensions of an individual or her environment may play multiple parts: both need and predisposing, predisposing and enabling, and so forth. Accordingly, ethnicity may be a predisposing factor, as described earlier. In addition, ethnicity may affect perceived need. Cultures associated with individual ethnic groups often contain definitions of health. A human quality that may be considered either predisposing or enabling is that of *self-efficacy*.[40] Self-efficacy refers to the individual's belief that he can be effective in pursuing improvements in conditions of life or human relationships. Self-efficacy both militates against acceptance of an adverse health condition and promotes the individual's ability to overcome any barriers to health care that he may encounter.

Table 4.4 presents a summary list of factors that can affect an individual's use of health services. However, the model also has a dynamic feature.[41] This feature is illustrated in Figure 4.1.

Unlike earlier versions, the version of the Behavioral Model of Health Care Utilization shown in Figure 4.1 highlights the importance of factors outside the individual. Need, predisposing, and enabling factors remain important, referenced as "population characteristics." However, this version also includes the health care system itself and the individual's external environment. The schematic in Figure 4.1 illustrates the manner in which the constructs in the model interact. Thus, characteristics of the health care system (such as cost and cultural bias) may have negative effects on individual predisposing and enabling factors (namely, wherewithal and self-efficacy), ultimately affecting utilization.

FIGURE 4.1   *A dynamic model of health care utilization*

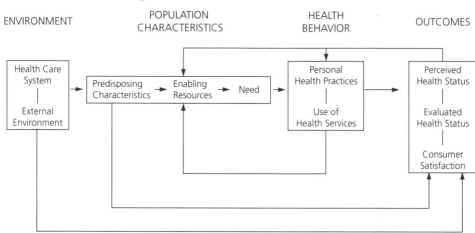

Source: Andersen R. Revisiting the behavioral model and access to medical care: does it matter? *Journal of Health and Social Behavior.* 1995;36(1):1–10.

ADVERSE PATIENT BEHAVIOR

Although the Behavioral Model of Health Care Utilization and associated research are of great practical value, they provide an incomplete understanding of health behavior. Requirements for favorable consumer behavior extend beyond making visits to providers and receiving prescriptions and recommendations. Meeting the health care system's goals require that the consumer act in a manner consistent with the prescriptions and recommendations of providers. Health professionals use the terms *nonadherence* and *noncompliance* to denote deviation from medical advice. The term *nonadherence* is preferred today, since it does not imply fault or shortcoming on the patient's part. The two terms are used interchangeably from now on.

Adverse patient behavior may be observed throughout the health care system. Its forms include not taking medications according to instructions or not at all, failing to follow through for recommend or scheduled procedures, and leaving the hospital without having been officially discharged. Express refusal of care may represent unfavorable patient behavior in some instances, but reasonable prudence and wisdom in others.

Nonadherence or Noncompliance

Failure to follow medication regimens represents the most widespread form of noncompliance. It has been estimated that up to 50 percent of patients do not take the medications they are prescribed or do not take them as directed.[42] Patients may fail to take medications for a number of reasons. They may think that the medications will be ineffective, produce adverse effects, are not necessary, or cost too much money.

Communication with health care providers makes a difference in patient behavior. Patients who report better general communication with their doctor, better instructions on how to take a medication, and who receive more medication information are more likely to take medications as prescribed.

A smaller but potentially significant percentage of patients who receive recommendations for intrusive procedures fail to follow up. According to one report, about 5 percent of patients for whom angiograms and coronary bypass surgery are recommended do not ultimately receive these procedures.[43] A study released in 2006 reported that about 18 percent of scheduled surgeries are ultimately cancelled, 30.1 percent of these because the patient did not show up. Almost half of the cancellations could be attributed to noncompliance, including patient nonappearance, patient or guardian refusal, and failure of patients to abstain from food or water by mouth shortly before the scheduled surgery.[44] Nonappearance for surgery was in part predictable, occurring most often among individuals who had not regularly kept prior clinic appointments.

Premature departure from the hospital represents not only a hazard for the patient but financial loss to the hospital. According to a study of adult hospital admissions, 1.4 percent of those admitted on an urgent or emergency basis eventually left the hospital against medical advice.[45] Although the percentage may seem small, it represents hundreds of thousands of self-discharges in every year. This study did not cover psychiatric, substance abuse, or federally operated hospitals (such as facilities of the Veterans Administration), in which patient-initiated departures might have occurred at a higher rate.

Research has demonstrated that factors identified in the Behavioral Model of Health Care Utilization may help identify individuals at risk of nonadherence. Predisposing factors associated with race and ethnicity can be important. Caucasian patients, for example, are 50 percent more likely to leave the hospital against medical advice than Latinos. Enabling factors are also clearly applicable. Patients responsible for their own medical bills are over three times as likely to leave the hospital against medical advice as those with private health insurance. As late as 2005, over 15 percent of Medicare beneficiaries did not follow medication regimens due to the cost of the required drugs.[46]

The greatest impact of need, predisposing, and enabling factors, however, may take the form of a feedback cycle. A favorable experience with the health care system increases the individual's predisposition to use health services when new needs arise. The opposite is also true. A history of unfavorable encounters with the system lowers predisposition to utilize services and, even when services are utilized, promotes noncompliance. A study of patients in whom signs of cancer had been detected at a screening facility illustrates the feedback cycle. Individuals who had had weak linkages with the health care system or experienced poor service prior to screening tended not to follow up the facility's findings to obtain definitive diagnosis.[47]

Refusal of Care

A patient's refusal of potentially beneficial care represents an extreme form of adverse behavior. Religious beliefs are perhaps the most visible reason for refusal of medical intervention. Some thirty different religions currently practiced in the United States prohibit or restrict widely used medical procedures. Because of the frequent need for blood and blood products, members of the Jehovah's Witnesses often refuse surgery or other procedures that may require transfusion. Refusal or delay of care occurs among Christian Scientists and other religious communities who believe that prayer should be the primary or sole intervention in time of illness.[48]

Patients may refuse care because they believe the proposed intervention will be ineffective, prove excessively burdensome, or fail to achieve desired results. A study of patients with life-threatening illnesses provides facts about the preferences of patients among whom such decisions clearly matter. These patients were strongly inclined to express positive sentiment if success seemed highly likely or assured. However, positive sentiment declined if the treatment involved substantial pain or discomfort. Relatively little acceptance of treatment was expressed if it was assumed that the treatment might preserve life but result in physical or mental impairment.[49]

Like many features of health behavior, refusal of care has causes and implications beyond the individual patient's bedside. Ethicists ask whether the rising cost of health care may someday result in widespread efforts by health professionals and managers to persuade the desperately ill or elderly to refuse treatment. In recent times, broader issues have emerged surrounding refusal of or noncompliance with treatment of tuberculosis. This disease, endemic among homeless individuals, poses threats to life and well-being in the broader community. When treated, the street resident with tuberculosis often fails to take her entire course of antibiotic medication. This practice has promoted the development of drug-resistant strains of tuberculosis, a potential peril to thousands. In response, public health authorities in some places have resorted to forced confinement and medication of homeless patients. While this issue raises both ethical and civil libertarian concerns, the practice continues in the tradition of quarantine established in earlier centuries.

HEALTH LITERACY AND CULTURAL COMPETENCE

Thus far, the present chapter has concentrated on individual thinking and behavior with only minor attention to the organizations, institutions, and professionals who deliver health care. Factors outside the individual, however, strongly influence his thoughts and actions. Race, socioeconomic status, and culture exercise powerful influences. But so do the structures, operating procedures, and outlooks of organizations and individuals involved in health services delivery. The individual's experience with the health care system helps mold his outlook and behavior as a consumer of health care. Negative outcomes from this process create barriers to achievement of the health care system's goals regarding personal or population health. An understanding of these barriers can lead to development of means for surmounting them.

Two areas of concern in the health care industry—**health literacy** and **cultural competence**—have arisen from observation of the consumer's interaction with the system. Often tied to race, socioeconomic status, and culture, concerns with health literacy and cultural competence expose some of the basic cleavages in American society. More generally, these concerns reflect disconnection from the health care system capable of producing negative outcomes for both the individual and society. Health care providers are becoming increasingly aware of health literacy and cultural competence as necessary for appropriate consumer behavior. Many organizations concerned with health services have made significant efforts to build capacity in these areas.

Health Literacy

According to a definition used by the Institute of Medicine, health literacy refers to "the degree to which individuals have the capacity to obtain, process, and understand basic health information and services needed to make appropriate health decisions."[50] Traditionally, health literacy has meant a patient's ability to understand communications from health professionals and written medication or self-care instructions. But the concept may be extended to an understanding of reports on disease outbreaks and other health risks in mass and specialized media.

Lack of health literacy affects areas other than communication between clinicians and patients. It prevents people from obtaining health benefits for which they may qualify and understanding the range of treatment options that may be appropriate for them. In the role of citizen, only adequate health literacy enables people to assess policy positions and options affecting their community and nation.

According to some, the problem has its roots in the degree of general literacy possessed by many in the United States. One researcher[51] has reported that half the U.S. population has deficiencies in reading and computation sufficient to inhibit full participation in "what we might consider normal daily activities." But even the well-educated may fare poorly in interpreting arcane language in medical and insurance-related communication. In even the best-educated individuals, level of comprehension may decline with age, particularly likely among people with chronic diseases or deficits in vision or hearing.

It would be a mistake to attribute lack of understanding of medical communication solely to deficits in comprehension by consumers. Medical professionals today are not consistently trained to communicate well. Communication with even the best-educated patients requires translation of technical terminology into everyday language. Many clinicians today lack the time required to make this translation, and some are not temperamentally fitted to do so. Clinicians in different specialties, moreover, do not always understand the procedures, objectives, or terminology (much less the cultures) of clinicians in other specialties. Clinicians are not trained to understand the language or technicalities of management and policy analysis, two fields increasingly important in health care.

Clinicians and health services researchers have increasingly experimented with interventions to remedy low health literacy since the beginning of the twenty-first century. One important action group in health literacy, the Partnership for Clear Communication, combines interests including the AMA, Pfizer, Inc., the American Public Health Association, the American Pharmacists Association, the American College of

Nurse Practitioners, and several other professional and industrial groups. Interventions include a campaign called Ask Me 3, which encourages patients to press their caregiver for clear, useful information via three simple questions:

- What is my main problem?

- What do I need to do?

- Why is it important for me to do this?

Other interventions attempt either to increase the patient's level of health literacy or bypass its effects on comprehension. Interventions often encourage clinicians to substitute simple, everyday words for medical terminology—some, of potential value for nonspeakers of English, utilize cartoons, pictographs, and other nonword-based communication modules associated with medical procedures, prescriptions, and prevention; others introduce health-related material into elementary school reading curricula. Laws in several states ensure that pharmacists are available to instruct patients receiving new prescriptions. A particularly innovative experiment has involved reading to children waiting for their appointments in pediatricians' offices.[52]

Cultural Competence

A concept relevant to many fields other than health, cultural competence can be thought of as an individual, organizational, or systemwide capacity. At all levels, cultural competence requires acknowledging and incorporating into practice "the importance of culture, assessment of cross-cultural relations, vigilance toward the dynamics that result from cultural differences, expansion of cultural knowledge, and adaptation of services to meet culturally unique needs."[53] *Culture,* an often misused word, comprises ethnically and historically transmitted beliefs, values, ethics, and general conceptions about how the world works. Cultural competence involves a person or organization's appreciation of the culture of others and willingness to adjust one's practices accordingly.

Culture differs from socioeconomic status. Ethnic minorities may typically be poor. But important cultural differences prevail among Latinos, African Americans, and Chinese Americans, to name only a few. Even among Latinos overall, Cuban immigrants and their descendants in Florida differ in history and outlook from Puerto Ricans in New York and immigrants from Central America in Los Angeles. Urban homeless people and migrant agricultural workers may both be itinerant but have vastly differing experiences and cultures.

Elements of culture relevant to health care include conceptions of illness. The preceding chapter has identified diseases recognized in one culture (*mollera caida* and *empacho*) but not in others and nonacknowledgement within some cultures of diseases that are widely recognized in the United States (such as depression). In an era when ethnic distinctions in the United States were very strong, recognition of pain and its implications seemed to differ strongly among ethic groups.

Expectations regarding health services stand out among important cultural differences. The health care system embodies the mainstream of U.S. institutions and professions. While some cultures may view the health care system as friendly and helpful, others may view it as distant and sinister. The Tuskegee experiment, in which African American men were allowed to suffer and die from untreated syphilis, remains in the memory of many in the African American community. Even among Latinos settled in the United States for many generations, fear of the authority represented by mainstream institutions remains strong. Across many ethnic groups, then, an atmosphere of mistrust and avoidance prevails regarding health care providers.

Lack of cultural competence among health professionals and organizations is often visible in a number of areas. Most obvious is language. With increasing immigration in the United States has come a growing proportion of health care consumers lacking English fluency. No health care organization can serve these individuals well without adequate translation services. Hours of clinic operation may be incompatible with work patterns in the community. Clinic intake procedures and hospital visitation rules may prove antagonistic to some groups. The use of home or traditional remedies may be kept secret by minority patients who fear embarrassment or criticism.

Of special importance is prevention of ethnic stereotyping by providers. According to one study, minority race was associated in the minds of physicians with disregard for the patient's intelligence, weak feelings of affiliation with the patient, and pessimism about patient's risk behavior and compliance with medical advice.[54] Other research suggests that stereotyping, in the worst cases, may lead to less aggressive or effective treatment decisions by providers.[55]

Following are several steps widely viewed as essential for achievement of cultural competence by a provider organization:

■ *Adequate translation services.* Services of this kind are widely available today through specialized firms or via real-time telecommunication.

■ *Ethnically representative staff.* Most health professions in the United States today underrepresent ethnic minorities other than Asian Americans. A more appropriate balance, it has been reported, would facilitate better communication and adherence to medical regimens.

■ *Cross-culturally trained providers.* Doctors, nurses, and other health professionals aware of the health beliefs of all their patients and the effects these have on perceptions and behavior provide better care.

■ *Monitoring processes and outcomes.* Systems that provide information on potentially disproportional waiting room times, successful referral, and outcomes of treatment enable provider organizations to ensure high quality of care for all consumers, regardless of social background.

Outcomes of Health Literacy and Cultural Competence

Association of health literacy and cultural competence with actual health outcomes has not yet been demonstrated in a consistent fashion. Some researchers have found low health literacy to be associated with adverse health outcomes. Diabetics with low health literacy, for example, are less likely to achieve high glycemic control than their more health-literate counterparts. Other studies have failed to detect relationships of health literacy to outcomes such as control of blood clotting conditions.[56] Some relationships between cultural competence and patient outcomes have been reported, including improvement in diabetes control among Latinos. These were attributed to increased cultural awareness among providers and use of Spanish-speaking diabetes educators.[57]

Neither health literacy nor cultural competence has yet been established as a strong, causal element in health outcomes. However, circumstantial evidence suggests that relationships exist. Difficulty in measurement of health literacy and cultural competence may mask important relationships between health literacy, cultural competence, and health outcomes. Large-scale attempts by health professionals and organizations to promote health literacy and cultural competence are historically recent phenomena. Development of more effective means of building these capacities among both consumers and providers may well help establish stronger relationships of cause and effect.

COMPLEMENTARY AND ALTERNATIVE MEDICINE

Although allopathic medicine predominates in the United States, the public still consumes a substantial volume of services involving different principles and interventions. The term *allopathic* denotes what is traditionally thought of as Western medicine, which is based on factual observation, scientific experimentation, and disciplines such as anatomy, physiology, immunology, and pharmacology. Medical care based on other theories and traditions is known today as **complementary and alternative medicine (CAM)**.

Table 4.5 provides an overview of the use of CAM by U.S. consumers based on a federally supported survey conducted in 2002. Consumption of products and services associated with CAM is clearly quite widespread, with approximately 127 million U.S. adults using CAM in some form.[58] About 35 percent of U.S. adults used one or more of the therapies included in the table. U.S. consumers spend billions of dollars on CAM every year. The percentage of U.S. adults using CAM in the early years of the twenty-first century differs only slightly from the percentages found in earlier surveys.[59] Use of some practices has changed over the years. Chiropractic, for example, declined between the 1990s and the early 2000s; use of herbs and yoga for the individual's "health or treatment" increased.

The demographic profile of CAM users has several distinct characteristics. Individuals forty to sixty-four years of age are most likely to have used CAM in the past year. In this age category, 39 percent reported having used CAM, compared with 25 percent of individuals sixty-five and over. Women (39 percent) were more likely to have used CAM, compared with 31 percent of men. Non-Hispanic whites (37 percent) and "others" (41 percent)—presumably including many Asian American individuals—were most likely to have used CAM, compared with 27 percent of Hispanics and non-Hispanic African Americans.

TABLE 4.5 Frequency of use of complementary and alternative medicine (CAM), United States, 2002

Type of Therapy	Percentage Used in Past Twelve Months	Estimated Number of Users (Thousands)
Herbs	18.6	38,183
Relaxation techniques	14.2	29,220
Chiropractic	7.4	15,226
Yoga	5.0	10,386
Massage	4.9	10,052
Diet	3.3	6,765
Megavitamins	2.8	5,739
Homeopathy	1.7	3,433
Tai chi	1.2	2,565
Acupuncture	1.0	2,136
Energy healing or Reiki	0.5	1,080
Qi gong	0.3	527
Hypnosis	0.2	505
Naturopathy	0.2	498
Biofeedback	0.1	278
Folk medicine	0.1	233

(Continued)

TABLE 4.5 *(Continued)*

Type of Therapy	Percentage Used in Past Twelve Months	Estimated Number of Users (Thousands)
Ayurveda	0.1	154
Chelation	0.03	66
Total		127,046

Source: Tindle HA, Davis RB, Phillips RS, et al. Trends in use of complementary and alternative medicine by U.S. adults: 1997–2002. *Alternative Therapies.* 2005:11(1):42–49.

CAM users are often socially and economically advantaged people. Relatively high income strongly predicts CAM use: 44 percent of people with annual household incomes of $65,000 or more reported using CAM, compared with 29 percent of those with incomes below $20,000. U.S. citizens were more likely to use CAM than noncitizens (36 versus 25 percent).

CAM has been found to have a place in disadvantaged communities as well. A study of African American asthmatics in a disadvantaged community found that some use of CAM was associated with nonmainstream theories of illness in a disadvantaged community.[60] It is certain that some of the originally Asian practices appearing in Table 4.5 are practiced in disadvantaged immigrant communities, but it would be incorrect to conclude that disadvantaged CAM users had abandoned mainstream care. Most of the African American asthmatics who used CAM said they trusted their allopathic physicians and followed their advice. The use of traditional healers in perhaps most ethnic communities today would appear a rarity. The *curandero,* or traditional Mexican American healer, is often mentioned as an important resource in the Latino community. However, a study of employed California Latinos, about two-thirds of whom were immigrants, found that less than 1 percent identified a *curandero* as their usual provider of health care.[61]

A number of studies have shown that U.S. consumers use CAM to supplement, rather than replace, conventional medicine. A study of cancer patients in the 1980s, for example, found that about one-third used some form of unconventional care.[62] Such care included procedures believed to arrest cancer, including visualization and meditation. This study did not find that consumers substituted unconventional for conventional cancer treatment. Most continued to see their regular doctors and undergo mainstream therapies; however, they would receive unconventional interventions as well. The authors of this study speculate that more emotive care, better communication, and opportunities to take make decisions regarding therapy contribute to the attractiveness of unconventional care. The use of CAM, moreover, has been interpreted as a means through which patients frustrated with chronic or intractable conditions attempt to exercise control over their lives.[63]

CONSUMER PREFERENCES AND HEALTH CARE MARKETING

Emerging only in the late twentieth century, the field of health care marketing plays an increasingly visible role in the operation of professional practices, health plans, and hospitals. **Health care marketing** aims to enable providers to offer services that best meet the consumer's needs in a convenient and affordable manner. Health care marketers conduct surveys, mine publicly available databases, conduct focus groups, and study regional maps to determine which products, services, and facilities are most attractive to the public. Two of the principles emerging from a generation of health care market research—insistence on quality and valuation of choice—provide final insights on the health behavior of Americans. These principles also raise issues for management and policy.

Insistence on Quality

Despite differences between rich and poor in the United States, people from all walks of life insist on quality in their health care. Every day, consumers are reminded of products and services that exceed their capacity for purchase. Americans may accept lack of access to top-quality automobiles, clothing, and education, but will not explicitly acknowledge acceptance of health care they feel is inferior to that available to the better situated.

This fact was illustrated in a series of focus groups conducted to learn how the public assesses quality of managed care plans.[64] The groups were composed of women ages thirty through fifty-five, a demographic that plays the central role in selection of family health care providers. Of special interest were responses to a question about how the women would view a health plan that would be 50 percent cheaper than their current plan, but would clearly not be of top quality. It was explained to the women that providers in the plan would be licensed and otherwise qualified, but would not be the best in their fields. The plan, it was explained, would have equipment that was adequate, but not the most advanced.

Very few of the women considered the inexpensive plan attractive. This was especially true in a focus group whose members were predominantly members of minority groups. These women expressed strong feelings about not accepting care at a level of quality lower than that provided to the more advantaged members of society.

The public's concern with quality raises a challenge to health care management. Measures of quality are difficult to standardize in health care. Critics have commented that the public confuses quality in medical care with convenience, cleanliness, and courtesy. Measures of quality widely accepted by professionals are in widespread use today. But these measures are not widely known to the general public and may not fully address consumer concerns.

Valuation of Choice

The American public places great value on choice. Perhaps the best evidence for this assertion is the decline in popularity of health maintenance organizations (HMOs) since the end of the twentieth century. HMOs are health plans that typically place tight restriction on the providers and facilities of which subscribers may make use. The public, however, has expressed preference for less restrictive plans and options. Thus, the preferred provider organization (PPO) has become the predominant type of health plan in the United States, surprising many pundits who had predicted a health marketplace composed largely of competing HMOs.

Concern with choice has bedeviled policy makers as well as HMO managers. Fear of reduction in choice has been a barrier to widespread acceptance among Americans of policy changes aimed at extending health insurance to more people. According to some, the American consumer's concern with choice has an ironic feature. Relatively few Americans actively shop for their doctors. Few ask where their doctor received her training, and many may not even know their physician's specialty. Though a value strongly expressed by the public, choice in health care may be exercised by only a few.

KEY TERMS

Sick role

Health literacy

Cultural competence

Complementary and alternative medicine (CAM)

Health care marketing

SUMMARY

This chapter identifies aspects of human thinking and behavior that affect health and the use of health services. Individual choice ultimately determines utilization of health services and in some cases health itself. People differ in the value they place on health services and the extent to which they accept risks to their health. Individual behavior and thinking are affected by culture, community, and broad social forces.

The Behavioral Model of Health Services Utilization specifies factors that affect consumer behavior. Elements of the model include *need* factors (comprising dimensions of perceived need, such as physical symptoms, pain, and dysfunction); *predisposing* factors (including age, education, and ethnicity); and *enabling* factors (such as income, wealth, insurance, and physical and linguistic access).

Consumers often do not utilize health care appropriately and hence fail to obtain its potential benefits. *Noncompliance* or *nonadherence,* in which the patient receives care but does not follow provider recommendations, may render the value of health services negligible. *Health literacy,* or the ability of the consumer to understand treatment and provider instructions, is required for maximum benefit from health care. Both individual understanding and system-level accommodation contribute to favorable consumer behavior. Cultural competence by the provider is believed to promote favorable consumer understanding and behavior.

Many consumers today are attracted to complementary and alternative medicine (CAM), products and services outside the medical mainstream. The popularity of CAM may be explained in part by consumers' desire to exercise more direct control over their care and avoid the perceived aloofness of mainstream providers.

DISCUSSION QUESTIONS

1. To what degree are health risks among Americans today voluntarily accepted versus imposed? What implications may be drawn for health care management and health policy?

2. Age can be regarded as the most important (and least preventable) health risk. Why might this be considered true, and can steps can be taken to reduce age-related risk?

3. This chapter has characterized neighborhood-level and occupational risks as imposed, rather than voluntary. To what degree is this true?

4. Can the Behavioral Model of Health Care Utilization be used to explain not only use of health services but behavior, such as noncompliance with medication instructions and leaving the hospital against medical advice? Explain your answer.

5. Does the popularity of CAM suggest widespread deficits in consumer understanding of medicine and science? Does CAM's popularity raise issues regarding conventional health care in the United States?

PART

2

MEANS OF DELIVERY

The U.S. health care system employs a large number of organizations and a vast labor force to accomplish the tasks that were outlined in Part One. Health care organizations include ambulatory practice settings, hospitals, mental health facilities, nursing homes, and many more. Most significant business in the United States is conducted in *formal organizations*, recognizable by physical facilities, specialized job descriptions, and organizational charts. Health care organizations, however, encounter distinct challenges in carrying out their tasks. The professional independence enjoyed by physicians and nurses reduces the ability of managers to exercise command and control. Health care organizations are highly visible institutions, and public expectations regarding standards of behavior and community benefit are high.

Health care workers in the United States comprise a key segment of the labor force. *Professionalism*, the possession specialized knowledge and independently formulated codes of behavior and ethics, distinguishes health care workers from other personnel. Examples of key health professionals include physicians, nurses, and health administrators, each of which has a unique history and set of contemporary challenges.

The U.S. health labor force is marked by uneven distribution of personnel. This is particularly true of physicians, who locate predominantly in economically advantaged urban areas. Racial minorities are strongly underrepresented in medicine and other health professions. Policy makers have had difficulty determining the optimal number of health professionals needed in the United States, and policy interventions have periodically resulted in surplus or shortage.

An elaborate financing system drives health care in the United States. Most health care bills are covered by *third-party payers*, which are usually private employers and public agencies. Rising health care costs in the United States have caused health care finance to become a key public issue. Cost accelerators in the United States include the continuous development of new technology and expectations by the public that their requirements will be met expertly and promptly. Lack of health insurance has placed a growing number of Americans in a position of health care insecurity. The high cost of health insurance is largely at fault, discouraging employers from offering insurance to their workers and making it impossible for individuals to afford private plans.

Research constitutes a key feature of the health care system in the United States, and research personnel are an important segment of the health care labor force. Research is essential for development of new technology and has clearly contributed to the well-being of Americans. Managers, clinicians, and policy makers require an understanding of the methods used by researchers and the pressures under which they operate to assess the validity and applicability of their findings. Politics, ideology, and competition are important features of the world of research. Decision makers, then, must review research findings with attention to methodology and detail. This principle is particularly relevant to determining whether costs of procedures are justified by benefit to the patient and whether innovations in the delivery of health care have been effective.

CHAPTER

5

HEALTH CARE ORGANIZATIONS

LEARNING OBJECTIVES

- To obtain an overview of organizations that deliver health care in the United States
- To appreciate the connection between organizations and the market segments they serve
- To understand the structure, characteristics, and challenges of health care organizations
- To distinguish differences among managed care organizations
- To recognize the policy issues raised by the organization of health care in the United States

THE IMPORTANCE OF ORGANIZATIONS IN HEALTH CARE

Effective delivery of health services requires an understanding of human organization. Health care today usually involves coordination of large numbers of diverse individuals. "Diverse" in this sense signifies not only differences in the racial, cultural, and religious backgrounds of individuals, but also differences in professional training, personal experience, and individual values. A few providers of health care today may work alone. But the most important entities providing health care combine the effort of hundreds, if not thousands: health professionals, management staff, and support personnel, to name only a few. Medical science, management philosophy, and public policy can affect the consumer and society as a whole only if they are implemented by effective organizations. Organization amounts to assignment and supervision of people for the purpose of maintaining cooperation and focusing effort on defined objectives.

Modern society achieves this level of cooperation and focus through the so-called **formal organization.** According to one definition,[1] a formal organization is "a body of individuals working under a defined system of rules, assignments, procedures, and relationships designed to achieve identifiable objectives and goals."

In another perspective, formal organizations (*organizations* for short) may be recognized by certain distinct properties. They have *boundaries,* enabling outsiders to join or engage in commerce with those inside only by demonstrating distinct qualifications. To become members of a health care organization, providers must have specific professional credentials. Formal organizations also have a recognizable **structure**. Established patterns of command and control, information exchange, and resource allocation help define the structure of an organization. The familiar organizational chart, featuring lines of communication stemming from the chief executive officer (CEO) to department heads and finally to production workers, reflects a key dimension of structure.

For generations, management courses and textbooks have highlighted the importance of organizations and provided instruction on how they should be run. Today's top executive in business, government, or the nonprofit sector is more likely an expert in running an organization than in manufacturing, medicine, or any other technical field. Required expertise in organizational management includes setting strategy, financing operations and expansion, ensuring favorable relations with the public and other organizations, resolving internal conflict, and promoting productivity and morale. The strategy, structure, and management of an organization determine its ability to serve the public.

Organizations involved in health care in the United States include ambulatory care practices, hospitals, mental health facilities, skilled nursing facilities, nursing homes, managed care organizations, and many others. The variety of U.S. health care organizations has given rise to a plethora of abbreviations and acronyms, an "alphabet soup" including MSOs (managed services organizations), PPOs (preferred provider organizations), and IPAs (independent practice associations). By describing the most important types of health care organizations in operation today, the present chapter highlights the system's key players. By addressing structural features and sources of stress and conflict within some of these organizations, this chapter illustrates major challenges taking place in U.S. health care today.

HEALTH SERVICE INDUSTRY SECTORS

Before focusing on health care organizations themselves, it is important to examine some divisions into which health services are often placed. Marketing language provides a basic framework. A **market sector** is composed of similar types of organizations offering similar products—for example, the hospital or HMO sector. A **market segment** refers to a group of consumers with common characteristics, such as age, gender, or level of disposable income. Health care organizations comprising a particular market sector may specialize in serving a particular market segment.

Other marketing terminology promotes an understanding of divisions within the health care industry. **Mass market** health services include those that anyone throughout society may find useful. Among mass market services, some are used regularly by many people, others rarely and by only a few. **Niche services**, by contrast, constitute those used by only restricted segments of the population. Services of this kind are often *elective* in nature, utilized by choice rather than on the basis of immediate necessity. Understanding the sector in which a particular health care organization specializes helps explain the challenges with which it must deal.

The Mass Market: Levels of Service

Mass market services may be grouped under the labels *primary, secondary,* and *tertiary care.* The term *quaternary care* is also sometime used, but the term is often misused, and true quaternary care is rare.

■ *Primary care.* Primary care is the first line of services in the health care industry. A primary care provider (PCP) is the first practitioner a consumer normally visits in response to illness or injury or for preventive services. Primary care is typically of routine nature. PCPs provide diagnosis and treatment for such common concerns as ear aches, sprains, and sore throats. They may manage blood pressure medication or perform school examinations. Among physicians, PCPs typically include family practitioners, general internists, and pediatricians. Sometimes, obstetricians/gynecologists may provide primary care to women for whom reproductive or female health is a predominant concern. Nonphysician health providers, including nurse practitioners and physician assistants, also function as PCPs. The ability to provide services for a wide range of day-to-day complaints is the hallmark of primary care practice. Traditionally, consumers have sought primary care within their neighborhood or close to their workplace.

■ *Secondary care.* The term *secondary care* describes services beyond the scope of general medical practice. Services in this category include general and some specialized fields of surgery and specialized fields of internal medicine such as gastroenterology, rheumatology, and oncology. Unlike primary care, consumers typically reach secondary care providers via referral from PCPs. Though psychiatry is technically a secondary care specialty, it is often obtained via self-referral. As in the case of primary care, consumers usually obtain secondary care within or near their own communities.

A great deal of secondary care is delivered in hospitals, where patients receive such typical surgical interventions as appendectomy, gall bladder removal, skin lesion excision, and mastectomy. Such surgeries more often take place in community hospitals than in regional medical centers. As yesterday's advanced science becomes today's routine care—in the case of coronary artery bypass graft, for example—more services are received in secondary care settings. The area from which secondary care hospitals draw their patients—known in hospital administration lingo as the *catchment area*—includes a number of adjacent neighborhoods, zip codes, or census tracts.

■ *Tertiary care.* Tertiary care denotes services of greater specialty than would be available in most communities. Services of this kind may include highly specialized and advanced interventions, such as complex heart surgery or unusual or scientifically advanced cancer therapies. Tertiary care is available only in major cities with populations large enough to generate sufficient volumes of unusual cases. Large medical centers or university-operated or -affiliated facilities predominate among providers of tertiary care. It is not unusual for consumers and their families to commute long distances for tertiary care or to temporarily reside close to the facility in instances where treatment requires an extended time period. It is not unusual to find wealthy or politically powerful people from far-distant countries occupying the beds of U.S. tertiary care centers.

Of thousands of hospitals in the United States, only a few hundred are true tertiary care facilities, such as the University of Chicago Medical Center, the Texas Heart Institute in Houston, and the Fred Hutchinson Cancer Research Center in Seattle. Often tertiary care is delivered in connection with clinical trials—experimental procedures through which biomedical scientists determine whether treatments still under development have true therapeutic value. Tertiary care is almost always obtained on referral. Self-referral, however, is not unknown, as desperately ill patients shop among facilities and providers for acceptable financial terms or services that are of uncertain benefit.

Quaternary Care

Although everyone is potentially a consumer of *quaternary care,* services in this category cannot be considered mass-market products. This category of services includes interventions that are at once highly specialized and rarely used. Quaternary care is delivered only in the most specialized facilities. Outstanding examples include the National Institutes of Health Clinical Center in Maryland and the Hospital for Tropical Diseases in London. Quaternary care may include diagnosis of rare or evasive disease entities or extreme interventions for the gravely ill or injured. The catchment area for quaternary care spans the entire world.

Diagnosis and treatment of a case of *trypanosomiasis* originating in South Africa and seen at the Hospital for Tropical Diseases in London provides an illustrative instance of quaternary care. This disease, a form of sleeping sickness, is caused by a parasite, *Trypansoma brucei rhodensiense,* spread to humans via mosquitoes. In addition to a wide array of imaging and standard tests, diagnosis requires distinction of the causative parasite from other organisms via genetic analysis. A multidrug regimen plus intensive life support intervention enable the patient to survive despite relapses.[2]

Another illustration involves a surgical procedure known as *translumbar amputation* (TLA), also known as *hemicorporectomy.* TLA is a radical surgical procedure used as a last resort for patients with a life-threatening diagnosis (such as intractable cancer or severe traumatic injury) but good health in other respects. The procedure entails removal of the entire body from the lower lumbar vertebrae downward, and involves loss of the pelvis, rectum, bladder, genitalia, and both legs. Continued survival and functioning requires an elaborate system of tubes, prostheses, and devices. At least one treatment center, however, reports long-term survival with a significant measure of independence.[3]

Niche Markets in Health Care

The health care market covers additional areas that, though important, are utilized largely by people with special interests, unusual needs, or nonmainstream lifestyles. Marketing professionals often refer to these consumer populations as niche markets. As in the plant and animal worlds, the term *niche* reflects a limited range of operation, specialized resource base, and a restricted universe of competition. Participants in a niche market evolve in a manner adapted to these restrictions and opportunities. Health services of this kind are difficult to fit into the traditional categories of primary, secondary, and tertiary.

Niche markets may be based on a number of dimensions, including disease category, ethnicity, age group, geographical residence, and lifestyle. The sociological term *status group* can also define a market niche. Status group in this sense refers to individuals of similar socioeconomic status whom society regards and honors (or dishonors) in a special way. Corporate CEOs and U.S. senators belong to distinct status groups, as do homeless individuals and incarcerated criminals. Health care organizations offer distinct products adapted to the needs and resources of these status groups. Status group–related niches have attracted the interest of both mainstream health care facilities and specialized entities. Private groups of physicians offer their services to the advantaged on a concierge basis, maximizing convenience to these individuals.

On the opposite end of the spectrum, private health care organizations are providing an increasing proportion of health services received by prisoners: in 2006, member organizations of a private industry trade group received a $3 billion share of the $7.5 billion budgeted for correctional health care nationwide.[4]

Some services in niche markets are highly population-specific, but widely familiar. These include substance abuse treatment venues, weight reduction clinics, and many of the complementary and alternative treatments referenced in the preceding chapter. Lifestyle-related niche products include relatively limited interventions such as plastic surgeries to reduce, enlarge, or reshape lips, buttocks, and stomachs. More extensive procedures of this nature include surgical interventions providing male and female transsexuals with genitals that conform to those of the desired sexual identity.[5]

Intrasectoral Competition

The structure and internal operations of health care organizations will receive detailed attention in the pages to follow. Internal matters of this nature have dominated the attention of managers and researchers for generations. But the external environment in which a health care organization operates is also quite important. Rival organizations constitute a crucial dimension of the external environment. Competition for both business and the means of doing business is the most readily visible result.

Providers of primary, secondary, and tertiary care tend to practice in different types of organizations. Primary care providers most often practice in small professional organizations. Less often, they work in clinics or HMOs whose workforce may have up to a thousand physicians and other providers. Much of the work of secondary and tertiary care personnel takes place in similar settings. However, the most distinct forms of secondary and tertiary care, such as imaging and surgery, are carried out in hospitals. Hospitals differ in their mix of secondary and tertiary care. Community voluntary hospitals predominate among providers of secondary care. Large metropolitan or regional medical centers, often university-affiliated, provide most of the hospital-based tertiary care consumed in the United States.

Competition among health care organizations occurs predominantly within the market sectors described earlier. The competitive picture for primary care providers and their organizations resembles that of small business everywhere. Traditionally, peers (either individuals or organizations) have competed against each other. Increasingly, solo practitioners and small professional organizations have faced competition from large, lower-cost providers such as closed-panel HMOs much in the way that mainstreet merchants face supermarket chains and big-box outlets.

Community hospitals face competition from nearby peer institutions. Competition among hospitals may take the form of underbidding each other in hopes of obtaining managed care contracts. Hospitals add capacity that, though unprofitable, demonstrates service offerings equal to those of its competitors. Industrial espionage is not unknown. In the last few decades, freestanding facilities owned by physicians or health care management companies have begun to compete with hospitals. These facilities offer services once available only in hospitals, such as imaging, surgery, and emergency care.

Tertiary care facilities engage in major regional or worldwide competition. They cultivate vast networks of physicians in far-flung locations as potential sources of referral, providing these individuals with free or low-cost education and consulting services. Tertiary care hospitals compete for the most influential physicians to upgrade their services or to start new ones. Intense competition occurs over funds obtained from sources other than patient care for construction and equipment. Most, if not all, hospitals of significant size maintain development offices and staffs to cultivate potential donors. University medical centers engage in fierce competition for research grants from both government and private sources.

Cross-sectoral competition also occurs. Rivalry between university medical centers and local community doctors serves as an example. It has been observed that community physicians hesitate to refer patients to highly specialized and prominent doctors for fear that their work will be criticized or that the patient will not be returned to the original doctor's care. A study of referral of cancer patients to the University of Chicago Medical Center found that out-of-state physicians were more likely than local doctors to refer to the facility. One observer explained that local doctors feared that their patients would stay with the university even after the specialized work was completed. Doctors in other states had no such fear, knowing that their patients would return home and back to their care after treatment in the far-off city.[6]

Battle of the Giants: Tertiary Care Facilities Square Off over Liver Transplant

The University of Washington Medical Center tried to keep a rival hospital from competing for liver transplant cases through an appeal to the courts. Hospitals may reap substantial profits from transplanting livers. In 2008, a liver transplant could cost $500,000, plus the expenses of follow-up care.

Since the procedure was introduced, the University of Washington Medical Center, located in Seattle, had enjoyed a liver transplant monopoly in a service area comprising the states of Washington, Alaska, Montana, and Idaho (collectively known as WAMI). Swedish Medical Center, a rival tertiary facility in Seattle, wanted into the business.

In order to offer liver transplants, Swedish Medical Center had to obtain approval from the Washington State Department of Health. State legislation dating from the era of federally mandated health planning (see Chapters One and Eleven) required that organizations wishing to establish a new transplant program apply for a certificate of need (CON) prior to entering the market. The certificate of need law was intended to keep excess capacity out of the health care market, believed by many to increase costs and lower quality.

(Continued)

(Continued)

> The University of Washington vigorously opposed Swedish Medical Center's CON application. Its representatives argued that the university already met all the region's needs. An additional facility, they argued, would lead to relatively low transplant volume at both the university and Swedish facilities, as available cases were split. It is well known that high volume for a number of surgical procedures corresponds to high rates of success.[7]
>
> The Department of Health approved Swedish Medical Center's CON application in 2004. State officials reasoned that relatively few liver transplants occurred in the WAMI region, that patients often had to travel to other regions for transplants, and that donor livers were often not used for the benefit of local residents but were exported for transplantation in other regions.
>
> Aided by both private attorneys and the state attorney's office, the university appealed the CON award to the state supreme court. In 2008, after four years of argument, litigation, and delay, the court finally rejected the university's appeal. Swedish Medical Center planned to begin transplanting livers within a few months.[8]

AMBULATORY CARE ORGANIZATIONS

Organizations that deliver ambulatory care function as the basic units of the health care system. Derived from the Latin root *ambulare* (to walk), the term *ambulatory* is traditionally used to describe a class of patients with the ability to walk. In modern usage, ambulatory care refers to services delivered in a physician's office—to which the patient has presumably walked—rather than a hospital or an emergency room. The terms *office-based care* and *outpatient care* are nearly synonymous with *ambulatory care,* except for the fact that many physicians who see patients in their offices treat these same patients in hospitals. A surgeon or interventional radiologist, for example, generally requires hospital-based resources for key treatment procedures.

Internal Organization

The types of practice organizations in which ambulatory care takes place are numerous. Solo practice, the most traditional, is not an organization in the strict sense. In past generations, many physicians practiced alone, frequently in offices that were part of their homes. They were often assisted in practice by their wives in the manner of a small family business. Solo practice is still important in the United States, but today's solo practitioner usually works in a setting closer to that of a formal organization. He is likely to maintain an office away from home, employ an office staff for matters such as scheduling and billing, and retain one or more aides such as physician assistants or nurse practitioners.

Several types of formal associations involving multiple physicians are notable. Seen from the perspective of physicians, lawyers, and others involved in the delivery of health services, key classifications are *associations, partnerships,* and *corporations.*

■ *Associations.* Physicians share the expenses of maintaining common facilities such as offices, equipment, aides, and the like, while maintaining their own panels of patients. Under such arrangements, physicians may establish relationships with others to care for their patients during vacations or other absences.[9] Physician associations often involve real estate investment, with each member, for example, owning shares in title to the building that houses the offices of the members. Real estate deals of this kind provide considerable income to U.S. physicians as mortgages are successively refinanced.

■ *Partnerships.* This form of organization involves a high level of member commitment. Income from all patients may be pooled and distributed according to formula. New members may buy into the partnership. Current members wishing to sever their relationship for retirement or other reasons may sell their shares to newcomers. In this fashion, a mechanism for turnover of personnel is established, enabling the capture of a pool of patients as a stable asset of the partnership irrespective of which members remain or depart. Partnerships may involve only two individuals, as when an established physician allows a newly licensed individual to buy into her practice. Partnerships may include hundreds of members, however, sometimes practicing (individually or in clusters) at separate locations throughout a geographical region.

Partnerships are legally organized according to devices such as the limited liability partnership (LLP). Organizing as an LLP enables the entity to make contracts with outside parties such as managed care and other insurance carriers. LLPs can bring suit and be sued. Entities known as group practices are generally organized under the LLP mechanism.

■ *Corporations.* In some instances, physicians wishing to practice in a collaborative fashion are best served by a corporate structure. A legal mechanism often found convenient by physicians who wish to incorporate is the professional limited liability company (PLLC or LLC). Professional corporations have advantages over partnerships in providing greater protection of members from malpractice liability of other members. As applied to medicine, state limited liability corporation laws—those of Iowa, for example—allow only physicians to own voting shares. The LLC mechanism provides offers several features convenient to small entities. Compared with other types of corporations, LLCs do not have to hold regular ownership and management meetings and are taxed in a manner more convenient to individuals. As do LLPs, LLCs serve as the legal underpinnings of many group practices.

It is important to note that organization under a partnership or corporate charter (via LLP or LLC) does not necessarily signify group practice. Substantively, group practice means participation in a common patient pool, coverage during absences, potential pooling and redistribution of income, and, increasingly, collective obligations under managed care contracts. The LLP or LLC mechanism may be just as valuable to physicians in "associations" as the term is used earlier. Individuals wishing to share only a real estate venture (typically the building in which they practice) often find the LLP model useful. Solo practitioners often incorporate. Larger practices, though, must adopt a formal partnership or corporate structure. Selecting the most advantageous partnership or corporate format is a job for attorneys. Criteria vary by context and may change as the practice develops or as external conditions affecting practice alter.

Most health care organizations are small in comparison with the entities of corporate America. Some, such as those providing medical services for Kaiser Permanente and other large HMOs, may have a few thousand physician members. However, a great many physician organizations are similar in size to their counterparts of the 1950s. Of the group practices active in the late 1950s, for example, those with three to five full-time physicians comprised 57 percent.[10] According to data from the National Center for Health Statistics, almost 75 percent of nonsolo and nonpartnership practices active in 2005 and 2006 had between three and five members.[11] These same statistics indicated the continuing importance of solo practice, with 36.8 percent of all ambulatory care physicians working in solo practice settings as late as 2006.

The limited size of most ambulatory care physician organizations reflects a professional culture of independence. For over a hundred years, representatives of physicians such as the American Medical Association have fought the establishment of corporate delivery of health care. For a long time, group practice itself was frowned upon. As late as the beginning of the twenty-first century, only about 25 percent of U.S. physicians were employees.[12]

Organizations involving patient care professionals other than physicians may employ the same mechanisms described above for doing business collectively. Partnerships and corporations of nurse practitioners, physician assistants, podiatrists, perfusionists, and technicians in many specialties often make contracts with hospitals and medical groups for providing services. Firms that serve the health care industry in areas such as law and consulting are often structured similarly. In addition, partnerships or corporate structures are widely used by physician entities that, while not having their own patients, contract with health plans to provide specialty services. These "unbedded" specialists include diagnostic radiologists, anesthesiologists, pathologists, hospitalists, and emergency physicians.

Practice Setting

The internal arrangements involved in ambulatory practice organizations are of great concern to professionals. But they hold little interest for the consumer, for whom the suffix LLP or LLC on the door usually means nothing. Consumers, though, readily grasp the setting in which care takes place and choose the places where they seek care according to related preferences. Ambulatory care settings correspond to specific types of organizations or organizational subunits.

Settings in which ambulatory care is widely practiced include

- Private physician offices

- Integrated delivery systems

- Community health centers

- Urgent care centers

- Retail clinics

- Hospital emergency facilities

According to the federal National Health Interview Study of 2007, 76.2 percent of Americans who had a usual source of care identified a private physician's office (including HMO facilities) as the place they went when sick. Nearly 20 percent named the clinic or health center as their usual source, and 1.2 percent the hospital emergency department. The remainder were scattered among a wide variety of health care outlets.

The Private Physician's Office. The private physician's office is likely familiar to most readers. Consumer surveys indicate a strong preference for treatment in such facilities.[13] Private medical practice, however, has encountered serious challenges in recent years. The most traditional forms of private office–based service delivery— solo practice and practice in small partnership settings—have been in decline. Doctors who practice in small office settings face challenges of dealing with government programs, private insurance, and increasingly expensive necessities such as the computerized health record.

Among the most noticeable trends in ambulatory care practice organization in the early twenty-first century has been growth in *single-specialty* at the expense of *multi-specialty* practices. At one time analysts thought that multispecialty practices would predominate in U.S. health care. Multispecialty practice includes both primary care doctors and specialists practicing under a single roof. It was reasoned that this mix of physicians could readily exchange information, provide convenient one-stop shopping for consumers, and help restrain costs by reducing avoidable specialty care. However, specialists such as cardiologists, orthopedic surgeons, and oncologists have increasingly banded together in moderate to large group practices (six to fifty physicians). Such groups attract procedure specialists due to their profitability. Single-specialty practices are able to buy the expensive equipment required by "procedure-oriented" physicians and bill at high rates for their utilization. Single-specialty practices are also better able to negotiate with hospitals and health plans, ensuring still higher billing rates. Single-specialty practice frees the specialist from having to share income or governance with primary care providers, who bill at lower rates.[14]

Integrated Delivery Systems. The integrated delivery system (IDS) is distinguished by formal linkages among individual health care providers and shared resources supporting the delivery of medical care. The centerpiece of the IDS is a large, multi-specialty group practice. Like the large single-specialty practice, the IDS is able to use pooled resources to purchase equipment. Pooled resources include shared services such as physician recruitment, regulatory compliance, and financial management. An IDS today is likely to have a computerized health record system. The IDS is also capable of facilitating communication among health professionals for determining best practices and supporting patient referrals. The IDS model can be found in both managed and nonmanaged care environments, government agencies, and private organizations such as policlinics. Well-known IDS examples include organizations as diverse as Kaiser Permanente, the Veterans Administration, and Intermountain Health Care.

The IDS encounters challenges in fulfilling its potential for controlling cost and promoting patient convenience and favorable outcomes. The relatively large size of the IDS raises organizational concerns such as faulty communication and interunit rivalry. Consumers may encounter feelings similar to those of HMO patients, sensing that service is insufficiently personal. A great deal more will be said about HMO and other managed care outlets in this and later chapters.

Community Health Centers. The *term community health* center denotes several types of provider organizations that deliver ambulatory care to underserved populations. These populations may be urban core or rural. Both tend to have high rates of poverty and a shortage of health professionals. Community health centers typically provide services at reduced fee or free of charge. Because they often provide services to the poor and uninsured, community health centers are important *safety net providers.*

The so-called *free clinic* is a type of community health center. Originating in the 1960s to care for the transient and drug-oriented, these clinics in the early years of the twenty-first century numbered over 1,700 and treated 2.5 million people, largely uninsured and Medicaid clients.[15] They are formally free-standing but often affiliated with hospitals or faith-based organizations. They provide health services directly and refer patients to networks of physicians willing to provide services for low or no fee. Free clinics face a recurring cycle of funding shortages and are heavily dependent on private donations. Physicians and other health professionals typically serve on a vol-unteer basis.

Federally qualified health centers (FQHCs) provide a greater volume of services within the safety net, reportedly treating 14 million people per year. Most people receiving care from FQHCs are uninsured or insured through Medicaid.[16] In the early twenty-first century there were over one thousand FQHCs, most of which served patients at multiple sites.[17] These organizations rely heavily on federal grants, receiving close to 60 percent of their income from the federal Bureau of Primary Health Care and Medicaid.[18] FQHCs are governed by boards on which clinic users are strongly repre-sented, comprising an unusual degree of consumer presence.

Most physicians working at FQHCs are in primary care specialties. These doctors rely heavily on RNs, nurse practitioners, and physician assistants, who are strongly represented in FQHC staffing. Although federal funding for FQHCs has remained strong, these organizations have had increasing difficulty recruiting physicians and finding specialists willing to see their patients on referral.[19]

It is notable that hospital outpatient departments and clinics operated by local health departments share the safety net mission with FQHCs.

Urgent Care Centers. Urgent care centers represent a relatively recent development in U.S. health care. The Urgent Care Association of American defines the services these facilities offer as "ambulatory care outside of a hospital emergency department on a walk-in basis without a scheduled appointment, [treating] many problems that can be seen in a primary care doctor's office, [but including] some services that are generally not available [such as] X-rays and minor trauma treatment." The number of urgent care centers in the United States was estimated to be as high as twenty thousand in the early 2000s.[20] According to the Urgent Care Association, nearly half were owned by private profit-seeking firms, 26 percent by hospitals, and 8 percent by multispecialty group practices or clinics. Under certain types of managed care contracts, large multispecialty practices can save money by routing patients after hours to urgent care centers. Physicians and other health care personnel may be salaried, but are often retained on contract.

The urgent care center serves a market niche of the convenience-oriented customer. Urgent care centers serve this need by not requiring consumers to make appointments and staying open on evenings and weekends. According to some, the urgent care center's popularity stems from the public's frustration with doctors' office scheduling. Consumers often report having to wait several weeks for a regular doctor's appointment. For many, the hospital emergency department does not provide an attractive alternative. As described earlier, these facilities are often overcrowded and require long waits for all but the most emergent cases.

Critics of urgent care centers dismissively describe them as "doc-in-the-box" facilities. In this fashion, the critics liken urgent care centers to inexpensive, drive-in, presumably low-quality fast food outlets. However, consumer satisfaction with services received at the urgent care center compares well with other medical outlets.

Retail Clinics. Among the organizations involved in health care delivery, retail clinics represent the most recent development. If "doc-in-the-box" describes the urgent care center, "mall medicine" applies to the retail clinic. Retail clinics are small facilities located in supermarkets, big-box stores, and shopping malls. Like urgent care centers, they draw consumers primarily on the basis of convenience, by not requiring appointments. The retail clinic's scope of service is smaller than that of the urgent care center, and care is more likely to be given by a nonphysician health professional.

Retail giant Wal-Mart has actively adopted the retail clinic model in its facilities. In 2007, clinics operated in seventy-six Wal-Mart stores; plans were afoot to open four hundred more. In this enterprise, Wal-Mart established partnerships with local hospitals hoping for downstream business. A majority of the Wal-Mart clinic consumers were uninsured.[21]

Both retail clinics and urgent care centers occupy the convenience niche in health care. They share this niche with hospital emergency departments. The hospital emergency department, though, is a much more important part of the health care system. Its functions extend well beyond the needs of the distressed or convenience-seeking, ambulatory patient. The hospital emergency department raises key issues for health care management and policy. It will receive in-depth attention later in this chapter.

THE HOSPITAL

Today's hospital descends from an era when hospitals were usually charitable organizations dependent on private donations. The majority of U.S. hospitals are still classified as community nonprofit; only about 20 percent are for-profit. This history has led the public to expect hospitals to act in a more charitable manner than they are sometimes perceived to act.

History and Impact of the Hospital

Some of the earliest hospitals in the United States were federal public health institutions. Dating from the late 1700s, these hospitals were established in seaport cities to observe and quarantine seamen stricken with potentially contagious diseases. These hospitals continued to function until the 1980s, when they were decommissioned under the administration of President Ronald Reagan.

During most of the nineteenth century, hospitals in the United States and elsewhere had minimal science and technology on the basis of which to offer services. In this era, they functioned largely as *almshouses* and *pesthouses*. As almshouses, hospitals provided custodial care to sick people who had no family and were too poor to hire others to care for them at home. As pesthouses, hospitals served as quarantine facilities for people with contagious diseases. Exceptions to these were hospitals such as New England General and Johns Hopkins University, which conducted research leading to major medical advances.

Many hospitals in the late nineteenth and early twentieth century were founded by private charities. During this period, one of high immigration to the United States, numerous ethnic groups formed benevolent societies for the purpose of helping community members who became ill and the families of those who died. The same forces established hospitals, often led by successful members of the ethnic community who contributed start-up funds. Hospitals in large U.S. cities still bear the imprint of their ethnic origins. These include Mount Sinai Hospital in New York, Cabrini Hospital in Chicago, and Swedish Hospital in Seattle. Also in this category are hospitals founded by religious orders, such as the Sisters of Charity in New York, Florida, and Ohio, and the Sisters of Mercy in California. Because these hospitals received support from voluntary donations, they were know as *voluntary hospitals,* a synonym for the designation of *community hospital* in common use today.

By the early twentieth century, hospitals began to benefit from the development of medical science. They were able to offer surgery that was made safe by sterile technique and tolerable due to the availability of anesthetics. Such offerings attracted paying customers from the middle class seeking services such as assisted childbirth and formerly dangerous and excruciating procedures such as appendectomy and gall bladder removal. Ownership of the hospitals included physicians, a practice that gave rise to the name *doctors' hospital* in a number of municipalities.

The 1950s and 1960s began another era in the history of U.S. hospitals. By that time, health insurance had become widespread, and most hospital payments were made by health insurers. The movement toward hospitalization insurance was furthered by Medicare and Medicaid legislation in the mid-1960s, which provided generous benefits for care in the hospital.

A number of milestones are notable in this development, involving legislation, payment, and management. Federal and state legislation made major changes in the hospital industry. The Hill-Burton Act of 1946, also known as the Hospital Survey and Construction Act, provided financial support for refurbishing old and building new hospitals. The legislation intended to make up for years of neglect to the sector due to the Depression and World War II. The measure resulted in a large increase in the number of hospitals operating in the United States and obliged hospitals receiving funds under the measure to provide a specified amount of care to indigent persons.

Later federal legislation had both a direct and an indirect impact on the manner in which hospitals were paid. In the early 1980s, the Tax Equity and Fiscal Responsibility Act mandated a prospective payment system structured under diagnostic-related groups (DRGs) for Medicare payments. A 1983 California law mandated that a selective contracting procedure be used to select a small number of hospitals eligible to receive payment under Medi-Cal (the California Medicaid program). A law that passed in close sequence allowed private insurance companies to also engage in competitive contracting. Due to these laws and related regulatory decisions, hospital payment changed markedly. Earlier, hospitals had billed on a cost-plus basis, charging payers the cost of the services they delivered plus a negotiated rate of profit. Afterward, hospitals had to bill under a DRG (or its equivalent in the private sector), according to a negotiated schedule with insurance companies.

Legislation and resulting billing changes created a more competitive market for hospital services than had previously existed. Important management changes followed. Although private donors had ruled the roost in the early days of U.S. hospitals and physicians assumed this role later on, professional hospital administrators were now needed in leadership roles. These trained specialists were best equipped to conduct newly important negotiations and manage the paperwork associated with the hospital's insurance and regulatory environment.

Changes in the Hospital Industry

Table 5.1 presents an overview of hospital ownership in the United States today. The information in this table is consistent with data presented earlier (see Chapter Two). The majority of hospitals in the United States are of the nonprofit community variety. Such hospitals operate beds in far greater numbers than all government agencies and for-profit entities combined. They are governed by a board of trustees that holds the hospital's assets in trust for the public.

TABLE 5.1 Distribution of hospital beds and occupancy rates in the United States, 2006

Ownership	Number of Beds	Occupancy Rate
All hospitals	947,412	68.9
Federal	46.691	66.4
Nonfederal	900,721	69.1
Community	802,658	67.1
Nonprofit	559,216	68.8
For-profit	115,337	58.7
State-local government	128,105	67.4
6–24 beds	6,446	32.9
25–49 beds	34,217	47.2
50–99 beds	69,408	57.6
100–199 beds	160.426	63.0
200–299 beds	148,541	67.7
300–399 beds	121.747	69.4
400–499 beds	79,732	71.1
500 beds or more	182,141	75.2

Source: National Center for Health Statistics. *Health, United States, 2008.* Table 116. Hyattsville, MD: National Center for Health Statistics; 2009.

A look at changes in the hospital industry over time supplements the view presented in Table 5.1. The picture is one of consolidation. The number of hospitals operating in the United States dropped from 7,156 in 1975 to 5,747 in 2006. The number of beds operated by these organizations declined from approximately

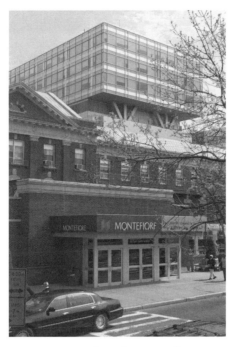

Montefiore Medical Center, Bronx, New York, early twenty-first century. Varied architecture reflects over one hundred years of change in the U.S. hospital industry. The copper-roofed brick structure in the left foreground is the original Montefiore Hospital. Dating from the late 1800s, the facility offered limited services to neighborhood residents. Serving a worldwide clientele, the Montefiore complex today includes several specialized hospitals, research and educational facilities, and housing for patient families.

1.5 million 947,412 in this period.[22] These declines occurred as a consequence of adoption of DRGs in Medicare and Medicaid and their equivalents in private plans. From the hospital point of view, DRGs and analogous private systems turned lengthy hospital stays from money-makers to money-losers. Shorter stays in turn meant lower occupancy rates and pressure on the bottom line. Between 1975 and 2006, almost 20 percent of U.S. hospitals closed their doors or were acquired by hospital management firms or other hospitals.

Contemporary Challenges

Although it occupies a dominant position in the U.S. health care system, the hospital today faces many challenges. Hospitals are visible institutions in their communities; hence, public expectations of them are high. They operate in a tightly regulated environment. Most must maintain accreditation from the Joint Commission on Accreditation of Healthcare Organizations; without such accreditation, hospitals may not bill for services under Medicare and Medicaid. Licenses from the state must be sought and maintained. Requirements of local agencies such as the fire marshal must

FIGURE 5.1 *Simplified structure of a community hospital*

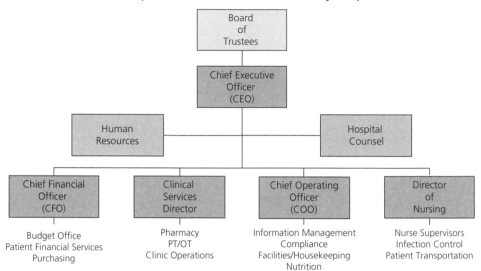

be met. Constructive ties with physicians, who alone can admit patients, must be cultivated. Strategic planning and marketing must be carried out with great accuracy in today's intensely competitive environment. Three challenges facing hospitals merit special attention: internal organization, finance, and public image.

Internal Organization. Everyone who has worked for a large organization has seen an *organizational chart.* Usually, this illustrates a hierarchical structure with a single chain of command. Thus, the organizational chart of most private firms depicts a chief executive officer on top, with a number of department heads reporting to her. Under these department heads may be individual programs, functions, or support units. Continuous subdivision of authority continues downward until it reaches the ranks of the operatives, employees who do standardized work and have no supervisory responsibility. The administrative hierarchy of a typical community hospital is illustrated in Figure 5.1.

The structure shown in Figure 5.1, however, tells only part of the story. Hospitals differ from most other work organizations in that they have a duel hierarchy. The management hierarchy mirrors the traditional structure of most organizations, and a separate medical hierarchy exists as well. The *attending staff,* comprising fully trained physicians, usually has an outside office–based practice and admits patients to the hospital. These physicians work outside the authority of the management. Physicians maintain a separate hierarchy, supervising *house staff;* among house staff itself, more experienced residents supervise newer ones. Nurses, it may be argued, constitute yet another hierarchy. It is notable that highest-ranked members of the management hierarchy cannot issue orders to the lowest member of the medical hierarchy.

The dual (or tripartite) character of the hospital creates problems for management. No single individual has the authority to direct the entire organization. Negotiation must take place across hierarchies to get things done. Cleavages open between doctors and managers, often over resources for building or acquiring new equipment. During the 1990s, it was said that a hospital CEO could expect to hold his job for no longer than three years.

Financial Management. Selective contracting and a general trend toward competitiveness among payers has created significant difficulty for hospital managers. Hospitals, for example, must admit patients under a DRG for Medicare and Medicaid or its equivalent for privately insured patients. Under this mechanism, hospitals are assured a fixed payment for admission under each DRG category. Thus, hospitals take a risk with each admission. If the patient stays a short amount of time and uses relatively few resources, the hospital makes money. If the patient exceeds the average reflected in the DRG, the hospital incurs a deficit. The hospital, then, must manage patients with great care. Hospitals hire personnel to determine the specific DRGs under which they can operate profitably, and expand (or reduce) the hospital's capabilities accordingly.

Hospitals are also active in the bond market. They borrow from this source to purchase equipment and finance expansions and retrofits (as is now required in earthquake-prone California). In some states, hospital charges are regulated, adding to the complexity of financial management.

Public Image. Because they are part of a regulated industry, hospitals are concerned with their public image. An unfavorable public image can attract the attention of regulatory agencies that oversee hospitals. Hospitals are extensive users of public resources, such as land in congested urban areas, local streets, and the local labor force.

The amount of public benefit that hospitals deliver has recently become controversial. As nonprofit organizations, community hospitals have a legal obligation to contribute to the public good. Both politicians and academics have criticized the nonprofit hospital sector for contributing too little in this area. In a famous critique, economist Regina Herzlinger presented evidence suggesting that for-profit hospitals provide as much public benefit (including primarily charity care) as nonprofits do.[23]

Today hospitals of all types face limits on their ability to provide charity care. Most, if not all, hospitals have fully discharged their responsibilities under the Hill-Burton Act. For many years, hospitals were able to cover the cost of charity care by cost-shifting: well-insured patients could be charged enough to cover both their care and that of charity cases. Competition and prospective payment today, though, have reduced both operating margins and the hospital's ability to shift costs.

As a consequence of these factors, hospitals try to avoid admitting charity patients. Those seen in the emergency department may be stabilized and released while still obviously impaired. Some hospitals have moved aggressively to recover bad debt. These actions sometimes give the hospital a highly uncharitable appearance, a perception that has drawn the attention of legislators.

How Charitable Are Nonprofit Hospitals?

The degree to which nonprofit organizations operate in a manner consistent with public expectations has become a major policy issue. The public expects nonprofit organizations, from churches with worldwide membership to local food banks, to have warm hearts and offer a helping hand to the community. Hospitals are among the most visible institutions in the nonprofit world.

Many people have been shocked to find that hospitals today behave like businesses. It is even more shocking to discover that hospitals that legally incorporate as nonprofits can be as aggressive and tight-fisted as any profit-seeking firm.

Here are a few recent examples:

In 2004, Richard Scruggs, the lawyer who with great success sued tobacco firms for billions of dollars on behalf of state governments, led a class-action suit against nonprofit hospital systems in eight states. The suit argued against allowing these systems to keep the exemption from taxes they had long enjoyed by virtue of their nonprofit status.

Scruggs alleged that nonprofit hospitals overcharge uninsured patients. Hospitals often bill individual patients without insurance at substantially higher rates than they have negotiated with insurance companies. They are also said to engage in aggressive collection tactics, such as placing liens on homes and assessing interest, fines, and legal fees.

The suits charged that nonprofit hospitals had violated "an explicit or implicit contract with the government to treat needy patients with compassion in return for significant tax breaks."[24]

In its issue of July 14, 1997, the *Wall Street Journal* published an article entitled "Nonprofit Hospitals Sometimes Are That in Little but Name." Nashville's Baptist Hospital was reported to have leased a skybox at the Houston Astrodome for $75,000 per year. As the Houston Oilers' official health care provider, Baptist was reported to give discounts to injured players. The football connection was part of Baptist's marketing strategy, which implied to the public: If Baptist is good enough for the Oilers, it's good enough for you.[25]

Especially striking was a report on the Daughters of Charity, an international order of nuns involved in the delivery of health care. In 1998, the order owned forty-nine hospitals in the United States. The order's movement of its capital from hospitals to more profitable investments excited the attention of the business world. The tendency of Daughters of Charity Hospitals to locate in affluent suburbs and treat fewer Medicaid patients than other hospitals drew public criticism. The nuns' financial acumen led Wall Streeters to coin the nickname Daughters of Currency.[26]

Even so, the order reported that it spent 86 cents of every dollar it earned on charity health care and other community work. Representatives of the order summarized their approach as "No margin, no mission" or, as a spokesperson put it, "We don't say we'll take care of the poor until we run out of money."

Key U.S. Senators and other public officials have expressed doubt that nonprofit hospitals deserve their favored tax status. Facing the possibility of adverse changes in tax laws, community hospitals have instituted systems to audit and report the value of the community benefits they generate. Such reporting is mandatory in California. Determination of public benefit, however, is complex and uncertain. A 2007 report by the California state auditor indicated that nonprofit and for-profit hospitals provided charity care of equal value. Operators of nonprofits, however, have argued that they generate benefits to the community other than charity care. These benefits are alleged to include medical research, physician training, and wellness promotion.[27]

The Hospital Emergency Department

The hospital emergency department (ED) has long been an important resource for consumers. Once operating in highly confined spaces adjacent to the hospital entrance, the so-called emergency room has evolved to an extensively staffed, expensively equipped department, or profit center, in many places. Glamorized in movies and television, EDs serve functions ranging from the most heroic to the most mundane. Of all the health care organizations discussed in this chapter, today's ED combines the greatest breadth of access and service offerings. EDs are open virtually all the time. They serve as an intake mechanism for the full range of professional and hospital care. Issues regarding access, quality of care, and health care cost crystallize in the context of the modern ED.

Types of Emergency Facilities. Hospital EDs today differ significantly in resources and capacity. Best known are *trauma centers*. A system comprising three categories of trauma centers is used by the American College of Surgeons (ACS) and state-level agencies:[28]

■ *Level I.* Facilities that deliver the highest level of emergency care available are designated level I trauma centers. The level I trauma center serves as a regional resource for teaching and research as well as patient care. It is required to be open twenty-four hours per day, have immediate access to trauma surgeons, and be able to obtain at short notice the services of specialists in fields such as orthopedic surgery, neurosurgery, anesthesiology, emergency medicine, radiology, internal medicine, oral and maxillofacial surgery, and critical care. The ACS stipulates volume requirements for level I trauma centers, including 1,200 admissions per year, 240 major trauma patients per year, or an average of 35 major trauma patients per surgeon.

■ *Level II.* A level II trauma center supplements level I centers in its area or provides trauma services in areas less densely populated than an urban core. Level II trauma centers provide twenty-four-hour service and must have ready access to essentially the same personnel and equipment as level I centers. There are no minimum volume requirements and the unit is not expected to maintain a teaching or research program.

■ *Level III.* A level III trauma center does not have full availability of specialists, but does have resources for emergency resuscitation, surgery, and intensive care of most trauma patients. Level III centers have transfer agreements with level I or level II facilities. Typically, level III facilities serve communities that do not have immediate access to a level I or II center.

The designations level IV and level V trauma centers are sometimes used to denote facilities capable of providing life support to trauma patients prior to their transfer to facilities with superior emergency resources. Hospitals as a whole, rather than EDs themselves, are designated by the ACS as trauma centers. In the first decade of the twenty-first century there were 190 level I trauma centers, 263 level II trauma centers, and 251 level III trauma centers operating in the United States.

Most EDs are not trauma centers. Trauma centers have special capacity to treat immediately life-threatening conditions such as serious traffic injuries and gunshot wounds. Cases such as these arrive by ambulance. Nontrauma EDs specialize in emergent cases such as sudden illness, burns, lacerations, fractures, and poisoning. Conditions such as these may threaten function or survival, but they are generally less severe than the cases seen in trauma centers.

ED Utilization. EDs, and particularly trauma centers, are best known for the urgency and intensity with which they can provide care. Historically, however, people have used EDs for nonemergent, primary care purposes. Nonemergent in this context signifies the likelihood that a complaint could be taken care of without adverse consequences after a delay of a day or so—when the consumer could often find care in the community. Nonemergent conditions include such everyday complaints as toothaches and earaches. But they may also include examination of potentially cancerous growths and blood tests for diabetes.

Poor access to health care in the community contributes to use of the ED for nonemergent conditions. Those with poor access are most often economically disadvantaged or members of minority groups. Looking to the ED as a usual source of care is one index of utilization for nonemergent needs. The 2007 National Health Interview Survey asked Americans whether they could identify a place where they usually went when they got sick. Of those who could identify such a place, only 1.8 percent named a hospital emergency room. Among employed Latinos in California, a group whose members often lack health insurance, this percentage increased to 3.5.[29]

Repeated ED visits in a single year is another index of use for nonemergent needs. Table 5.2 illustrates the relationship between social background factors and repeated

TABLE 5.2 Percentage of U.S. children and adults with two or more emergency department visits, 2006

	Children (Under 18)	Adults (18 and over)
All Americans	7.7	7.4
Race		
White	7.5	7.0
African American	9.9	11.3
American Indian or Alaska Native	(not available)	10.5
Asian	5.8	3.8
Latino background		
Latino (any race)	7.7	5.7
Not Latino	7.7	7.3
Percentage poverty level		
Below 100%	10.1	13.0
100 to 199%	8.8	10.6
200% or more	6.4	5.5
Health insurance		
Private	6.3	5.3
Medicaid	10.8	20.7
Uninsured	7.0	6.9

Source: National Center for Health Statistics. *Health, United States, 2008.* Tables 91 and 92. Hyattsville, MD: National Center for Health Statistics; 2009.

ED visits. This table presents percentages of individuals in each racial, ethnic, and socioeconomic category who made two or more visits to an ED in 2006.

Table 5.2 indicates that members of some minority racial groups (African Americans and American Indians or Alaska Natives) are more likely than others to make repeated ER visits. The table presents evidence for a strong relationship between poverty and repeated ED use. Americans below 100 percent of the federal poverty line are more than twice as likely as nonpoor Americans (with incomes 200 percent or more above poverty) to repeatedly use the ED.

However, poverty and minority group membership do not tell the whole story. People covered by Medicaid, a joint federal-state health insurance program for poor people, are the most likely of those represented in Table 5.2 to report repeated ED use. Some physicians do not readily accept Medicaid patients, leaving them to seek primary care in the ED. White and nonpoor Americans, moreover, make a significant number of repeat visits. Some of these individuals may not have primary care physicians or may find doctors' or clinic hours inconvenient.

Public Policy Regarding Duties of Emergency Departments. Use of the ED for non-emergent purposes is encouraged by the open access EDs provide. EDs are required to see (though not necessarily treat) all comers. An important federal law known as the Emergency Medical Treatment and Active Labor Act (EMTALA) mandates this access.

Explicitly, EMTALA requires that all emergency departments in hospitals receiving funds under Medicare must treat anyone with an emergency medical condition and may not transfer such a patient unless he has been stabilized. In practice, however, EMTALA requires an ED to see any individual who presents herself for any condition. Regulations associated with EMTALA define an "emergency condition" as a medical condition manifesting itself by acute symptoms of sufficient severity (including severe pain, psychiatric disturbances, and/or symptoms of substance abuse) such that the absence of immediate medical attention could reasonably be expected to result in

- Placing the health of the individual (or, with respect to a pregnant woman, the health of the woman or her unborn child) in serious jeopardy

- Serious impairment to bodily functions

- Serious dysfunction of any bodily organ or part

Stabilized means that no material deterioration of the emergency condition is likely, within reasonable medical probability, to result from or occur during the transfer (including discharge) of the individual from a facility.

Quality of Care. The quality of care that people receive for nonemergent needs is thought by many to be variable. The ED's staffing, configuration, and mandate are inconsistent with the best primary care. ED physicians focus on the patient's most emergent condition and are not obligated to look for underlying diseases or health risk. Thus, a patient who routinely seeks care in the ED may never receive screening tests for diabetes or cancer. He is unlikely to receive advice about staying well. ED physicians are often highly focused and rushed.

Continuity of care is also a classic problem in the ED. Because visits are unscheduled, no attempt can be made to obtain patient records, even if the patient has been seen in the same ED beforehand. This denies the physician baseline data on any presenting condition and information about potentially important features of the patient's history.

Crowding and Queuing. Both health professionals and consumers often express concern about crowding of emergency facilities and resulting delays in care. It is not unusual for a patient with a condition that is not clearly urgent to wait several hours before seeing a provider. Such delay is a major source of consumer dissatisfaction. Health professionals worry that delayed care for people who need prompt treatment may result in avoidable morbidity, dysfunction, or mortality. *Triage,* a process in which patients are sorted by urgency of their needs, is an integral part of ED functioning. But the process is not infallible, nor is it always possible to treat urgent cases with the desired promptness.

A large number of studies reveal the following factors as the most important in causing ED crowding and delay:[30]

- *Nonurgent care,* as described earlier.

- *"Frequent fliers,"* or people who made four or more annual visits; these individuals have been estimated to account for 14 percent of all ED visits.

- *Seasonal complaints and outbreaks.* Flu season brings more people to the ER, as may episodes of air pollution, which aggravates asthma and other lung diseases.

- *Insufficient staff.* An unfavorable ratio of staff to patients is an obvious cause of delay; this problem may be particularly severe in psychiatry, where lengthy interviewing and examination are sometimes needed.

- *Insufficient community resources.* Unavailability of primary care providers in the community may lead people to seek nonemergent care in the ED. Of great importance may be the lack of sufficient trauma care in a catchment area. Ambulances may be redirected from an emergency facility of choice when that facility is filled to capacity, a process known as *diversion.*

Despite these issues and challenges, EDs can function as profit centers for hospitals. The mix of emergent and nonemergent patients seen in most EDs facilitates this process. A recently published comment by a specialist in this field summarizes the logic by which queuing of nonemergent cases may contribute to the bottom line: "When patient influx ebbs and flows, an overstaffed department inevitably sees quiet times when costs surpass revenue and employees sit idle. The easiest way to remedy this problem is to lop off the peaks in patient flow by stockpiling them in waiting rooms to fill the valleys."[31]

This comment helps explain the experience of many consumers seeking care for emergent as well as nonemergent complaints in the ED. A crowd of seated patients waits. Slowly, individuals are called one by one to be seen by a provider. Suddenly, the routine is punctuated by the arrival of an ambulance, perhaps accompanied by a police car and trailing relatives. The victim of an accident or shooting is rushed into the treatment area. The room quiets. Again, seated patients are called slowly, one by one. The cycle repeats throughout the night.

Costs. Health care managers and policy makers often remark on excess cost of nonemergent care in the ED. The ED's primary mission is to treat and stabilize emergent conditions. The staffing, equipment, and physical plant required for emergent cases greatly exceeds that usually found in a doctor's office. This is particularly true of a trauma center. Bills issued by EDs for nonemergent care reflect the presence of resources unnecessary for such services.

THE MANAGED CARE ORGANIZATION

The increasing proliferation of managed care in the United States has given rise to a variety of organizations of distinct types. *Managed care* refers to an arrangement under which an administrative entity intervenes between the consumer and the provider. This administrative entity may take the form of a scheduling bureaucracy, case manager, or utilization review agency. The administrative entity has been viewed in a number of ways, including a means for ensuring optimal care and a rationing device. Large managed care organizations (MCOs) emerged in the 1940s, serving a restricted but stable market. Federal legislation enacted in 1973 (the Health Maintenance Organization Act) and numerous state laws in the 1980s, though, moved managed care onto center stage among U.S. health care organizations. Table 5.3 summarizes the characteristics of the major organizational forms found in managed care.

Health Maintenance Organizations

MCOs, first, include the health maintenance organizations (HMOs). HMOs often own physical facilities such as office buildings and hospitals. Typically, they retain physicians under exclusive contract. They provide care under *capitated* contracts—prospective agreements to care for a specified population for a fixed time period. HMOs tend to have tight utilization review and practice a conservative style of medicine. Physicians are paid a salary or its equivalent, plus a small bonus in some plans if costs have been adequately restrained.

Several distinct organizational forms exist under the general label HMO. The Kaiser Permanente HMO, predominant in the states of Hawaii, Oregon, and California, has an unusual yet apparently effective and enduring structure. Kaiser Permanente is really a cluster of three organizations, separately incorporated: the Kaiser Health Plan, Kaiser Hospitals, and the Permanente medical group. The health plan acts as an insurance company, and the hospital system owns and operates hospitals. A Permanente

TABLE 5.3   **Types of managed care organizations**

	Health Maintenance Organization (HMO)	**Independent Practice Organization (IPA)**	**Preferred Provider Organization (PPO)**
Legal status	Nonprofit	For-profit	For-profit
Relationship with physicians	Exclusive engagement, staff or group	Open engagement: physicians may join multiple IPAs	Open engagement: physicians may join multiple PPOs
Physician payment	Salary with risk sharing bonus and/or withholding	Capitation, possible risk sharing	Fee-for-service, no risk sharing
Relationship with hospitals	Owns and/or contracts with hospitals	Contracts with hospitals	Contracts with hospitals
Utilization review, practice management, and practice guidelines	Frequent (over 75 percent)	Frequent (over 75 percent)	Occasional (60 percent or less)
Relationship with payers	Prospective contracting	Prospective contracting	Prospective contracting
Patient access	Normally limited to plan physicians and hospitals	Normally limited to plan physicians and hospitals	Available from large network of providers
Patient costs	No charge beyond small copayment for within-plan care; no coverage outside plan	Small copayment for visits and prescriptions	80 percent coverage within plan; higher copayment outside plan

medical group is incorporated separately in each state where Kaiser Permanente operates. Each Permanente medical group negotiates exclusive contracts with the health plan. Members of the medical groups receive salaries, sometimes accompanied by bonuses for economical operation.

Independent Practice Associations

Independent practice associations (IPAs) combine individual physician practices into entities that contract independently with health plans or MCOs. Under this arrangement, the individual physician keeps her practice and sees patients in her own office. The IPA structure serves as an entity capable of negotiating contracts on behalf of individual physicians. IPAs pay their physicians primarily on a capitation basis, with some services being reimbursed on a fee-for-service basis. It is important to note that an individual physician may join multiple IPAs and at the same time retain his private practice. Although an IPA may have a strong utilization review mechanism, membership in multiple IPAs may attenuate its impact.

Preferred Provider Organizations

Preferred provider organizations (PPOs) are entities that contract with independent physicians to provide discounted care to large purchasers of health care. Under these arrangements, the physician or physician group practices fee-for-service medicine, according to a discounted fee schedule. Utilization review is less frequent and less stringent than in the HMO or IPA. Like IPA members, individual physicians or groups may join multiple PPOs. During the past decade, the PPO emerged as the predominant form of MCO, propelled by the desire of consumers for choice. PPOs typically carry out less extensive utilization review and thus cannot control costs as effectively as HMOs.

Some researchers and commentators have contended that, among all MCO structures, the HMO is best suited to economical operations. The typically strong utilization review mechanism of the HMO, it is said, contributes to this objective. The exclusive contracts (or employment relationships) accepted by HMO physicians may also contribute to cost restraint. IPA and PPO physicians, it should be remembered, may contract with multiple MCOs. These physicians are less dependent on, and less acutely conscious of, the cost control objectives of their individual contracting partners.

OTHER HEALTH CARE ORGANIZATIONS

Other organizations involved in health care include nursing homes, mental health facilities, free-standing surgical operations, and research agencies, both public and private. The numbers of these organizations have waxed and waned as the U.S. health care system has changed, and their structure is continuously evolving. Only a few of the remaining types of organizations will be described here.

Mental Health Facilities

As Table 5.4 indicates, residential mental health facilities maintained approximately 212,231 beds in 2004, about 15 percent of all inpatient beds operated in the United States. Although of considerable importance, the number of residential mental health beds operated today represents a mere fraction of the number a few decades ago. As recently as 1986, there were 111.7 mental health beds per 100,000 Americans; in

TABLE 5.4 Mental health organizations, beds, and beds per 100,000 civilian population in the United States, 1986 and 2004

Ownership	1986			2004		
	Organizations	Beds	Beds per 100,000	Organizations	Beds	Beds per 100,000
All organizations	3,512	267,613	111.7	2,891	212,231	71.2
State and county mental hospitals	285	119,033	49.7	237	57,034	19.1
Private psychiatric hospitals	314	30,201	12.7	264	28,422	9.5
Nonfederal general hospital psychiatric services	1,351	45,808	19.1	1,230	41,403	13.9
Department of Veterans Affairs medical centers[a]	139	26,874	11.2	—	—	—
Residential treatment centers for emotionally disturbed children	437	24,547	10.3	458	33,835	11.4
All other organizations	986	21,150	8.8	702	51,536	17.3

[a]VA facilities not surveyed as of 2004.

Source: National Center for Health Statistics. *Health, United States, 2008.* Table 117. Hyattsville, MD: National Center for Health Statistics; 2009.

2002 there were 71.2 per 100,000. The decline in number of beds has resulted from a deinstitutionalization movement in mental health, as well as the development and widespread use of antipsychotic medications. This is particularly true of the public institutions that once housed large numbers of mentally ill people, often hospitalized involuntarily. In the eighteen-year period represented in the table, the number of state and county mental health beds declined by about 60 percent.

Despite these decreases in inpatient capacity, the mental health market is not in decline. The number of mental health beds maintained by private, general hospitals declined by a little over 25 percent during the period covered by the table. But most hospitals that had psychiatric services in 1986 still had them in 2004. New means of delivering psychiatric services also evolved. Nonhospital mental health services have become popular, delivering outpatient, nonresidential care. MCOs often provide mental health care through "carve-outs" to companies that specialize in providing and managing mental health and substance abuse services. Known as managed behavioral healthcare organizations, these agencies typically contract with fee-for-service behavioral health care providers.[32]

Long-Term Care Facilities

Long-term care facilities provide a mix of health and nonhealth personal care services for the elderly and disabled. In the first decade of the twentieth century, about 16,000 long-term care facilities certified as eligible for Medicaid or Medicare funding operated in the United States. The majority, about 10,000, were operated by private profit-seeking firms or individuals. Another 5,000 were operated by nonprofits, and the remainder by government and other entities.[33] About 1.5 million people lived in long-term care facilities in 2005.

Many types of long-term care facilities exist today. These types of facilities serve the needs of people with differing levels of medical and service need. Following are some of these types of facilities:

■ *Continuing care communities.* Continuing care communities (also known as *assisted living facilities*) offer a continuum of living options—including independent living, enriched living, assisted living, and skilled nursing home care—on one campus. Residents can move from one level of care to the next as needs change.

■ *Adult homes.* Adult homes are small residential facilities intended for people who are unable to live independently. They usually include supervision, personal care, housekeeping, and meals. Facilities such as these are sometimes called *board and care* homes.

■ *Skilled nursing facilities.* Skilled nursing facilities (SNFs) provide twenty-four-hour medical attention by trained nurses, therapists, or other health care professionals. People may reside in SNFs on only a temporary basis, following operations or illnesses. Patents are managed according to intensive treatment plans developed by physicians.

- *Intermediate nursing facilities.* These facilities provide care for individuals whose condition is stable and does not demand twenty-four-hour attention, but who still need daily care. A physician creates the treatment plan, but it is likely to be carried out by certified nursing assistants and supervised by nurses. The nursing assistants manage the patient in daily issues such as bathing and eating.

- *Custodial care facilities.* Custodial care comprises a basic array of services to maintain patients who can no longer bathe, eat, or dress without assistance. Because it does not require concentrated medical care, those performing custodial care are generally without medical skills.

Full discussion of long-term care and associated issues must be sought in a more specialized source than this text. In a surprising observation, however, the number of nursing home beds in the United States declined between the late twentieth and early twenty-first century. The number of total beds was reduced from about 1.48 million in 1995 to 1.45 million in 2003. In that period, the occupancy rate of U.S. nursing homes declined from 84.5 to 82.6 percent. This decline can be attributed in part to greater maintenance of function among the elderly. This has been particularly true among the very old. In the period 1973 to 1974, more than 25 percent of Americans eighty-five years of age and over resided in long-term care facilities; in 2004, the percentage had fallen to 13.9.[34]

Practice Management Organizations

Practice management organizations represent a departure from the ambulatory care organizations covered earlier in this chapter. Practice management organizations accumulate large volumes of physician service capacity under the control of a single management structure. Theoretically, advantages accrue to both physician members and practice management organization operators and owners. Practice management organizations promise physicians leverage with insurance entities and a guaranteed patient flow. Initiators and owners of practice management organizations seek business for hospitals and other facilities in which they have an interest. They also obtain profits from delivery of physician services.

Physician hospital organizations (PHOs) represent one type of practice management organization. A hospital or system of hospitals is the centerpiece of the PHO. Under one model, hospitals buy physician practices, contract with medical groups, or directly employ physicians. Under these arrangements, they may finance physician office development or equipment purchase. PHOs offer hospitals a way to promote admissions and compete effectively with other hospitals.

Physician practice management (PPM) organizations constitute another mechanism for large-scale accumulation of medical practice capacity. PPMs are organized independent of hospitals and may seek hospital resources for their patients from a number of hospitals through a selective contracting process. Like PHOs, PPMs purchase individual physician practices and medical groups. They also form or purchase IPAs, which in turn contract with physicians or employ them directly.

While most U.S. hospitals and associated PHOs are nonprofit, PPMs are typically profit-seeking and owned by shareholders. Shares of PPMs are often traded on stock exchanges.

The late twentieth century saw a strong spurt of growth in practice management organizations. PPMs grew to significant size. MedPartners, for example, employed or contracted with thousands of physicians and provided services to hundreds of thousands of patients. Like other PPMs, MedPartners grew by merging with or acquiring smaller PPMs.[35] By the first decade of the twenty-first century, however, serious problems began to appear in the practice management organization sector. Disputes over payment to physicians developed, lawsuits ensued, and several key organizations downsized or disintegrated.[36]

Health Networks and Systems

Health networks and health systems represent the organization of health services on the largest scale. Like physician practice organizations, health networks and systems accumulate large volumes of assets and capacity under one management roof. Organization via health networks and systems, however, primarily involves physical facilities rather than professional personnel. The most visible feature of these organizations is coordination among or ownership of multiple hospitals. But health networks and health systems may also include mental health, long-term care, and insurance components.

Health care organization specialists Gloria J. Bazzoli and Steven M. Shortell distinguish health networks and health systems according to how tightly their components are linked.[37] *Health networks* are linked in a relatively loose fashion. Networks of this kind fundamentally amount to strategic alliances among hospitals. Linkages are maintained among hospitals (as well as other types of health care organizations) through contracts. Health networks are sometimes referred to as *virtual organizations.*

Health systems involve stronger linkages among hospitals and other units. In health systems, one corporation owns, leases, or operates associated hospitals and other health care units. Key health systems today include corporations such as Tenet and Community Health Systems, Inc. Both companies are worth billions of dollars and are publicly traded.

Health care executives seek to establish networks and systems for purposes such as control of costs, leverage with insurance companies, and bargaining power in local or national insurance markets. *Integration* of operations—coordination of resources under one decision-making structure—is the general objective of both networks and systems. Networks and systems are said to be *horizontally integrated* if they concentrate on acquiring or contracting with similar entities, such as hospitals. They are said to be *vertically integrated* if they acquire or contract with entities that provide a variety of services and address multiple levels of care. Under vertical integration, for example, a hospital (or hospital system) may acquire mental health and long-term care facilities. Networks and systems may be both horizontally and vertically integrated.

Other Types of Health Care Organizations

A number of other types of health care–related organizations are clearly worthy of attention. Free-standing imaging and surgical centers have become an important part of the U.S. health care scene. Research organizations such as those operated by the government, pharmaceutical companies, and independent nonprofit and for-profit entities play a basic role. Home care agencies attend to the daily needs of people with severe chronic illnesses. Hospices provide care and comfort to people approaching the end of life. Public health departments, ubiquitous among county agencies throughout the United States, provide vital services in disease surveillance, toxicology, and facility inspection. They play an important role in providing health services to the uninsured in some localities and are being looked to for disaster preparedness everywhere.

ORGANIZATIONAL MANAGEMENT IN HEALTH CARE

Even the brief overview presented here demonstrates the wide variety of organizations involved in delivery of health care in the United States. The diversity of health care organizations described here reflects the complexity of the health care system itself, as represented in Chapter One. Figure 1.3 depicts the U.S. health care system as a jumble of triangles and quadrilaterals representing functions such as hospital care, ambulatory practice, and long-term care. Actual formal organizations are required to carry out the functions depicted in Figure 1.3. Thousands of organizations may participate in performing each of these functions. An individual organization may combine the efforts of thousands of individuals.

The effectiveness with which each organization operates ultimately determines the degree to which the public benefits. Challenges faced by hospitals—strategy, financing, public relations, interpersonal conflict—also apply to MCOs, mental health facilities, and the numerous other organizations concerned with health care. Additional challenges are widespread in the health care industry. Following are some examples:

■ *Recruitment, retention, and motivation of personnel.* Every health care facility requires qualified and reliable staff. Adequate monetary compensation is a basic necessity. However, other considerations are important as well. An organization must be viewed as a desirable place to work. Desirable features include acceptable expectations regarding patient care volume, presence of up-to-date and well-maintained equipment, and high professional standards. The importance of women in health care organizations should not be underestimated. Employed women today often have disproportionate responsibility in caring for children and elders. Health care organizations must take steps to help women both carry out their job duties and meet family needs.

■ *Maintenance of communication.* All organizations depend on effective communication. Communication linkages enable top management to understand changes occurring at ground level and operations personnel to carry out the directives of the top ranks. People in different specialty areas must coordinate their actions. Faulty communication, however, frequently occurs in organizations with hierarchical structures.

Transmission though extended channels of communication reduces both the volume and accuracy of information. Individuals in separate specialty areas often lack the opportunity or motivation to communicate.

■ *Adaptation to change.* All organizations operate in a continuously changing social, economic, technological, and legal environment. The history of business abounds with once-prosperous enterprises that failed because they were unable to perceive or adapt to changes in the world around them. Health care changes more rapidly than perhaps any other industry. Effective strategic planning in health care organizations requires not only perception but anticipation of change.

■ *Avoidance of malfeasance.* Any industry characterized by high cash flow and insufficient accountability is predisposed to financial malfeasance. At times, health care organizations have shared these features with mafia-operated casinos in Los Vegas. The uncertainty that characterizes diagnosis and cost of care, as well as the presence of uninformed and vulnerable clients, creates opportunities for fraud. In 2006 alone, the FBI conducted 2,400 investigations of billing by health care organizations for unnecessary interventions or services never delivered.[38]

■ *Effectiveness of leadership.* Perhaps the most popular topic in management science, leadership is an indispensable element in any organization. **Leadership** can be summarized as the ability to develop a program of action and enlist the energy of others to carry the program forward. Leaders initiate action when it is called for. They set the cultural and ethical tone of an organization. People exercise leadership in a wide variety of ways, but organizations without leadership have difficulty meeting any of the challenges listed earlier.

KEY TERMS

Formal organization	Mass market
Structure	Niche services
Market sector	Leadership
Market segment	

SUMMARY

This chapter describes the operating components of the health care system and the internal and external challenges they face. Health care organizations—doctors' offices, hospitals, and many others—constitute the venues where the actual work of health care takes place. Organizations such as these make application of professional skill and technology possible on a large scale. Organizations are systems of human relationships that are designed through recognizable rules, assignments, and procedures to achieve identifiable objectives and goals, directs individual efforts toward shared goals. Health care organizations range in size from solo professionals working with a few aides to corporations that employ thousands. Effective and efficient health services depend on the structure and leadership of the organizations that deliver them.

Hospitals are the most visible type of organization in the health care industry. They differ from other large organizations in that they have multiple hierarchies, including separate administrative and medical chains of command. This organizational structure creates challenges for management and has led to instability within top leadership ranks. The hospital emergency department, where particularly intense and expensive care takes place, raises additional issues. Managed care organizations (MCOs) have taken their place alongside hospitals as key facilities for delivering health services.

Both hospitals and MCOs today face significant challenges in areas such as financing, competition, regulation, and public image. They compete fiercely, yet form alliances ranging from loose and flexible to firm and centralized. The degree to which the operations of health care organizations may affect the cost and quality of care is a continuing concern among both managers and policy makers.

DISCUSSION QUESTIONS

1. In comparison with traditional, small-scale health care organizations, what benefits (if any) might large-scale organizations provide?

2. Urgent care centers and retail clinics represent relatively new practice settings for physicians. On balance, do these innovations benefit or harm the consumer? Explain your answer.

3. What leadership challenges result from the unusual organizational structure of the modern hospital?

4. To what degree are today's tax exemptions for nonprofit hospitals justified by the community services they render?

5. EMTALA was originally intended to protect the public from being "dumped" when seeking emergency care. What unanticipated consequences have occurred from this legislation?

6. Is there evidence that increasing size and complexity in health care organizations correspond to an increased likelihood of ethical and legal transgression among professionals and managers? Explain.

7. What are the prospects for future growth in the long-term care sector? In which segment of the industry is growth likely to be the most pronounced?

CHAPTER

6

THE HEALTH CARE LABOR FORCE

LEARNING OBJECTIVES

- To attain an overview of the health care labor force
- To appreciate the histories of selected health professions and their impact on present-day management and practice
- To distinguish professionalism from other occupational orientations
- To understand the challenges posed by health professionals to management
- To become familiar with policy issues associated with the size and distribution of the health care labor force

HEALTH CARE LABOR FORCE ISSUES

The preceding chapter identified health care organizations as the operating units of the system. Whatever system of health care a country adopts, formal organizations are necessary as the venues for providers to exchange services for payment. The individual health professional represents an even more fundamental element of the heath care system. The quality of services available to consumers can be no better than the skill, motivation, and availability of individual health professionals.

From a systems perspective, society requires mechanisms that ensure sufficient numbers of readily available and appropriately qualified health care providers. Policymaking tasks include determining the supply of health professionals and exercising oversight. Policy makers carry out these functions by initiating and supporting training programs, establishing licensure and oversight machinery, and adjusting immigration policy to help alleviate shortages.

Ideal public policy would aim at a fine-tuning of the supply of health professionals, since either under- or oversupply of such personnel has undesirable consequences. Undersupply of health professionals, for example, may result in excess and expensive hospitalization. If access to appropriate health professionals is available in the community, many widespread illnesses can be treated in the doctor's office and not require hospital care. Examples of such illnesses, known as *ambulatory care–sensitive conditions,* include asthma, diabetes, and congestive heart failure. People with these conditions who cannot get a medical appointment or who wait long periods of time for an appointment are more likely to be hospitalized than those with ready access to health professionals.[1]

Alternatively, oversupply of health professionals does not necessarily result in a benefit to society. Excess physicians may schedule patients more often than they really need to be seen. Specialists with unfilled practices may recommend procedures of marginal value.

The professional character of the health care labor force creates challenges for managers. Traditional management tools such as command, control, and supervision, for example, are difficult to apply, if not prohibited by law. Routine management tasks in the context of health care personnel include the following:

- Recruiting personnel, often within a competitive market

- Verifying professional credentials

- Scheduling personnel to ensure that all services are covered when consumers require them

- Maintaining a professional community in which providers share information, make referrals to each other when needed, and continuously improve their level of practice skills

To illustrate the policy and management issues regarding the health care labor force, this chapter concentrates on three health professions: physicians, nurses, and health service administrators. Physicians make key clinical decisions and thus direct many of the system's resources. Nurses constitute the largest number of health professionals and have become the subject of much administrative concern due to issues of supply. Health service administrators, who comprise a relatively new profession, hold much of the responsibility for both operating and shaping the health care system. Personnel such as X-ray technicians, perfusionists, physician assistants, and many others are no less important to the industry. But detailed examination of physicians, nurses, and health care administrators well illustrates the range of policy and management challenges raised by health care personnel.

THE CONCEPT OF PROFESSIONALISM

The term professionalism itself raises issues for management and policy. In popular usage, professionalism signifies simply a high degree of training and specialization. But social scientists add a number of key dimensions regarding mission, self-identity, actions, and power. According to this thinking, true professionals belong to a community of fellow practitioners united by common beliefs, values, and economic interests. In theory, membership in such a community is sufficiently powerful to counteract the demands of the organizations in which professionals work.

The Hippocratic Oath

Attributed to the ancient Greek physician Hippocrates, the Hippocratic Oath is the best known of all professional credos. Generations of modern physicians have taken the oath upon graduation from medical school. Elements of the oath emphasize the obligation to serve humanity and to refrain from doing or assisting in harm. For example, those who take the oath swear to

> Benefit of the sick, remaining free of all intentional injustice, of all mischief and in particular of sexual relations with both female and male persons, be they free or slaves.

> Neither give a deadly drug to anybody who asked for it, nor will I make a suggestion to this effect [nor] give to a woman an abortive remedy. [Keep to myself] what I may see or hear in the course of the treatment or even outside of the treatment in regard to the life of men, which on no account one must spread abroad.

Notably, the oath emphasizes respect for fellow professionals and loyalty to the professional community. The oath requires the physician to "hold him who has taught me this art as equal to my parents and to live my life in partnership with him, and if he is in need of money to give him a share of mine and to regard his offspring as equal to my brothers . . . and teach them this art without fee and covenant."[4]

According to some well-known formulations,[2,3] the characteristics of a profession include the following components.

Service Orientation and Ethical Obligation. Professions typically embody a sense of mission. The professional mission comprises obligation by the individual practitioner to help those in need and contribute to the general social well-being. Perhaps every true profession has a written code of ethics. These codes typically emphasize the duty to help others, refrain from dishonest or harmful behavior, and practice according to the technical standards of the professional community.

Dominance over Knowledge and Technology. A true profession is said to exercise ultimate control over knowledge and technology relevant to its area of competence. In the health field, physicians exercise strong dominance over both development of knowledge and instruction of people seeking to enter the field. Physicians play the lead role in biomedical research, occupy most teaching positions in medical schools, instruct medical students and residents, and exercise oversight and discipline in a peer-review process.

Independent Organization. No body of individuals constitutes a true profession without a formal organization. Although the American Medical Association (AMA) has the highest visibility, all health professions have similar organizations. These organizations express their members' professional identify and serve a variety of individual needs. Professional organizations contribute to development of knowledge and technology by holding conferences and publishing journals. Of potentially greater importance, professional organizations advocate for the profession's rights and privileges. The AMA has served as a powerful voice for American medicine since the nineteenth century. Organizations representing nurses, pharmacists, optometrists, chiropractors, and many other health professionals also act as advocates. These organizations exercise political influence in both state legislatures and at the national level.

Legal Recognition. The most successful professions stake out legally protected spheres of practice for their members. The legal requirement of a license to practice represents an important milestone in the development of a profession. Nascent professions push state legislatures to require licenses for practice and to empower members of the profession to write and administer licensure examinations. The developing profession also seeks to dominate boards and commissions responsible for surveillance and discipline of its members. Legal recognition includes the privilege of practice without supervision from outside the profession and the right to independently bill insurance companies and government programs for services.

Laws passed at the state level known as practice acts specify procedures that members of a particular profession may carry out and the areas of the body over which they have jurisdiction. Professional organizations perennially dispute limitations on their scope of practice. Georgia podiatrists, for example, have contested state law that permits them to operate on the ankle, but not to amputate toes.[5]

Professionalization can occur by degrees. Medicine, the oldest of the health professions, is the most strongly professionalized. Physicians are represented by strong professional organizations, hold licenses, and enjoy an extensive scope of practice. Medical doctors dominate biomedical research and medical education. Many states prohibit nonphysician corporations and hospitals from employing physicians—the so-called **corporate practice of medicine.** States that do not expressly prohibit such practice restrict the liberty of corporate supervisors to direct physician's decision making.[6]

Nursing, though a well-established professional field, is not as strongly professionalized as medicine. Like physicians, nurses hold licenses and teach in professional schools. They have professional organizations that publish journals, hold conferences, and lobby for the interests of their members. The scope of practice of nurses, however, is limited in comparison with that of physicians. Usually, nurses do not practice or bill independently, but carry out instructions of physicians and are employed by hospitals. *Advanced practice nurses,* discussed later in this chapter, are an exception.

The most successful health service administrators can enjoy higher earnings than any physician or nurse. Yet health service administration is a weaker profession than either medicine or nursing. Organizations such as the American College of Health Executives (ACHE) provide voluntary certification. But no licensure requirement exists. Universities have offered professional health administration programs since the 1930s. However, hospitals, HMOs, and other health care organizations can hire administrators with any background or training they find desirable. The most prominent university health service administration programs today base their curricula on master of business administration (MBA) requirements, with relatively minor contributions from epidemiology and medical sociology.

Professionalism as considered here has both a positive and a negative dimension. By asserting their independence from corporate superiors and politicians, professionals achieve the liberty to concentrate on the patient's best interests. Licensure excludes unqualified individuals from practice. However, professionalism also reduces the range of services available to the public and raises costs. From the administrative perspective, restriction on corporate practice of medicine reduces the range of organizational options available for the delivery of health care. The independence inherent in professionalism constitutes a barrier to supervision of any kind. The standard setting and self-discipline that characterize professionalism reduce public accountability. In this respect, the famed author George Bernard Shaw once remarked that the professions are "all conspiracies against the laiety."[7]

HISTORY, BACKGROUND, AND CHALLENGES IN THREE KEY FIELDS

The professions whose members participate in the health care industry are too numerous to address in detail. Examination of three professions helps identify a range of issues associated with the professional labor force from a management and policy perspective. Two of these, medicine and nursing, dominate the health professions numerically and are familiar to everyone. A third, health administration, is less publicly visible. But this profession is indispensable for the delivery of health care and is increasing in importance.

Medicine

While a great many patient care professions have attained significance, medicine occupies the central position. This is true even though physicians composed well under 10 percent of the health care labor force in the first decade of the twenty-first century (see Chapter Two). One hundred years earlier, two out of every three people who made their living in health care were doctors.[8]

Still, medicine deserves more attention than any other segment of the health labor force. The importance of doctors arises from their domination of clinical decision making, rather than their gross numbers. This dominance has key ramifications for both the content and cost of care. Economist Victor Fuchs has written in a classic book:

> *The dominant role of the physician is particularly important with respect to the problem of the cost of care. This is not primarily because physicians' fees are too high, though they are in many instances, but because physicians control the total process of care. Typically, this process begins when a patient seeks help. From then on, the initiative passes to the physician, whose decisions significantly influence the quantity, type, and cost of service utilized.*[9]

In this fashion, the physician exercises great influence over the pharmaceutical products purchased by the patient, laboratory and imaging studies, referral to other physicians, and procedures such as biopsy and surgery. All of these involve costs, and the appropriateness of their application affects quality of care and ultimate outcomes.

Like other features of modern health care, modern medicine developed only in the late nineteenth and early twentieth centuries. Today, medical training is time-consuming and highly standardized. Licensure is required throughout the United States. Many hospitals and health care organizations require their affiliated physicians to hold an additional credential in the form of *board certification*, which must be periodically renewed. Hospital credentialing committees carefully verify whether physicians who apply for admitting privileges have actually attained the degrees and training they claim.

As recently as the late nineteenth century, however, patients could count on none of these features in their medical care. In the early days of the republic, some states had enacted licensure and practice laws. However, most people who practiced medicine or other forms of health care lacked formal education and were not licensed. Farmers and frontiersmen and -women who possessed a few medical skills would work as part-time practitioners. Because America lacked a system of roads between isolated farms and towns, it would have been difficult for even a well-educated provider to earn a living only from medicine.

During the early nineteenth century, medical science was itself primitive. Mainstream medicine provided few demonstrable benefits to patients. Fueled by egalitarian ideology and mistrust of elites, a movement arose to prohibit states from issuing medical licenses. Most, if not all, of the states that had instituted licensure repealed these laws. Proponents of open practice of medicine argued that licensure would be equivalent to establishment of a state religion. Among the forces that opposed licensure was the Thomsonian movement. Led by Samuel Thomson, a botanical practitioner, this movement paralleled the Jacksonian thinking of the early nineteenth century in its opposition to elite institutions.

Freed from a dominant model of healing, medical practice in the United States became highly diverse. In addition to **allopathic medicine**, the approach that predominates today, many physicians practiced in the botanical, homeopathic, or eclectic traditions. Much medical training took place under an apprenticeship model, under which aspirants to medicine took informal study with an established practitioner. Even formal medical schools often required no more than two or three years of study.

The late nineteenth century, though, brought economic and technological developments that enabled medicine to develop into its modern form. As noted in earlier chapters, this era brought basics such as antisepsis and anesthesia into medical practice. The public and policy makers began to recognize that medicine had achieved the ability to actually benefit patients. Led by scientific progressives in the medical profession, a movement arose to require rigorous scientific training and licensing of physicians. Established in 1893, the Johns Hopkins Medical School required all entrants to hold college degrees and to complete four additional years of study for graduation. Leading university-based medical schools throughout the United States adopted this model. Licensure laws were passed in every state by 1901.

A milestone in the development of modern medicine was passed in 1910. A historically significant study evaluating the quality of contemporary medical education appeared in that year. Initiated by the AMA and conducted by the Carnegie Foundation, the ensuing report was named after Abraham Flexner, the Carnegie Foundation researcher who conducted the investigation. The famed **Flexner Report** indicated that a high percentage of U.S. medical schools were inadequate beyond remedy. These schools lacked such essentials as qualified faculty, laboratories, and requirements for class attendance. Other schools were found to be wanting, but were encouraged to make improvements. Championed by the AMA, the Flexner Report resulted in large-scale closure of medical schools that did not conform to the model established by Johns Hopkins and other leading institutions.

While a modernizing event, the Flexner Report greatly restricted entry into the practice of medicine. The 131 U.S. medical schools operating in 1906 had dropped to 81 by 1922; the number of medical school graduates had been 3,535 in 1915, but declined to 2,529 by 1922. Because the schools that admitted women and African Americans were largely those considered irremediable, new female and African American physicians ceased to be graduated. Fields such as naturopathy, homeopathy, and eclectic medicine, which had flourished in the nineteenth century, drastically declined.

Medicine at a Crossroads

The Flexner Report was instrumental not only in standardizing medical education but in standardizing medical practice itself. Medical schools approved in the report tended to emphasize the allopathic approach. As the twentieth century wore on, several important fields of healing went into eclipse, a process vigorously promoted by the AMA.

Homeopathy, for example, dates from the late 1700s. According to its practitioners, homoeopathy emphasizes activation of the body's natural healing mechanisms. Traditionally, homeopathic physicians have subscribed to the doctrine that "like cures like," according to which agents that produce the symptoms of a disease in fact cure that disease. As medications, modern homeopaths prescribe highly diluted solutions of agents believed to be curative. Homeopathic remedies also include water from which the agent believed to be active has been filtered, under the assumption that the water retains a memory of the filtered-out ingredient.[10]

Although many fewer than before the Flexner Report, schools of homeopathy still operate in the United States. A homeopathic diploma does not in itself lead to licensure. To legally practice homeopathy in most states, homeopaths must hold a license in another health profession. Homeopathic services are not generally covered by health insurance.

Naturopathy uses interventions such as therapeutic nutrition, botanicals, and lifestyle counseling to both prevent and treat illness. In 2001, there were five institutions of higher learning in the United States that awarded the degree of doctor of naturopathic medicine (ND). In that year, NDs were licensed in twelve states. Generally, neither private insurance nor government programs cover naturopathic medicine.[11]

A remarkable survivor of this historical shakeout has been *chiropractic.* First organized as a profession in 1895, chiropractic uses musculoskeletal manipulation to treat complaints such as back and elbow pain. Chiropractic operates its own educational system and formulates and conducts licensure examinations. An increasing number of Americans have used chiropractors in recent years, and some scientific research indicates that procedures such as spinal manipulation are effective. Unlike other nonallopathic fields, chiropractors may bill government and private insurance plans for services. A high proportion of managed care plans offer chiropractic. For a hundred years, allopathic medicine and chiropractic engaged in intense conflict. The AMA's code of ethics, for example, forbade physicians from making referrals to chiropractors, a provision that was finally deleted in response to a series of antitrust suits by the chiropractic profession.[12]

Another survivor has been *osteopathy.* Osteopathy distinguishes itself from allopathic medicine by including manipulative techniques in its practice. Similar in some respects to chiropractic, this approach, known as osteopathic manipulative medicine (OMM), is characterized by manual, rather than pharmaceutical or surgical, intervention. An osteopathic physician, for example, may apply manual techniques to increase the range of motion in a joint. In the United States, about three thousand doctors of osteopathy graduate from institutions specialized in that field each year. These individuals qualify for medical licensure, are welcome in mainstream residencies, and, despite the distinctive history of their field, are virtually indistinguishable from allopaths.

Over the generations, the AMA has served as the principal professional organization of U.S. physicians. The AMA began as a progressive organization. Its founding members championed modern scientific medicine. Founded in the 1840s, the association played an important part in both reinstatement of licensure and the requirements of medical education. AMA members worked the politics of their local state legislatures to pass such laws. As early as 1904, the AMA's Committee on Medical Education lobbied state legislatures to grant licenses only to people who had graduated from four-year postgraduate medical institutions and had completed internships.

The AMA became a conservative force in the twentieth century. Through most of the century, the AMA strove to keep the supply of physicians available to the public low. Despite an increasing U.S. population, the AMA opposed both expansion of medical education and immigration by foreign physicians into the United States. In addition, the AMA opposed health insurance when the concept first appeared. As recently as the 1950s, county medical societies—local units of the AMA with considerable independence and power—excluded physicians involved in HMOs. The AMA opposed the legislation that gave rise to Medicare and Medicaid in the 1960s.

Today, the AMA mixes some progressive policy positions with seemingly traditional positions regarding the medical profession's interests. In the first decade of the twenty-first century, for example, the AMA favored use of government funds to cover all uninsured Americans. But the organization also backed legislation to permit *balance billing* under Medicare.[13] This practice would allow physicians to charge patients the difference between the rates paid by Medicare and the higher rates that physicians often consider justified.

Professional organizations other than the AMA have become increasingly important. Organizations of specialists such as orthopedic surgeons lobby independently in the interest of their members. The American Association of Medical Colleges (AAMC) represents academic medicine. The American Medical Women's Association (AMWA), which focuses on women's health issues, refers to its charter members as the Founding Mothers.

Changes in the health care system have constituted challenges to the medical profession. Traditionally, medicine has been a highly paid profession whose members practice alone or in small organizations and enjoy significant autonomy. Managed care, utilization review, and practice in increasingly large organizations make autonomous practice more difficult. Physicians complain about restrictions on the fees they may charge imposed by Medicare and private insurance plans.

Yet career satisfaction among physicians remains high. A 2001 survey asked U.S. physicians how satisfied they were with their overall career in medicine. Over 80 percent answered that they were very satisfied or somewhat satisfied. About the same level of satisfaction was found among both primary care physicians and specialists. Satisfaction tended to be lower among primary care physicians whose working hours had recently increased, whose income had decreased, and whose practices included many complex cases. Among both primary care physicians and specialists, perceived lack of autonomy correlated with dissatisfaction. Neither the primary care physician's nor the specialist's degree of involvement with managed care was related to her level of satisfaction. But specialists whose practices included a large number of different managed care contracts were more likely to feel dissatisfied.[14]

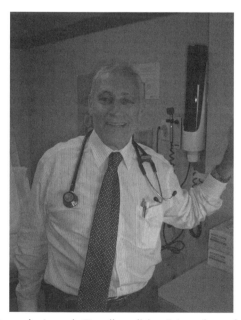

A U.S. physician completes a day's work. To call medicine "strongly professionalized" is not to characterize other health care personnel as less dedicated or skilled. Among the health professions, however, medicine is most strongly organized, politically powerful, and publicly esteemed.

Nursing

Nursing in its modern form developed even more recently than medicine. The first schools of professional nursing in England and the United States began in the 1870s. The field grew very rapidly after these beginnings. Although the medical profession initially opposed the development of professional nursing, physicians quickly realized the value of trained nurses. As surgery became popular and the hospital industry grew, medicine became increasingly reliant on nursing. The sick had always needed to be fed, bathed, and otherwise attended to. But patient needs became more complex and technical as medical science developed. Highly trained nursing personnel were required to meet these needs. The number of nursing schools in the United States grew from 3 in 1893 to 432 in 1900 and 1,129 by 1910.[15]

The fact that nursing developed after medicine had established itself as a profession is significant. Sociologist Eliot Freidson has observed that no other clinical field was able to claim the right to independent practice once medicine had begun to organize and gain respect.[16] Chiropractic, which was established contemporaneously with medicine, retained the right to practice without physician supervision. Chiropractic, moreover, exercised significant political efforts to retain its independence. Nursing, on the other hand, has only recently begun to assert a degree of independence. The subordinate status of women in society overall was mirrored in the subordinate status of nurses, who were preponderantly female.

The saga of Florence Nightingale provides insight into the development of nursing and some of its modern features. Born in 1820, Nightingale was an exemplar of upper-class, Victorian English women. As did others of her class in both the United States and England, Nightingale felt a calling to promote social well-being, particularly among the disadvantaged. At that time, family members usually attended to the sick. Hospitalized patients received "nursing" care from untrained women to whom society accorded very low social status. Training in skilled nursing techniques was available in Germany, however, and Nightingale went there to study.

Both Nightingale and the concept of professional nursing advanced markedly during the Crimean war (1854–1856). The British press began reporting horrendous conditions at hospitals for the British wounded. Resulting public alarm led Secretary of War Sidney Herbert to request that Nightingale lead a contingent of nurses to improve conditions at the facility. In the military hospital at Scutari, Turkey, Nightingale took on self-appointed administrative functions. She kept both administrative and clinical records. She detected malfeasance and fraud in the management of supplies. She took charge of dietary matters, using her own wealth to purchase foods more suitable to ill and wounded people than those the army had provided.[17]

Relationships between Nightingale and the military authorities were antagonistic. In Nightingale's achievements officials saw what they believed the public would interpret as evidence of their own incompetence. Strained relationships with military and civil authorities continued after the war's end, as Nightingale campaigned for hospital reform and modernization. She also founded the first professional nursing school in

England. Only Nightingale's personal wealth and connection with the English elite enabled her to retain her influence.[18]

Several of Nightingale's tenets appear consistent with nursing as it was practiced for one hundred years after her death. Her organizational and political skills are usually omitted in her altruistic and heroic portrayals. She knew that nursing would have to adapt to, rather than challenge, the power of medicine. The antagonism of medical men at Scutari to her personnel clearly demonstrated this fact. Principles emphasized by Nightingale at Scutari and afterward emphasized strict adherence to regulations and intervention with patients only according to doctors' orders.[19]

The challenges and forms of accommodation apparent in the early years of nursing remain evident today. A sociologist who studies nursing might characterize the field as marginal, but nursing is far from marginal in a practical sense. Modern health care could not function without large numbers of nurses. Nursing may be considered marginal, though, in the sense that important characteristics of the field are mutually inconsistent. Nurses are highly educated in comparison with many others who work in hospitals, yet they exercise little control over treatment decisions. Nurses hold a great deal of responsibility for the patient's well-being, but have little authority on the wards. The frontline position occupied by nurses exposes them to blame for unfavorable outcomes.

Although many pursue satisfying careers in nursing, dissatisfaction with nursing jobs and careers appears widespread. A survey by Linda Aiken, a specialist in nursing issues, found that 43.2 percent of nurses experienced high emotional exhaustion and 41.5 percent expressed dissatisfaction with their current job.[20] Comments by the U.S. Bureau of Labor Statistics suggest that the physical and emotional rigors of nursing work contribute to these negative feelings:

> *Nursing has its hazards, especially in hospitals, nursing care facilities, and clinics, where nurses may be in close contact with individuals who have infectious diseases and with toxic, harmful, or potentially hazardous compounds, solutions, and medications. RNs must observe rigid, standardized guidelines to guard against disease and other dangers, such as those posed by radiation, accidental needle sticks, chemicals used to sterilize instruments, and anesthetics. In addition, they are vulnerable to back injury when moving patients, shocks from electrical equipment, and hazards posed by compressed gases. RNs also may suffer emotional strain from caring for patients suffering unrelieved intense pain, close personal contact with patients' families, the need to make critical decisions, and ethical dilemmas and concerns.[21]*

The rigors of bedside nursing have led many in the field to seek employment that does not involve direct patient care. The practice of *utilization review,* for example, has opened an alternative career path for nurses. Insurance companies employ utilization review personnel to determine whether a patient's insurance plan should cover a particular procedure or medication for a given ICD code. Utilization review specialists formulate protocols for this purpose, and nurses have sufficient clinical background for making actual case-by-case decisions.

Recent developments suggest that important changes in outlook and opportunity within nursing are taking place. First, the emergence of **advanced practice nursing** constitutes an important development. Advanced practice nursing emerged in response to a shortage of primary care physicians in the 1950s. The label "advanced practice nurse" covers nurse practitioners (NPs), nurse anesthetists, and nurse midwives. Advanced practice nurses typically have baccalaureate degrees in nursing plus master's degrees and additional clinical training. The rise of advanced practice nursing was not universally hailed in either nursing or medical circles. MDs sensed potential for professional rivalry, while nurses voiced discomfort over potential divisions within their profession.

Today, over seventy thousand NPs, the largest division of the advanced practice nursing field, care for patients in the United States. Although many practice alongside MDs, NPs enjoy significant professional autonomy. Medicare permits NPs to bill independently, and fifteen states allow NPs to independently prescribe medications. NPs fought persistently and skillfully to obtain these privileges. Following the model of successful political action in the United States (see Chapter Eleven), NPs lobbied both in Congress and on the grassroots level with great success.[22]

Another movement in nursing intended to benefit these care providers has been unionization. If the advanced practice movement mimics the tactics of established professions such as medicine and law, unionization borrows tools used successfully for generations by teachers and blue-collar workers. Nurses resistant to unionization have argued that nursing unions are "unprofessional" and tarnish the image of nursing. However, unionization among nurses grew rapidly in the late twentieth and early twenty-first centuries. Professional organizations of nurses such as the American Nurses Association (ANA) have become collective bargaining agencies. Rivalries have sprung up between the AFL-CIO-affiliated ANA and the break-away Service Employees International Union, which has aggressively recruited nurses.

Health Administration

As a distinct occupational group, health administration dates from no later than the mid-1920s. In 1926, an organization was founded known as the National Association of Clinic Managers. This organization later became the Medical Group Management Association (MGMA), one of the most important of today's associations of health care managers. During the years prior to World War II, health care administration was simple and straightforward. Accordingly, topics covered in the National Association of Clinic Managers' initial meeting included such humdrum titles as "What Is a Business Manager Expected to Know?" "Better Collections," and "How to Stay Out of Trouble."[23] Subject matter of health administrator meetings in that era could include the desired temperature of dishwater in hospital kitchens.

The health care system in the early twentieth century was simple, technologically primitive, and cheap compared to the system that exists today. This simplicity and parsimony was reflected in core management functions such as accounting and billing. With neither a health insurance system nor significant government participation, financial management was straightforward. Large, publicly owned hospitals engaged in negotiation with municipal agencies and issued bonds. More routine finance-related tasks included working out agreements with revenue-producing departments (such as radiology and surgery) on overhead allocation.

The memoirs of George Bugbee, a pioneer in development of health administration as a recognized profession, offer a glimpse at the work of hospital administrators in the 1930s.[24] Hospital administrators interacted with elected officials and other representatives of the public, as well as the press. Yearly budgeting was a key responsibility, as was reviewing the functioning and costs of laundry, food service, and housekeeping. Hospital administrators received reports from nurses on shortcomings in care and emergency incidents. Matters that concerned health service managers in Bugbee's time remain important, but represent only a small segment of the modern health executive's scope of work.

Today, the dominance of private insurance and government programs in paying for health care has made billing and collection extremely complex. Prior to the widespread presence of third-party payment systems, however, health care providers enjoyed significant latitude regarding what to charge a patient. Hospitals, for example, could determine charges simply on a cost-plus basis, billing patients for what administrators believed their treatment had cost plus a percentage for margin. In addition, providers had the discretion to determine charges based on what they thought the patient could afford. Bugbee describes the process as he conducted it at the University of Michigan hospital in the 1920s and 1930s:

> Collection rules were strict. Non-emergency patients were required to deposit estimated costs for treatment, so I became quite adept at securing information from medical staff for such estimates. If patients were non-emergencies without funds, they were referred to local welfare officials before admission. We interviewed physicians, quizzing them about degree of emergency, before admitting a patient unable to pay.

Under a system adopted from the Mayo Clinic, a sort of sliding scale of charges worked as follows:

> We secured confidential reports on pay patients, particularly those occupying private rooms, and assessed those to some degree in proportion to ability to pay. With the advice of physicians, we developed a pattern for charges. Most patients paid the same fees, but where considerable wealth was evident, fees were increased.

In one celebrated instance the system backfired. As the story went,

> Dr. Canfield, Chief of Oncology in the early 1920s, removed Edsel Ford's tonsils. The patient's father, Henry Ford, obviously pleased, sent a check for $5,000 (a considerable sum for that era and greatly in excess of the standard charge). Dr. Canfield returned the check with a bill for $25,000! Henry Ford paid and then established the Henry Ford Hospital in Detroit (to compete with the University Hospital) with a full-time salaried staff and a $100 ceiling on professional fees.

The story could well have been mythical. Clearly, however, a hospital could charge whatever it considered justifiable and felt it might be able to collect.

In an atmosphere of such simplicity, top hospital management could be carried out by doctors, nurses, or, in the case of religiously affiliated hospitals, by clergy. Accountants with no health care experience could move readily in and out of the health care sector. During his time as superintendent of Cleveland City Hospital, Bugbee describes one such accountant who was recruited from an automobile dealership and later moved to a New York law firm. Health administration might have required considerable effort and talent, but was not distinguishable as a specialized field. As late as the 1950s, one observer commented that "the hospital manager, like managers of other types of enterprises, must be a jack of all trades—a planner of physical plant, a purchasing agent, a labor relations expert, a personnel manager, a cost accountant, not to mention a public relations man."[25]

Prominent individuals found fault with management in health care even before the system achieved the complexity it has today. As in medical education early in the century, a private foundation played an important role in identifying and remedying faults in health care management. Work on Michigan hospitals at the W. K. Kellogg Foundation, led by the pioneering Andrew Pattullo, found that many of these facilities were characterized by "uneven and unassessed quality, weak management and lack of personnel and control systems, poor medical staff relationships, obsolete and unsafe facilities, lack of support by diagnostic specialists, etc."[26]

As World War II came to a close, Pattullo organized a series of commissions under the W. K. Kellogg Foundation's auspices to examine and make recommendations for specialized education in health services administration. A handful of university health administration degree programs already existed. Patullo himself had attended the first such program, which had begun in 1934 at the Graduate School of Business, University of Chicago. Under Patullo's leadership, the commissions drew on the experience of the early university programs and the outstanding hospital administrators of the era. The commissions' work led to formulation of a basic university curriculum in health services administration. Becoming a major grantmaker in the postwar years, the W. K. Kellogg Foundation used its financial resources to support existing master of health administration (MHA) programs, launch new ones, aid health administration students, and provide resources to agencies such as the Association of University Programs in Health Administration (AUPHA).

During this era, the institutional resources typical of a profession grew and consolidated. Long-standing organizations supporting the interests of health administrators and providing for their educational needs played prominent roles as the health care industry boomed. These included the MGMA; the American College of Health Executives, founded in 1933; and the American Hospital Association, founded in 1898. A quasi-independent agency, the Commission on Accreditation of Healthcare Management Education (CAHME), examines and grants accreditation to health administration programs. As of 2008, approximately 67 master's degree-level health services administration programs held CAHME accreditation. According to the Bureau of Labor Statistics, just under 300,000 Americans worked as health administrators in that year.

Despite the prominence of specialized education and organized interest groups, health administration must be viewed as less professionally established than medicine or nursing. People without specialized education may work their way up career ladders such as external communication and marketing. U.S. health administration is a licensed profession only in Puerto Rico. Although several organizations represent the interests of health services administrators, the number of such organizations can be viewed as a sign of fragmentation.

Fundamentally, professional status is marked by a unique body of knowledge and exclusive jurisdiction over practice. Such is not the case with health care administration. It is not unusual for health care organizations to look for leadership to executives with substantially no health care experience. The appointment of Peter J. Ratican as chairman, president, and CEO of Maxicare Health Plans serves as an illustration. Ratican, a film and television industry accountant, was brought in to manage the firm after it had defaulted on its debts.[27] In medicine, leadership at this level would never have been given to a lay person.

Among the pressures facing health administrators are the need to respond effectively to a rapidly changing, highly competitive, and increasingly resource-constrained environment. Patient care professionals look to health administrators for leadership under these challenging conditions. However, health services administrators also take the blame for sacrifices required of clinical professionals for needed change. Boards of directors at hospitals tend to take the side of clinicians. According to a 2005 ACHE survey, the average hospital CEO held his job for 5.6 years. However, the median CEO tenure was 3.4 years, and 22 percent of the hospitals surveyed reported having had at least three CEOs in the preceding five years.[28]

CLINICIANS AS MANAGERS

Patient care professionals play an important part in management of health services. Physicians participate in management of the ambulatory care partnerships and professional corporations discussed in the preceding chapter. In such organizations, physicians may take on management responsibilities on a rotating basis or delegate such duties to colleagues who have a personal interest in or flair for management. In hospitals and health systems, physicians act as department heads. As *president of the medical staff,* a physician represents the interests of her colleagues in system governance. As a member of the top management team representing, for example, the interests of stockholders, a physician occupies the position of *medical director.* Nurses participate in management in a more hierarchical fashion: *charge nurses* supervise floor nurses, and *nursing supervisors* supervise charge nurses. Hospitals and health systems have *nursing directors* who report to top management.

The question of whether clinicians should play a greater part in management of health services should concern both professionals and the public. It is reasonable to think that only a person who has provided direct care to the sick and injured has a true understanding of health services. According to this reasoning, one might argue that health care management should be a specialty within nursing, medicine, or other health professions. Hospitals and health systems would then prefer or even require that managers be licensed patient care personnel. Consistent with this belief, most county health departments require their directors to be licensed physicians. Outstanding physician managers have included Thomas F. Frist, cofounder, president, and CEO of HCA; and Harvard's Eugene Braunwald.

For a number of reasons, however, clinicians have not dominated the ranks of top health care managers. In the case of physicians, temperament and training often militate against following an administrative career line. Medical training, for example, emphasizes the application of empirical science to problem solving. Management, however, often involves compromise and guesswork. Medical training casts the physician into the role of a decisive, often independent decision maker. Management typically requires negotiation and compromise. Technical capabilities increasingly required in health care management are absent in medical training. These include finance, accounting, strategic planning, public policy, and marketing.[29] Universities and professional societies today offer training programs specifically oriented to the needs of physicians desiring to become managers. But participation in these programs requires time away from an often lucrative practice, plus tuition, which physicians and their employers may be reluctant to pay.

In the early 2000s, only about two hundred physicians served as hospital CEOs. This figure represented only about 4 percent of U.S. acute care hospitals.[30] Looking into the future, nurses and pharmacists may predominate among patient care professionals in management. These professionals may be better adapted to teamwork and less likely to resist making career changes because of already high incomes.

THE HEALTH CARE LABOR FORCE: FACTS AND FIGURES

Basic statistics on health professions and related occupations illustrate the importance of the health care sector within the U.S. labor force. The number of individuals directly dependent on health care for their livelihood illustrates the importance of this sector to the U.S. economy. Growth in the number of American workers in health care reflects a marked increase in the percentage of U.S. GDP associated with health care over recent generations. An increase in the health care labor force of the magnitude illustrated here has in part resulted from public policy favoring growth. Viewed positively, the figures presented below indicate the burgeoning of an industry that has produced numerous and high-paying jobs.

Table 6.1 presents 2004 data on U.S. physicians. It is readily apparent from the table that large differences prevail among specialties in both numbers and income. The key primary care specialties, including family practice, internal medicine, and pediatrics, are by far the most numerous. They are also the least well paid. Top incomes go to "procedure-oriented" fields such as radiology, urology, cardiology, and anesthesiology.

TABLE 6.1 Number of active physicians in the United States, income, and income change from preceding year, by specialty, 2004

Specialty	Number Practicing in U.S.	Average Income	Income Change from Prior Year (%)
Radiology	7,010	$412,000	7
Urology	8,804	373,000	12
Cardiology (noninvasive)	17,301	362,000	6
Oncology	N.A.	347,000	N.A.
Anesthesiology	29,254	341,000	2
Pathology	10,209	325,000	10
General surgery	25,284	292,000	1
OB/GYN	33,636	261,000	1
Emergency medicine	17,727	227,000	1
Neurology	9,304	220,000	3
Internal medicine	99,670	172,000	3
Pediatrics	47,996	172,000	4
Psychiatry	25,656	172,000	5
Family practice[1]	73,508	166,000	1

[1]Includes general practitioners.

Sources: Physician numbers: *Health, United States, 2005,* Table 106 (data are for 2003). Physician income: Modern Healthcare.com. July 24, 2004. MGMA survey findings for 2004.

As is true of other labor force–related matters, the income disparities visible among physicians reflect management and policy decisions. A relevant decision involves adoption of the *resource-based relative value scale* (RBRVS) by Medicare in 1992. Practitioners in the highest paid specialties tend to apply invasive procedures, often involving machinery or technology, to the patient. Developed at the Harvard School of Public Health, the RBRVS system specifies payments for thousands of medical services. It was adopted for use by Medicare in 1992 and has been periodically modified since then. Private insurance companies have adopted the RBRVS for their own use or have developed similar systems. For each medical service, the Harvard team computed a payment rate according to the total work of the physician, associated practice costs (such as liability insurance), and the amortized value of the opportunity costs for specialty training. Preliminary RBRVS rates were intensely reviewed by independent teams of physicians for validity.[31]

Despite the rigor with which the RBRVS system was developed, many physicians consider the resulting differences in reimbursements unjust. The resulting system of payment parallels the payments traditionally made by private insurance firms. Private insurance has traditionally made higher payments for technically intense services than "cognitive" services such as history taking, lifestyle instruction, or psychiatric care. Whether prevailing payments to physicians reflect the time and resources invested by individual providers is open to dispute according to several criteria. The practice incomes of procedure-oriented physicians, for example, have been shown to represent high rates of return computed on the basis of years of study, expenditures for tuition, and foregone income while in training. The investment return to a general internist or family practitioner, however, has been reported to be lower than what he would have obtained by attending an elite business or law school.[32]

Table 6.2 provides information on numbers of individuals involved in the practice of health professions other than medicine and the incomes they earned in 2006. The table clearly indicates that the field of nursing is the largest of the health professions in the United States. In addition, there is significant diversity among nurses. The highest incomes are earned by advanced practice nurses, those with specialized training in fields such as midwifery and anesthetic procedures.

Among the nonphysician health fields, dentists earn the highest incomes, followed by pharmacists and physician assistants. Physician assistants belong to one of several professions that began in the late twentieth century as *physician extenders*—clinicians of considerable skill operating under the supervision of physicians.

Table 6.3 illustrates significant growth among health professions through the late twentieth century. Growth in some fields has been very large. The representation of physicians relative to the U.S. population has grown significantly, approaching 100 percent from 1970 through 2001. The representation of registered nurses (RNs) has more than doubled. Physical therapy, a profession that developed only in the 1960s, grew by over 100 percent between 1980 and 2001 alone. However, the fields of dentistry and pharmacy have grown significantly less. The relative lack of growth in these

TABLE 6.2 Number of U.S. nonphysician health professionals and income, by profession, 2006

Specialty	Number Practicing in U.S.	Average Annual Income
Nursing		
Registered nurse, not otherwise specified	2,201,000	$59,000
Licensed practical nurse[a]	726,000	37,000
Nurse anesthetist	NA	130,000
Certified nurse midwives	8,000	83,000
Other Professions		
Dentistry	168,000	120,000
Pharmacy	196,000	99,000
Occupational therapy	72,000	61,000
Physical therapy	130,000	68,000
Physician assistant	62,000	82,000
Respiration therapy	118,000	56,000
MRI technician	NA	67,000

[a]Includes licensed vocational nurses (LVN).

Sources: Numbers of professionals: *Health, United States, 2005,* Table 108. Incomes: Salary Wizard, available at swz.salary.com. Data on numbers of LPN/LVN, physician assistants, and respiration therapy: USBLS, 2004, www.bls.gov.

TABLE 6.3   **Growth of the health professions, late twentieth century: active personnel per 100,000 population**

Specialty	1970	1980	2000[c]
Physicians	155.7	189.8	274.0[a]
Dentists	46.5	54.0	59.5[b]
Pharmacists	55.2	62.5	69.5[b]
Registered nurses (all)	367.7	560.0	789.1[c]
Occupational therapists	NA	10.9	25.5[b]
Physical therapists	NA	21.8	46.1[a]

[a]Data for year 2001.
[b]Data for year 2000.
[c]Data for year 1999.

Sources: Data for 1980 and 2000: National Center for Health Statistics. *Health, United States, 2006.* Table 108. Hyattsville, MD: National Center for Health Statistics; 2005.
Data for 1970: National Center for Health Workforce Analysis: U.S. health workforce factbook. www .bhpr.hrsa.gov/healthworkforce/reports/factbook.htm.

fields may be attributed in part to technical advances that have reduced tooth decay and made retailing of pharmaceuticals more efficient. Alternatively, it may be speculated that these professions have deliberately restricted their growth to maintain professional dominance and income.

Table 6.4 presents income data for high-ranking health administrators. The job titles included in these tables are those most often found in hospitals. Income data are difficult to obtain in health administration. For this reason, the table presents salaries for top officials at the University of California, San Francisco (UCSF), Medical Center, which are public information. UCSF salaries are high because of the institution's location, but are lower than in some private-sector institutions. It is not uncommon for the CEO of a large health care system to earn an annual income in excess of $1 million.

TABLE 6.4 Compensation for selected executive positions, University of California, San Francisco, Medical Center, 2005 (excluding bonus)

Job Title	Base Salary
Chief executive officer	$434,400
Chief operating officer	355,400
Chief financial officer	309,600
Chief information officer	243,600
Chief patient care services officer	213,200

LABOR FORCE DYNAMICS IN THE HEALTH PROFESSIONS

Supply and compensation constitute basic facts and figures regarding the health care labor force. However, the actual benefit the public may realize from these health care workers depends on factors beyond these basics. These factors, described next, are more complex than simple numbers of human beings involved in a profession. These factors, moreover, are subject to unanticipated change.

Availability of Professionals

The dynamics of professional labor supplies present challenges for both management and policy. From a management point of view, quality health care cannot be delivered without an adequate number and appropriate mix of health professionals. Regarding policy, both scarcity and surplus create undesirable situations. Scarcity drives up prices and reduces access. According to some observers, however, surplus has undesirable economic consequences. Physicians act as consumer agents, ordering tests, prescribing medication, and recommending procedures. The existence of excess physicians, the argument goes, results in excess use of resources mobilized by physicians and acts as a accelerator to health care costs.

Several features of the professional labor force make it difficult to predict its features, even in the relatively short run. Classic economic models illustrate why this is the case. The producer of any commodity whose production requires a span of years can only guess at the price its output will bring when marketed. According to models with names like the **cobweb feedback cycle** or the *hog cycle,* scarcity (accompanied by high price) induces increased production. But the market cannot respond until the period required for production has passed. By that time, increased activity by many producers (responding to initially high prices) creates a surplus, driving prices to exceptionally low levels. Thus, the price of hogs fluctuates over a two- to four-year period.

Marketable hogs may take a couple of years to produce. But nurses require four years of professional education, and physicians twelve. Demand and starting salary (adjusted for inflation) has historically fluctuated over periods of four and twelve years. In addition, the medical environment changes, resulting in staffing cuts in some areas and increases in others. Government programs aggravate the fluctuations by artificially increasing production in response to public perceptions of scarcity.

Production of Services

In addition to the presence of health professionals in the labor force, the number of working hours they supply to the market is significant. Like supply of personnel, the number of hours worked over a week, month, or career affects both access and price. As indicated in the preceding tables, many clinicians are quite highly paid. The **backward-bending labor supply curve** model, depicted in Figure 6.1, suggests that such high pay may actually reduce hours worked. When an individual's hourly compensation reaches a certain point, he may decide to work fewer hours. After their material needs have been met, people make trade-offs between working and earning on one hand, and leisure, family, or other nonmonetary pursuits on the other.

Backward-bending curves such as the one presented in Figure 6.1 may be affecting the health labor force at present. Effects may take a number of forms. The female physician may reduce professional activity to care for children. According to one study,

FIGURE 6.1 *The backward-bending labor supply curve*

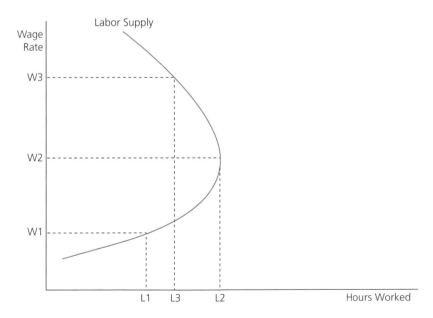

female OB/GYNs worked significantly fewer hours and conducted significantly fewer procedures than their male counterparts, resulting in an overall productivity among women that was approximately 85 percent of that achieved by men.[33] A nurse with the same family and child care responsibility as the female physician may choose to work part-time and thus be less professionally productive. Older health professionals in any field of either gender may choose to retire early. Thus, simple supply of personnel does not assure an adequate supply of services.

Deciding whether a health profession is in surplus or shortage is itself difficult. It may be argued that no surplus exists until all the public's needs are met. Although a shortage of nurses is talked about today, as recently as the 1980s there was evidence that nurses were in surplus. A study in the 1980s predicted that a physician surplus of 80,000 would develop by 1990; the most acute oversupply was predicted to occur among specialists. Conducted under the auspices of a commission known as the Graduate Medical Education National Advisory Committee, this study employed health services researchers of the highest caliber. By the late 1980s, however, it had become apparent that no surplus was developing.[34] At the beginning of the twenty-first century, both professional journals and the mass media had begun to express concern about shortages.[35, 36]

Because it is difficult to determine what the public may actually "need," price may serve as a better indicator of surplus versus shortage. Falling prices indicate the existence of a surplus, while rising prices reflect scarcity. During the early 2000s, prices of nursing services were on the rise, as would be consistent with the existence of a shortage. Prices of physician services themselves were steady or rising (see Table 6.1). This direction of price change suggests a shortage.

Juxtaposition of increasing supply (as measured by doctors and nurses per population) and rising price is an uncommon economic phenomenon. For most commodities, it is impossible for prices to rise while supply relative to demand increases. Additional factors, however, are at work in the medical world. Three explanations should be considered.

First, prices have risen despite increased supply of health professionals because the volume of medical work to be done has also increased. The health care system offers—and the public demands—a broader menu of services with each successive year. Services that seemed highly advanced and prohibitively expensive in the latter decades of the twentieth century are now commonplace. Technological innovation has produced more work for the health care labor force, requiring additional personnel in all fields for fulfillment of the associated tasks. Increasing *intensity of care* and its impact on costs will receive additional attention in Chapter Seven, which focuses on health care finance.

Second, physicians, dentists, and members of several other health professions have a great deal of control over the services that their patients receive. Unless they practice under strict utilization review or other constraints, health professionals tend to recommend or order whatever they believe may help their patients. Sometimes what is recommended has little proven value. Like most people, health professionals tend to act in a fashion that increases their incomes. Thus, at least some may consciously or unconsciously recommend or order interventions for which no compelling, objective justification exists. People in many fields are said to have *target incomes*. A target income is benchmark denoting how much money a person believes she needs to support a desirable standard of living. The uncertainty under which medical decision making often takes place (see Chapter One) increases opportunities for target income–driven behavior.

Finally, the power of the health professions may, through a variety of mechanisms, result in higher prices for care than would prevail if solely natural market forces were in operation. The medical profession is often singled out for fierce protection of its scope of practice. But professions such as nursing and pharmacy have used licensure laws and practice acts to protect their turf from lower-priced competition.

Surplus-Shortage Cycles in Nursing

The case of nursing deserves special attention in view of periodic fluctuation between surplus and shortage. Shortages in the early 2000s caused alarm in the health care industry. Estimates of unfilled hospital nursing positions in that decade reached over 100,000. Industry representatives and hospital officials called for increases in nursing school enrollment and pressed for generous visa allocations to facilitate immigration of nurses from abroad. Hospital-based nurse training programs were begun or expanded, often in collaboration with local educational institutions. Nurses flowed into the United States from countries such as Ireland and the Philippines.

The nursing shortage in the early years of the twenty-first century may have been acute and extended, but it was not a new phenomenon. Nursing has followed a cycle of shortage and surplus periods over the decades. Supply, conditions of work, and public policy have all contributed to the fluctuation.

The nursing shortage of the early 2000s may be partially explained in terms of supply. The opening of new opportunities for women (including medical school) had by that time depleted the traditional source of recruitment into nursing. At the other end of the life cycle, aging and retirement of nurses who had begun careers in the 1950s and 1960s took a toll. Supply issues were aggravated by state-mandated *nursing staff ratios,* requiring that nurses could be assigned to care for no more than a specified number of patients.

Factors related to working conditions in nursing help explain nursing shortages. Bedside nursing is physically and emotionally demanding. Most states do not mandate nurse staffing ratios, and hospitals have responded by increasing the number of patients for whom nurses must care. The greater volume of patient responsibility adds stress to the picture, a potential exaggerated by the fact that nurses may be blamed and disciplined for treatment error. The physical rigors of the profession have been referenced earlier in this chapter.

Low pay in comparison with competing professions, physical and mental stress, and family-related responsibilities have encouraged exit from the nursing profession. In past generations, a high proportion of nurses exited early in their careers. The higher salaries paid to nurses today may be slowing this exit, but the outcome in terms of supply remains uncertain. Replacement of exiting nurses is problematic. Nursing is not an easy-entry occupation. Admission to nursing school is competitive, and many motivated and qualified individuals are unable to attend.

However, supply of nurses does eventually increase as salaries rise. Several factors became apparent in the twenty-first century that seemed likely to accelerate the entry of new personnel or individuals returning to the nursing profession after exiting to start their families. Women, who predominate in the nursing profession, are much more likely to work outside the home for pay than in generations past. Today, a majority of women with children are employed, a revolutionary change from just a few generations ago. Finally, nursing has begun to attract entrants from an entirely new pool of potential entrants, as older women apply to nursing school and replace those who are lost to the profession due to new opportunities in other lines of work.[37]

The Distribution of Physicians: Origins, Ethnicity, and Location

A number of other issues regarding health professionals face managers and policy makers today. One concerns so-called foreign medical graduates (FMGs). The United States requires more physicians than its medical schools produce. To bridge the gap, the United States admits physicians trained by foreign medical schools and makes it possible for them to obtain licenses. FMGs are not always foreign nationals; thousands of U.S. citizens enroll in medical schools in places such as Grenada and Guadalajara. It has been shown that FMGs practice the same specialties and locate in the same places as graduates of U.S. medical schools.

The presence of FMGs raises a number of issues. It is asked whether FMGs are trained as well as graduates of U.S. medical schools. Medical schools, it seems, might be expanded to allow qualified and willing Americans to advance economically and to help fill demonstrated needs. Finally, the U.S. thirst for (and ability to attract) foreign doctors and nurses reduces the supply of such professionals in much more needy countries.

The ethnic distribution of health professionals in the United States raises very difficult issues. Today, some racial and ethnic minorities are represented in medicine in far lower numbers than the proportion they occupy in the general population. The racial and ethnic distribution of medical students today suggests that this picture will not change in the near future. In the period 2002 to 2003, white non-Latinos constituted 64.0 percent of the students and Asians 20.5 percent—both percentages exceeding their representation in the population. African Americans, Latinos, and Native Americans comprised 7.4, 6.4, and .9 percent respectively.

Solutions to this problem are evasive. Americans have found it hard to accept racial quotas for school admissions. An absence of health professionals who are racial minorities may not be effectively addressed at the professional school level. Effective remedies will likely require vast improvements in the elementary education given to minorities, as young people from disadvantaged groups must be able to win entry and succeed in professional training programs.

Another challenging issue concerns where health professionals tend to reside and practice. Geographic maldistribution of health professionals has remained an intractable issue for decades. Physicians in particular tend to shun underserved areas. The highly urbanized state of Massachusetts has 75 percent more physicians per capita than rural North Dakota. Some young physicians practice temporarily in rural areas, sometimes drawn by debt forgiveness programs offered by agencies such as the Indian Health Service, the Migrant Health Service, or the National Health Service Corps. But most are eventually drawn back to the cities, where quality of life is perceived to be higher.

Increasing production of health professionals has not eradicated the problem of geographic location. Testimony before the California state legislature asserted that the state's medical schools needed to produce ten doctors for every one who would practice in an underserved area. The ultimate solution may involve establishing health centers in underserved areas staffed by physician extenders, visited a few days a week by a supervising physician, and receiving advice and supervision at other times via telecommunication.

Finally, it is important to note that a definite pecking order prevails among physicians. The fact that an individual holds a license to practice medicine does not ensure that he delivers top-quality care. Physicians at the top and bottom level of this stratification system tend to practice in mutually isolated communities. Physicians with the best professional reputations hold privileges in the best hospitals and refer patients to each other. Physicians at the lower end of the spectrum often do not have hospital privileges. They are reluctant to refer patients to higher-end specialists for fear of incurring criticism from them.

When patients select a primary care physician, they entrust their care to a specific segment of the health care system, with definite implications for the quality of service they receive. This fact is particularly important because primary care physicians of different rank tend to treat patients of different social background. Some primary care physicians, for example, tend to have practices that include primarily nonminority patients, while the practices of others tend to include largely minorities. A high percentage of minority group members in the United States receive their primary care from physicians who have weak referral networks and lack hospital privileges.[38]

PROFESSIONAL ETHICS, OVERSIGHT, AND DISCIPLINE

Ultimately, the actions and decisions of health professionals determine the benefits, risks, and costs of the health care system to the public. Thus, it is essential that society ensure conduct by health professionals that is in the public interest. Departures from appropriate behavior may be ethical or legal in nature. As noted in Chapter One, ethics concerns obligations of an individual to act toward others in a manner consistent with socially reinforced values. All health professions have codes of ethics that reflect such values. The legal dimension of professional codes of conduct is more concrete. Laws and the actions of persons responsible for their interpretation and enforcement, however, are typically consistent with underlying ethical principles.

Codes of Ethics

Ethical codes formulated by professional organizations tend to be general and abstract. They are useful to practitioners as expressions of the culture of their profession. They may be distant from the practitioner's day-to-day concerns. But they reflect challenges and dilemmas that have repeatedly faced practitioners over the generations.

The AMA and the ANA code of ethics typify codes of patient care professionals.[39, 40] Common to both codes of ethics are provisions mandating that the practitioner do the following:

- Hold the patient's well-being as of primary importance

- Safeguard the confidence and privacy of patients

- Maintain competence through continuing study and communication with colleagues

- Protect the profession through personal conduct and by reporting colleagues who are deficient in character or competence or who engage in fraud or deception

- Respect the law, but seek changes to legal requirements that are not in the best interests of patients

- Advance the nursing profession through collaboration in education and research

Differences between the AMA code and the ANA code reflect concerns specific to each profession. The AMA code, for example, stipulates that "except in emergencies" the physician should be "free to choose whom to serve, with whom to associate, and the environment in which to provide medical care." The American College of Healthcare Executives (ACHE) differs from those of direct service providers and reflects the complexities of health administration. It addresses not only the patient's needs but those of the health care organization. The ACHE code includes provisions such as the following:

- Provide services consistent with available resources

- Lead the organization in the use of sound business practices

- Report negative financial and other information promptly and accurately, and take appropriate action

- Prevent fraud and abuse and aggressive accounting practices that may result in disputable financial reports

- Create an organizational environment in which both clinical and management mistakes are minimized and, when they do occur, are disclosed and addressed effectively [41]

It is important to remember from Chapter Two that ethics involve personal dilemmas. Provisions in the codes of the ANA, AMA, and ACHE provide no specific answers to concrete situations.

Oversight and Discipline

Legal machinery operating on the state level represents a more reliable safeguard for the public than abstract ethical principles. All state governments have **licensing and disciplinary agencies** that oversee the practices of physicians, nurses, chiropractors, and other health professionals. These agencies employ members of each profession as well as law enforcement personnel. They receive, investigate, and help adjudicate complaints from the public. In New York state, for example, the Office of Professional Medical Conduct, a subunit of the Department of Health, is responsible for investigating complaints about physicians and certain physician extenders. In Massachusetts, the Massachusetts Board of Registration holds similar responsibilities.

The Department of Consumer Affairs has jurisdiction over licensing and discipline in California. Specialized bureaus and boards operate within this agency. A unit called the Medical Board of California (MBC) has authority over physicians and several allied health professionals, including opticians, podiatrists, and midwives. In 2007, the unit was responsible for almost 100,000 physicians practicing in California and close to 30,000 additional physicians practicing in other states.[42] MBC's concerns and actions are typical of those in other states.

Reasons for administrative action taken by MBC illustrate the range of challenges and transgressions for which health professionals of any description may be at risk. These include the following:

- *Negligence,* including deviation from standards of medical practice, failure to keep records, and prescribing drugs without performing a physical examination

- *Incompetence,* as indicated by lack of knowledge or skills required for practice or for a particular procedure or specialty

- *Sexual misconduct,* in the form of sexual exploitation of patients or relationships with minors

- *Fraud,* as in invalid billing of private insurance companies or government agencies

- *Unprofessional conduct,* as in performing unnecessary tests and using inappropriate billing codes

- *Conviction of a crime,* whether related or unrelated to professional practice

In addition, MBC may take administrative action in response to finding that a health professional is mentally ill, is a drug or alcohol abuser, or has a medical condition affecting her ability to practice safely.

In response to these findings, MBC may apply a wide range of remedies. In the mildest of remedies, MBC can issue a public letter of reprimand. The board may suspend a license. In rare cases, a license is simply revoked. More often, the revocation is stayed, and the practitioner receives restrictions on his right to practice and stipulations to be followed until the period of probation ends. These stipulations may include performance of community service and receiving education in areas such as ethics, professional boundaries, record keeping, or practice skills. Conditions of probation may include refraining from using alcohol or working under the surveillance of a monitor.

Like many of its counterparts outside California, MBC operates a diversion program for impaired physicians. Under this program, the board allows the physician to continue practice under appropriate restrictions while undergoing treatment for alcohol abuse, drug use, or mental or behavioral problems. Many disciplinary bodies in the health field believe that remedial action is preferable to simple punishment.

Research suggests that remedial action is sometimes, though not always, effective. A study in Massachusetts reports that physicians who begin treatment for mental and behavioral health and substance abuse complete their programs about 75 percent of the time.[43] Another national study of physicians disciplined by state agencies, however, reports high rates of recidivism.[44] Critics have alleged that the percentage of physicians whose licenses are revoked is unrealistically low. The public, however, has recourse beyond state licensing and disciplinary boards, including malpractice suits. In addition, health professionals in any field who break the law are subject to criminal penalties.

Star Performers

Whatever the dynamics of the medical labor market may be, individuals of outstanding reputations can command extraordinary incomes and the envy of colleagues. Following are two late twentieth century examples.

J. Richard Steadman, MD. Steadman's office in the ski destination town of Vail, Colorado, is lined with testimonials from former patients, including quarterback Dan Marino, skier Marc Giardelli, and tennis star Martina Navratilova. At a time when Blue Cross paid $2,600 for repair of a common injury, a tear in the anterior cruciate ligament, he charged $5,000. In a practice that grossed $3.5 million in 1993, Steadman was in the top 1 percent of U.S. physicians in income. Steadman's net income in subsequent years was not made public, although he received additional fees as a director of ReGen Biologics, Inc.

Highly paid athletes and corporate executives flock to Steadman's clinic. But managed care plans and workers' compensation pay less than Steadman charges. People covered in this manner must make up the difference or seek treatment elsewhere.

Steadman maintains that the value he provides justifies his premium fees. He does far more surgery than the average in his field and has pioneered several surgical procedures and materials.

To a *Wall Street Journal* reporter, Steadman bristled at the suggestion that his rates might be too high, asking: "If you can do something faster and better than most people, shouldn't you be compensated for it? To me, it would be a shame if the system rewarded mediocrity."[45]

Jack O. Bovender, Jr., CEO. On multiple occasions, Bovender served as chairman and CEO of HCA, a Nashville-based corporate provider of health services, which provides about 5 percent of hospital services in the United States. Bovender received a master's degree in health care administration from Duke University in 1967, performed hospital administrative functions in the U.S. Navy, and worked his way through the ranks of HCA between 1985 and 1992. He left the company after a major merger, but returned in 1999 as a member of the board of directors.

Bovender's contributions have included determining which corporate assets to keep or sell, and leading the company as it transformed from a publicly trade to a privately held firm. He also represents the company in efforts to promote health care reform. Discounts for uninsured people and bad debts cost the company $5 billion in 2006.[46]

In 2006, HCA paid Bovender $3.74 million in salary and other compensation. These earnings placed him behind Wellpoint's CEO, who was paid $10.6 million in 2006, and distant from America's best-paid CEO, Richard Fairbank of Capital One Financial, who received $249.4 million in cash, stock, and other forms or remuneration.[47]

KEY TERMS

Professionalism	Advanced practice nursing
Corporate practice of medicine	Cobweb feedback cycle
Allopathic medicine	Backward-bending labor supply curve
Flexner Report	Licensing and disciplinary agencies

SUMMARY

This chapter presents key features of the health care labor force—including numbers, compensation, and distribution—and raises associated issues for management and policy.

In 2007, health care personnel represented over 10 percent of the U.S. labor force. Since the middle of the twentieth century, striking increases have occurred in the number of individuals in nearly all the health professions. Entirely new health care specialties emerged during that era.

Most members of the health care labor force may be characterized as professionals. Workers of this description possess specialized knowledge not shared by others. Professionals form independent organizations, seek freedom from supervision by nonprofessionals, formulate codes of ethics conduct, and pursue legal licensure. Professionalism protects the public from unqualified and unscrupulous practitioners, but creates challenges for cost control and management.

The American public depends on appropriate supply, utilization, and distribution of health care personnel. Concerns have arisen about both undersupply and oversupply of health care workers. Geographic maldistribution threatens public access, as physicians tend to practice in well-to-do urban communities and avoid disadvantaged and rural areas. Minority group members are strongly underrepresented in the health professionals.

Health care has provided desirable jobs for millions of Americans. According to some, however, an overabundance of health professionals increases costs without commensurate public benefit.

DISCUSSION QUESTIONS

1. Would licensing of health care administrators result in better public service?

2. If a young person asked you about career prospects in the health care field, what answer would you give? What health profession or specialty would you recommend?

3. How effective do you believe codes of ethics and the mechanisms that guide professional discipline are at present? Can you recommend means of improvement?

4. Should policy makers be taking steps in addition to those already in operation to increase the representation of racial minorities in medicine and other health professions?

5. What might the consequences be if the number of physicians per 100,000 residents in the United States were to increase by 50 percent? Overall, would such an increase be beneficial or detrimental to the interests of consumers?

6. What strategies can management use to promote optimal relationships with health professionals?

7. On balance, does "professionalism" as defined in this chapter benefit or harm the public?

8. Should nonallopathic health care be covered by private and public health plans?

CHAPTER

7

HEALTH CARE EXPENDITURES, FINANCING, AND INSURANCE

LEARNING OBJECTIVES

- To know where funds for health care in the United States come from and how they are expended
- To understand why U.S. health care costs are high and increasing
- To become familiar with health insurance practices and products
- To become conversant with Medicare and Medicaid
- To understand the economic rationale of managed care
- To learn about the problem of unsponsored care and associated issues
- To attain an overview of policy issues related to health care spending, financing, and insurance

HEALTH SERVICE FUNDING AND EXPENDITURES

A review of basic numbers presented in Chapter One highlights the financial importance of health care in the United States. Annual health care expenditures in the United States topped $2 trillion by late in the twenty-first century's first decade. Per capita health care spending was almost $7,000 in 2005, up from a mere $148 in 1960. Between 1960 and 2005, the percentage of U.S. gross domestic product (GDP) devoted to health care increased from 5.1 to 16.[1] Several European democracies experienced comparable or higher rates of increase during the same approximate period of time. Between 1960 and 2004, for example, the GDP share occupied by health care in Spain went from 1.5 to 8.4 and in Norway from 2.9 to 9.7.[2] But the United States has long spent the highest percentage of GDP on health care in the world. In almost every year, growth in per capita health care costs has outstripped general inflation in the United States.

The mechanisms by which health care is paid for in the United States have a major impact on associated costs. The vast majority of health care dollars changing hands in the United States do so through so-called *third parties* or *third-party payers.* **Third-party payers** disperse funds on behalf of the patient (the first party) to the health professional (the second party). Private insurance companies once predominated among third-party payers in the United States. Third-party payers, however, also include the public agencies that operate programs such as Medicare, Medicaid, the Indian Health Service, and the Civilian Health and Medical Program of the Uniformed Services (CHAMPUS). The amount of money paid for health care under these and related programs is now more than the amount paid by private insurance. In 2006, private health insurance paid 36.0 percent of costs for health care in the United States, government-sponsored insurance 45.3 percent, and out-of-pocket payments by consumers 14.6 percent.[3]

A majority of the dollars spent for health care in 2006 were paid to hospitals and physicians. Of every dollar expended on health in the United States in that year, 36.8 cents went for hospital care, 25.4 cents for physician services, 7.1 cents for nursing home care, 12.3 cents for prescription drugs, and 18.4 percent for a wide variety of other goods and services.[4] These percentages are graphically displayed in Figure 7.1.

Costs are unevenly distributed across the population. Of course, sick people utilize more health care resources than people who are well. It is no surprise, then, that costs are concentrated among a relatively small segment of the population.

Demographics and location also make a difference. In 2000, it was estimated that average Americans would spend $316,579 each in their lifetime. Women were expected to spend 34 percent more than men ($361,192 versus $268,697), due to the fact that women were expected to live six more years than men in 2000. Annual expenditures varied greatly by age. Of the lifetime expenditure expected of Americans, 7.8 percent were estimated to be spent by (or on behalf of) children (ages 0–19), 12.5 percent by young adults (20–39), 31.0 percent by middle-aged adults (40–64), 36.5 percent by seniors (65–84), and 12.1 percent by "old" seniors (85 or older).[5] Studies have consistently found that individuals in their last year of life are more expensive to the system than similarly aged individuals who survive.[6] For reasons that are not entirely

FIGURE 7.1 *Personal health care expenditures according to source of funds and type of expenditures, United States, 2006*

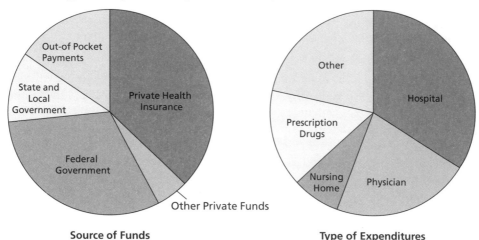

Source: Centers for Medicare and Medicaid Services, Office of the Actuary, National Health Accounts.

understood, location has a significant effect on costs. In their last six months of life, patients in Miami, Florida, are treated more intensively and expensively than anywhere else in the world.[7]

The astounding volume of resources expended for health care summarized here raises two interrelated questions. First, why have health care costs increased significantly in all industrialized democracies across the globe? Second, why does the United States spend more than other countries?

HEALTH CARE COSTS: A GLOBAL ISSUE

Several factors contribute to rising health care costs in all economically developed countries. First, economic prosperity itself leads to greater per capita health care spending.[8] As national economies grew in the latter half of the twentieth century, so did expenditures for health care. Second, groups with the strongest interests in health care spending tend to be among the most politically powerful in wealthy democracies. In the United States and elsewhere, powerful interest groups that favor health care spending include elders and providers of health services.

Growth in the intensity of treatment for individual complaints has occurred in the United States and other economically advanced countries. Changes in treatment for heart disease illustrate the growth in intensity and implications for costs:

Treatment has been transformed from one week of bed rest in the coronary care unit—with pharmacologic interventions to control cardiogenic shock, pulmonary

edema, and arrhythmias—to thrombolytic therapy, angiography, angioplasty, or coronary bypass surgery. The innovations require more capital (cardiac catheterization laboratories), more labor (the time of physicians, nurses, and other caregivers), and more expenses associated with spread of knowledge (fellowships in interventional cardiology)—all of which cost money that was not spent thirty years ago.[9]

New technology often involves more intensive treatment than was delivered before it became available. Joint replacement and organ transplant represent breakthrough therapies. Prior to their availability, treatment for severe joint disease and liver failure may have been limited to palliative measures. The newly available surgical procedures require personnel and facilities similar in magnitude to cardiac catheterization and coronary artery bypass. Pharmaceutical innovations do not require large increases in personnel and facilities, but add to costs nevertheless.

Increasing intensity of patient care, often involving increased advanced technology, is a worldwide trend. A close look at factors responsible for increasing costs in the United States illustrates the impact of intensity and technology. Except during periods of high inflation in the economy as a whole, increased intensity of patient care played the leading role in making health care costs higher. Between 2000 and 2005, for example, the average annual increase in personal health expenditures in the United States was 7.8 percent. According to U.S. government data, general inflation in the economy accounted for 32 percent of the increase. Inflation in the health care sector

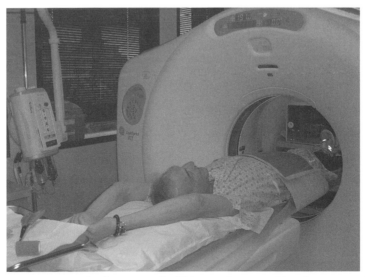

Patient receiving a computerized tomography (CT) scan. Once considered too expensive for general use, CT scanning is now a routine medical procedure. CT scanning is one example of the adoption of new technology driving up costs.

as a whole (based on prices of selected goods and services) accounted for 18 percent of the increase, and population growth another 13 percent. Increasing intensity of services was responsible for 38 percent of the increase.[10]

Another perspective on health care cost increases is provided by an analysis of hospital charges during a particularly expansive period of U.S. health care. Between 1965 and 1975, total hospital charges in the United States grew an astounding 382 percent from $9 billion to $39 billion. General inflation accounted for 36 percent of this increase, population growth 5 percent, aging of the population 7 percent, labor 24 percent, and capital 28 percent. Capital includes the cost of new construction (including costs of financing) and acquisition of equipment.[11]

The contributions of new technology and increasing intensity to the cost of care may be most apparent in the United States. But public expectations regarding access to care, often involving technology and intensity, are also important abroad. Sweden, the United Kingdom, the Netherlands, and New Zealand have set priorities and maintained waiting lists for services involving expensive, high-technology services. Yet public opinion in these countries often opposes explicit restriction. Public opposition is particularly visible in individual cases where denial of access is apparently responsible for loss of life.[12]

COST ACCELERATORS IN THE UNITED STATES

Although increasing health care costs are a phenomenon affecting the entire industrialized world, the United States clearly leads the trend. Researchers and commentators have identified a variety of potential explanations for the high costs that prevail in the United States. Illustrations of these appear below, some backed by strong evidence, others enjoying less factual support.

Values and Expectations

The values and expectations of Americans help explain why the United States spends more per capita on health care than other industrialized countries. As discussed in Chapter Two, maximization is an important American value. According to some measures, Americans have higher expectations than people elsewhere.

A study of service for urgent coronary artery bypass in the United States, Canada, and several European countries provides an example. This study reported that 20.3 percent of U.S. non-VA patients waited longer than twenty-four hours for urgent coronary artery bypass, the maximum delay period recommended by relevant specialists. Among patients in the United Kingdom, 88.9 percent waited longer than the recommended maximum, 80.0 percent in Canada, and 45.5 percent in Sweden. As a possible explanation, the study authors cite limited hospital budgets that "preclude immediate access to their facilities for expensive procedures such as cardiac catheterization or coronary artery bypass surgery or both."[13]

The longer wait times experienced outside the United States for cardiac procedures may signify more economical health care systems abroad. But the longer wait times place at least some patients in peril. Delay in coronary artery bypass surgery has been shown to increase mortality risk.[14]

Consistent with unacceptability of long waits for service among Americans is demand for access to new technology. Commentators such as Henry Aaron (see Chapter Two) have highlighted the diminishing gains in health obtainable from increasingly expensive innovations. Remedies for cost accelerators of this kind include empowering government to restrict deployment of new technology, a process known as **upstream resources allocation.** Americans, however, have hesitated to approve such measures.

The Prevalence of Health Insurance

The existence of insurance itself as the principal means of paying health care bills appears to play a part in the rising cost of health care in the United States. Health insurance puts purchasing power into people's pockets over and above what they could afford to buy with cash. All things being equal, prices of goods and services ultimately rise to the level that consumers are willing and able to pay. Insurance coverage adds purchasing power to the consumer cash supply. Prices should be expected to rise to the level made possible by the insured person's coverage *plus* the amount of cash she has available—and is willing to pay. An increase in the supply of medical goods and services, of course, may be expected to restrain price increases, as long as a free market actually prevails.

Some evidence suggests that health insurance has in fact increased the cost of health care. Enactment of Medicare in the 1960s created a vast new pool of purchasing power available to elders. A period of increased health care cost inflation characterized as a "firestorm" by a California lobbyist occurred in the years that followed. In the five years prior to Medicare's enactment, yearly health care expenditures in the United States had been increasing by 8.3 percent; in the five years after the program became operational, expenditures increased by 12.7 percent per annum. Three decades later, evidence suggests that expansion of Medicare benefits to cover pharmaceuticals had a similar effect. Inclusion of the pharmaceutical benefit coincided with large out-of-pocket payments by beneficiaries.[15]

The widespread practice by U.S. employers of providing health insurance as a benefit to employees has been cited as an accelerator of health care costs. Although such benefits have substantial cash value, they have not historically been subject to taxation. Much income that would be obtained from taxation of employee health benefits is forgone by the U.S. Treasury because employers deduct these dollars from their taxable income in the same manner as other business expenses. A number of analysts have argued that businesses should not be allowed to deduct health plan expenses or that employees should pay taxes on the benefits they receive.[16] According to these analysts, such tax changes would motivate both employers and employees to seek cheaper plans.

Consumption by the Disadvantaged

Other factors thought to be responsible for relatively high health care costs in the United States involve history and demographics. America's era of enslaving African Americans and displacing Native Americans has resulted in persistence of an economic underclass to the present. Millions of African Americans and Native Americans are born into poverty and remain there for their entire lives. Members of these groups usually receive substandard education. Many are consistently exposed to bigotry, adverse living conditions, and the threat of violence. These challenges contribute to poor health literacy, inadequate access to preventive resources (such as well adult care and healthful recreation), adverse health behavior, premature childbirth, and injury due to violence.

Costs associated with premature and low birthweight deliveries exemplify the economic impact of underclass membership on health. Economically disadvantaged African American women are at special risk for delivering prematurely. At great expense, medical technology has made it possible for many low birthweight infants to survive the perinatal period. Survivors are often later plagued with chronic disease, adversely affecting their quality of life and requiring expenditures for health care far beyond those of normal children.[17]

Aging Population

As noted earlier, older people have higher per capita health care costs than younger ones. In addition, elders are increasing as a proportion of the U.S. population. But the degree to which excessive health care costs can be attributed to an aging population is uncertain. The proportion of the population in every industrialized country represented by elders is increasing—often more rapidly than in the United States.

The U.S. population is indeed aging. But the rate at which the group of people sixty-five years and older is increasing as a percentage of the population is actually slow. Per capita spending for the elderly, moreover, is increasing less rapidly than per capita spending for the nonelderly. In a comprehensive review of current data, the noted economist Uwe Reinhardt concludes that the aging of the U.S. population will add "only about half a percentage point to the total annual increase in national health spending" in the coming years.[18]

Immigration

Some have attributed rising health care expenditures in part to immigration. In the late twentieth century, immigration into the United States (both legal and illegal) increased significantly. Undocumented immigrants are not eligible for most public insurance programs (such as Medicaid) except under emergency conditions. These individuals often seek care at emergency and maternity facilities and frequently lack personal resources for payment.

Facilities at which large numbers of undocumented immigrants seek care indeed face fiscal challenges. As a group, however, undocumented immigrants do not add significantly to the system's expenditures. According to an analysis published in 2006, the foreign-born, especially the undocumented, "use disproportionately fewer medical services and contribute less to health care costs in relation to their population share." Immigrants tend to be relatively healthy, and their frequent lack of health insurance decreases the volume of services they use. The study concludes that "the national medical costs of nonelderly undocumented immigrants are about $6.5 billion, and the publicly financed component is slightly larger than $1 billion—a small fraction of total U.S. health care costs."[19]

Administrative Costs

Finally, some of the blame for high costs has been attributed to the large number of administrative personnel involved in the health care system. Administrative personnel in health care organizations and the insurance industry cost money, but do not contribute directly to patient care. Based on 1999 data, researchers Steffie Woolhandler, Terry Campbell, and David Himmelstein argued that over $200 billion could have been saved if the United States had had a simpler, government-financed system such as Canada's.[20] Others have argued that administrative costs in the United States are actually closer to those of Canada.[21] Even by more conservative standards, however, administrative expenses in 1999 may have accounted for between 10 and 15 percent of U.S. health care spending. Administration of the decentralized, pluralistic U.S. health care system indeed increases costs. But the excess costs of health care in the United States compared with those observed elsewhere arise primarily from factors other than administration.

HEALTH INSURANCE

Only the existence of health insurance permits Americans to consume their present volume of health care. It is easy to think of insurance as a lackluster industry, peopled by clerks, bean counters, and bland sales personnel. But for many, availability of health insurance is a matter of life or death. The specifics of a person's insurance policy can do much to determine whether he maintains a desirable quality of life. Understanding the U.S. health insurance system is the key to grasping management and policy challenges that have prevailed for decades.

Insurance fundamentally amounts to a pooling of funds from many individuals to provide financial resources to those who experience a loss due to an unusual occurrence. In principle, health insurance differs from accident or life insurance only in the specific "unusual occurrence" for which the individual is insured—financial liability due to health care needs.

The health insurance industry illustrates the pluralism and lack of systematic integration that characterizes U.S. health care. A wide variety and huge number of non-profit and for-profit organizations offer health insurance of some kind. Organizations that have traditionally been nonprofit such as Blue Cross and Blue Shield have occupied a major segment of the health insurance business. In addition, hundreds of profit-seeking firms known as *commercial carriers* offer health insurance. Many commercial carriers are active in several lines of insurance. Publicly traded firms such as Aetna and Cigna are owned by stockholders, who receive dividends based on corporate profits. Other carriers, known as *mutual insurance companies,* have no stockholders. When these firms accumulate resources greater than their needs, the difference—which can be thought of as profit—is distributed to policy holders as rebates.

A large majority of Americans have health insurance. Table 7.1 shows the distribution of sources from which this insurance is obtained by individuals under sixty-five years of age. A majority of these individuals get health insurance through employment,

TABLE 7.1 **Percentages of individuals under age sixty-five with selected sources of health insurance**

	Year		
	1994	**2000**	**2007**
Employer-based coverage	64.4	68.4	62.2
Own name	33.2	34.6	32.1
Dependent coverage	31.3	33.8	30.0
Individually purchased	7.5	6.5	6.8
Public	17.1	14.6	18.2
Medicare[a]	1.6	2.2	2.7
Medicaid	12.7	10.7	13.9
Tricare/CHAMPUS/VA	3.8	2.8	2.9
No health insurance	15.9	15.6	17.2

[a]Although most Medicare beneficiaries are elderly, selected groups, such as end-stage renal disease patients, may qualify for the program at any age.

Source: Employee Benefit Research Institute. Sources of health insurance and characteristics of the uninsured: analysis of the March 2008 current population survey. *EBRI Issue Brief.* 2008;(321):1–33.

either their own or that of a family member. A comparatively small number purchase insurance on an individual basis.

Government provides financing for health services that in some respects resembles insurance. Medicare, for example, serves primarily elderly people. The program is funded by payroll taxes used to create a dedicated trust fund. Most Medicare beneficiaries have contributed to this fund during their years as working people. Medicaid, a program for the poor, is supported by taxation of individuals who may themselves lose their ability to pay for health care through private insurance or other personal resources. Consistent with long-term trends, Table 7.1 indicates a decline in private coverage (including employer-based and individually purchased) and an increase in government-operated programs.

Despite the importance of insurance, plans often do not cover the full range of consumers' needs or desires. Pharmaceuticals and devices often require out-of-pocket resources. Coverage for mental health tends to be severely limited. Consumers pay billions of dollars for unconventional medicine (see Chapter Four). Increasingly popular and not usually covered by insurance have been discretionary procedures ranging from cosmetic dentistry to modification of physical features such eyes, noses, lips, bellies, and buttocks.

Health Care and the Theory of Insurance

Insurance has existed as an industry for hundreds of years. Until the years following World War II, however, its availability and popularity was limited. Insurance today serves as the principal mechanism by which health care is funded in the United States. Differences among the traditional forms of insurance—property, casualty, and life—raise questions about the soundness and ultimate viability of this arrangement.

The purchase of insurance allows individuals to make claims on a pool of funds when they experience an unexpected loss. As do payments for repairs following accidents and fires, doctor and hospital bills represent losses that can be expressed in monetary terms. A *theory of insurance* established by Robert L. Mehr and Emerson Commack specifies the conditions under which an insurance plan may provide financial protection to members in a reliable and sustainable manner.[22] The most important of elements of the theory concern the events and losses that it is practical to insure. According to Mehr and Commack, insurable losses are restricted to the following types:

- *Definite.* The event that gives rise to the loss should take place at a known time, in a known place, and from a known cause, as in the case of fire, automobile accidents, and worker injuries.

- *Accidental.* The event should be outside the control of the beneficiary of the insurance. The loss cannot be a result of action that might have, under difference circumstances, produced gain. Ordinary business risks, for example, are not insurable.

- *Large.* The size of the loss must be of major proportion. The administrative and overhead costs incurred by an insurance company in coverage of small losses are proportionally larger than those incurred in coverage of large losses. Insurance against small losses requires a company to charge higher premiums that offer little real value to a buyer.

■ *Calculable.* The insurance company must be able to estimate the likelihood that an adverse event will occur and make an objective evaluation of the financial loss associated with the event.

■ *Affordable to the insurer.* Maintaining sufficient funds to pay claims is a fundamental challenge of insurers. In writing policies, insurers try to protect their assets by avoiding the possibility of very large claims by individual participants or simultaneous claims by many beneficiaries. This is why insurance companies hesitate to offer hurricane insurance in Florida and earthquake insurance in California, or charge high prices for these policies.

By insuring only losses with the characteristics listed above, an insurer may serve the public for many years in a reliable manner. Shipwrecks and automobile accidents clearly meet the criteria of insurability. Disparities between these criteria and key characteristics of health care, however, help explain why financing of health care in the United States has become problematic.

Health Insurance Challenges

Insurance of health care does make sense according to some dimensions of the theory of insurance. Definite diagnosis can be made of most, if not all, diseases. Occurrence of much disease, and certainly its timing and severity, is outside the control of individuals.

Predominantly Small Claims. According to some criteria, however, funding of health care through insurance appears practical and sustainable to only a limited degree. The theory of insurance states that losses must be large to be insurable. Many consumer expenditures for health care, however, are small. For most consumers, doctor visits and limited-time prescriptions resemble nuisance expenses much more than catastrophic ones.

Relatively small expenditures for health, moreover, are regularly made by numerous consumers. Under the theory of insurance, events covered by a plan should be not only costly but infrequent. Insurance against shipwrecks, storms, and fires provides resources to help individuals who encounter such rarely occurring occurrences to recapitalize or rebuild. Coverage of routine, expectable losses (as much health care utilization involves) raises cost of insurance far beyond what it would be if only rare, costly events were covered.

Incalculable Risks. From an insurer's point of view, health care expenditures are less calculable than losses in the property and casualty field. Unanticipated increases in the cost of care due to newly available technology occur regularly. Insurance plans may limit the services that are covered and specify caps on their financial liability to individual consumers. But entities providing health care coverage have less power to limit their liabilities through these means than in more traditional insurance. Refusal to cover a newly proven intervention, even if outside existing policies, can result in legal or public relations challenges.

Unfavorable Risk Pools. Another challenge to the funding of health care through insurance involves construction and management of *risk pools*. A risk pool is the technical term for the set of individuals whose financial contributions or *premiums* are added together and made available for use by those who incur a loss. To be financially sustainable, an insurance company requires a risk pool in which the presence of people at high and low risk is balanced. In a risk pool of this nature, the financial needs of those who get sick will be offset by the lack of need among those who stay well. Such a balance enables the insurance company to offer attractive premium rates to the public.

A *large* risk pool is desirable from both the insurer's and consumer's perspective. Health care experts have developed models that allow insurers to anticipate the needs of an individual based on her age, health status, and past use of services.[23] But the accuracy of these models is limited. Among individuals, random variation in incidence of disease or injury is likely to prevail. The larger the risk pool, however, the more likely it is that balance will occur in any given year.

Large pools balancing high- and low-risk individuals are clearly the most desirable for many insurance carriers and consumers. Such risk pools are necessary for health insurance to serve as the predominant funding mechanism for health care in any country. But market dynamics do not favor construction of such pools. High-risk members raise costs for the pool in its totality. Individuals at low risk and companies providing insurance plans for employees avoid buying into such pools. Most private insurance carriers operate under business models that avoid sales to high-risk people. High-risk pools, then, are typically mandated, operated, or subsidized by government agencies. Medicare itself is a large pool containing many individuals at high risk of incurring significant medical expenses.

Insurance carriers seek to capture large, favorable risk pools by selling plans to large employers. Employed individuals are relatively young, healthy people. A large employer, then, furnishes a risk pool ready-made with the most desirable characteristics. Insurers must accept greater risk when they operate smaller pools. Such pools may be constructed by putting together packages of individual policies or contracts with small business firms. In the absence of large numbers to balance random fluctuations in claims, insurance companies must charge high premiums to offset their risks. The cost of joining a small insurance pool helps explain why relatively few people in the United States obtain insurance on an individual basis and why small businesses often do not offer plans to their employees.

Adverse Selection and Moral Hazard. Health insurance shares a number of challenges with the traditional insurance industry. Of special note are *adverse selection* and *moral hazard*. Some evidence suggests that the nature of health risks and health care make adverse selection and moral hazard even more troublesome than they have traditionally been.

Adverse selection occurs when the people especially likely to incur a loss obtain insurance against that loss. In the broader insurance industry, the term is sometimes used in connection with concealment of facts by the person seeking insurance about his risks. A life insurance seeker, for example, may be able to conceal a family history of heart disease. If successful, this individual represents an adverse element in the risk pool.

In health care, the term adverse selection is often used to denote attraction by people at especially high risk to a particular plan. Insurance against burglary in a hypothetical city illustrates the process. A person who has never been the victim of burglary is unlikely to include insurance against such a misfortune among her unavoidable purchases. But a person who has experienced repeated burglaries is likely to show great interest. Eager purchasers of burglary insurance may be more likely to expose themselves to burglary by not locking their doors and windows, living in houses not readily seen from the street, or residing in neighborhoods frequented by felons. All things being equal, the greater the representation of these "adverse" individuals in the burglary insurance pool, the greater the premiums for everyone will have to be.

Adverse selection of consumers into health insurance plans is widely feared by plan operators. People who anticipate the need for repeated and extensive health services are not always adverse risks. They may be intelligently prudent. They may be hypochondriacs. But they often are people with genuine health risks. Examples include those with preexisting conditions or high-risk lifestyles. Health plans may try to bar such individuals from the pool, but cannot always do so. It is feared that predictably high-volume users will have substantial claims. Individuals of this description, it has been said, gravitate to plans with generous benefits and managed care arrangements that place no fixed dollar limit on benefits.

Insurance plans of any kind introduce the possibility of moral hazard into the consumer's thinking and behavior. Moral hazard involves people's temptation to incur a loss when they know they will receive payment for that loss. A worker, for example, may intentionally expose herself to injury in hopes of receiving a workers' compensation payment. Health insurance does not increase the likelihood of intentional injury by the insured. People with health insurance, however, are said to consume unnecessary care because they know that a third party will cover the associated expenses.[24] This possibility is particularly important in instances involving high-cost interventions of infrequent efficacy or unproven value.

Of perhaps greater importance is moral hazard among physicians. Physicians are exposed to moral hazard when they have the opportunity to profit by providing care of speculative or marginal value. Moral hazard is also present when physicians are able to choose between profit-yielding high-cost interventions and cheaper treatments resulting in lower financial returns. Use of certain chemotherapies provides a historical example. Until Medicare and private insurance companies restricted the practice, oncologists purchased chemotherapeutic agents directly from the manufacturer and charged patients significantly more for the agents than they had paid.[25] Insurance promotes moral hazard among physicians because patients with coverage are unlikely to question costs.

Expectable Losses. According to the traditional theory of insurance, it would make most sense for the health insurance industry to offer coverage primarily against *catastrophic* health care costs. Under such plans, only very high financial losses could be recovered. As recently as the 1950s, many U.S. families purchased "major medical" insurance, protecting themselves against financially disastrous misfortunes. But since that time, benefits under most policies have become increasingly broad. Most health insurance policies today cover everyday needs such as well adult exams and prenatal care. Many cover selected complementary and alternative services such as chiropractic and incidentals such as eyeglasses. Catastrophic plans, however, are making a limited comeback, as will be discussed later in this chapter.

Because regular and numerous losses are expectable, it is far from certain that insurance as it has traditionally operated can continue to serve as the predominant mechanism for funding health care in the United States. Virtually everyone will eventually encounter health problems and associated costs. All are at risk of misfortunes that cannot be accurately predicted. One might argue, then, that health care should be paid for from a pool of resources upon which everyone may potentially draw and to which all who are able contribute. In its National Health Service, the United Kingdom attempts to operate a risk pool that includes all citizens.[26] But values such as personal choice, meritocracy, and the free market inhibit development of such a system in the United States. Strongly vested industry interests, moreover, make it unlikely that health insurance as it now exists in the United States will fundamentally change in the near future.

Intense Regulation. Like other parts of the insurance business, health insurance in the United States is subject to regulation on the state level. State agencies grant insurance companies the privilege of doing business within state borders. State regulations specify how (and at what level) insurance companies set their rates. They determine the level of reserves insurance companies must maintain and how these reserves may be invested. It is not surprising that insurance company and interest group lobbyists are among the most important in state and national politics.

Evolution of Health Insurance in the United States

Health insurance as it actually exists in the United States has evolved over a period of over eighty years. Early pioneers in health insurance could not have predicted the direction taken by the evolution of health insurance. The manner in which the insurance industry has developed raises issues for consumers and for policy makers.

Private Health Insurance. Like many features of the U.S. health care system, health insurance is a historically recent development. Odin Anderson, an early heath services researcher, had an opportunity in the 1970s to interview participants in a movement that had given birth to health insurance in the United States forty years earlier. He also had the opportunity to review records of the Blue Cross plans that provided an important model for health insurance as it became part of everyday life.

According to Anderson, the earliest forms of health insurance in the United States were probably plans instituted by business operators for workers in remote locations such as lumber camps and railroad installations.[27] These were followed in the second decade of the twentieth century by efforts in several states to institute compulsory health insurance systems. The industrial practices did not spread to mainstream America, though, and the state movements never gathered sufficient support to achieve success.

The successful model that eventually became Blue Cross began as a plan that allowed consumers to prepay for services at individual hospitals. Around 1930, such plans existed in several U.S. cities. The most famous involved an arrangement initiated in 1929 between Baylor University Hospital and public school teachers in Dallas, Texas. Under this arrangement, the teachers paid fifty cents a month to the university hospital. Though seemingly low by today's standards, this premium represented a generous payment to the hospital. According to records of previous hospitalization experience, the teachers had incurred an average of fifteen cents a month in hospital bills.

Word of the Dallas plan spread to other communities through the American Hospital Association and other professional forums. County-level plans were established involving relationships with multiple hospitals; statewide plans followed, including most, if not all, of the hospitals in the individual states. Supported by dues from the local plans, a national agency was established within the American Hospital Association to support and coordinate the local plans. Among the agency's key activities was lobbying for passage of laws favorable to Blue Cross plans on the state level. Under this legislation, Blue Cross plans were considered community benefit corporations, relieved from some of the regulatory requirements of for-profit insurance companies and from tax liability. The name Blue Cross and the famed Blue Cross logo, first used in 1934 to designate nonprofit hospitalization plans, became the property of the American Hospital Association.

During the 1940s, Blue Cross plans began adding physician service benefits. Physicians themselves, under the auspices of state medical societies, developed Blue Shield plans to cover payment of professional fees. In some localities, Blue Cross and Blue Shield plans competed with each other. In other locales, Blue Cross and Blue Shield plans collaborated, with Blue Cross providing resources to help Blue Shield plans establish themselves and sharing administrative facilities with them.

Inspired by the success of the Blue Cross movement, commercial carriers entered the field of health insurance in the 1940s. These companies had several advantages over Blue Cross in the ensuing competition. Of greatest ultimate importance, the commercial carriers did not share the Blue Cross tradition of setting fees via *community rating*. Under community rating, Blue Cross plans set rates for *unitary risk pools* defined by the geographic boundaries of their service areas. Under such an arrangement, all participants in the geographical area pay approximately the same rate. Rate setting for a pool of this kind ignores variations in risk of illness (and associated financial requirements) among individuals. Of course, risk among individuals varies considerably, as illustrated in Chapter Four. The Blue Cross tradition, however, emphasized a public service ethic under which plans strove for wide accessibility.

In contrast, the commercial carriers used a system of *experience rating.* Under this system, insurance companies identified groups (chiefly employers) composed primarily of younger, relatively healthy employees as business prospects. Because these groups required less care (and hence less expense) than the population at large, the commercial carriers were able to offer them plans at relatively low rates. To remain competitive, Blue Cross was forced to abandon its traditions and accept experience rating.

In the decades that followed, most insured people held conventional indemnity policies. Consistent with traditional insurance, **indemnity policies** in health care allow consumers to obtain services from any provider available and receive reimbursement for associated expenses. During this era, care was typically delivered on a fee-for-service basis, according to which providers billed patients separately for each episode of care. Promoted by an expanding economy and increasingly generous union contracts, health plans came to include coverage of an increasing range of services.

Under the typical indemnity plan, insurance paid 80 percent of the billed amount, leaving patients responsible for the balance. As late as the 1970s, though, a significant proportion of Americans had plans that provided *full* or *first-dollar* coverage. In this expansionary period, health plans were often free to employees, with employers paying 100 percent of the premium.

But by the 1980s, employee plans and most other types had begun to require increasingly significant cost sharing. **Cost sharing** includes, first, payment of a portion of the premium. This provision had been part of many health plans in prior decades, but became nearly universal as the twentieth century came to a close.

In addition to payment of part of the premium, cost sharing includes partial payment for specific elements of service—including, for example, a visit to a doctor, admission to a hospital, receipt of a medication from a pharmacy. Such cost sharing includes, first, *deductibles.* A **deductible** is a dollar amount that the consumer is required to have paid before his insurance makes payments. Second, cost sharing includes *copayments.* **Copayments** *are applied to* the cost of each specific unit of service. A copayment may be a flat fee or a percentage of the cost of the service or medication.

A number of new methods of providing insurance have been added to the options available to employers, employees, and individuals purchasing plans on their own. The following cluster of interrelated insurance products and arrangements is of special interest:

- *High-Deductible Health Plans (HDHPs).* High-deductible health plans are insurance products with deductibles higher than those traditionally imposed but with proportionally low premiums. In 2006, the Kaiser Family Foundation defined an HDHP as a plan with a deductible of at least $1,000 for single coverage and $2,000 for family coverage. Employers seeking means of controlling employee health care costs have increasingly embraced such plans. A 2006 survey found that over five million workers were covered under such plans.[28] HMOs have developed their own version. Kaiser Permanente, the largest HMO in the United States, began offering high-deductible plans in 2006. The plans were instituted to make Kaiser Permanente, which has traditionally provided very rich benefits, more attractive to younger, lower-risk consumers. In 2006, a twenty-nine-year old male in Southern California was able to buy Kaiser Permanente coverage with a $1,500 deductible for $73 per month, about half the cost of its traditional plan.[29]

■ *Consumer-Driven Health Plans.* Many people covered by HDHPs are beneficiaries of employer-provided, consumer-driven health plans. Under a consumer-driven health plan, the employer puts cash in a tax-exempt health account for the employee. The beneficiary uses funds in her account to pay some of the deductibles for the high-deductible health plan. When funds in the account are exhausted, the beneficiary must pay any remaining deductibles out of pocket. If any funds are left over at the end of the year, the beneficiary may roll them over for the next year's health expenses or, under some arrangements, use them for other purposes. Consumer-driven health plans do not require employees to buy the high-deductible plan—they may opt for a lower-deductible plan or HMO with higher premiums. Consumer-driven health plans have proven attractive to employers because they place more responsibility for health plan selection and payment on employees than conventional insurance or managed care plans.

■ *Health Savings Accounts (HSAs).* Health savings accounts are tax-free programs for paying health care charges not covered by insurance. Companies may establish HSAs in connection with consumer-driven health plans, but people who have high deductible plans can also establish them as individuals. Under tax laws as they stood in 2008, a high-deductible plan for an individual was defined as one with a deductible of at least $1,100 and an out-of-pocket cap of $5,600.[30] Banks have been eager to enter the HSA business and offer account holders a variety of investment options for their funds. Unspent funds in an HSA in a given year may be rolled over.

■ *Medical Savings Accounts (MSAs).* Medical savings accounts are similar to HSAs in that they allow individuals with high-deductible health plans to establish tax-free funds to pay for those deductibles and other medical expenses. Such accounts may be established by people who are self-employed or work for firms with fewer than fifty employees. Under certain conditions, Medicare beneficiaries may establish MSAs.

Blue Cross, which provided the original model for health insurance, remains very important in U.S. health insurance. Blue Cross and Blue Shield plans are the largest health insurers in almost every state. They have at least half the individual market in thirty-three states and more than one-third of the group market in twenty-eight states. In some states, Blue Cross units have served as Medicare fiscal intermediaries.

Blue Cross has undergone changes no one could have expected in the 1930s. Generations ago, the Blue Cross movement championed the nonprofit sector as best fitted to provide health insurance to the American public. Over the decades this movement accommodated itself to changing market conditions; at present, it shows signs of having gone into reverse. In the late twentieth and early twenty-first centuries, some of the largest Blue Cross plans were transformed by their boards into private for-profit firms. Wellpoint, a huge holding company, now controls several formerly nonprofit Blue Cross organizations. Outcomes of these conversions have not been fully determined, but increases in premiums and reduced access to insurance within traditionally served populations appear possible.[31]

Public Programs. Public programs for the indigent have existed for generations. Many of these have been locally based. City and county hospitals today operate clinics for people of limited means, as they have for many years. In most states, counties have the legal responsibility for providing services to the local poor. In California, the state constitution requires that each county serve as the health care provider of last resort and that the state provide counties with funding for this purpose. The quality, generosity, and convenience with which services have been provided have varied from place to place. In some localities, health departments have collaborated with medical schools in the area. According to one observer, such collaboration has improved the quality of services delivered.[32]

In its modern form, public participation in health care began with the enactment of Medicare and Medicaid in 1965. Medicare funds health care primarily for people sixty-five and over. Medicare itself receives funding through taxation of working people. Individuals who have been employed for ten years, are citizens or permanent residents of the United States, and are sixty-five or older are eligible for Medicare. People under sixty-five who develop end-stage renal disease or end-stage liver disease or who become disabled may also be eligible for benefits.

Medicare resembles private insurance in that people contribute to a trust fund upon which they draw when they are elderly and ill. In this respect, Medicare is similar to other key *social insurance* programs in the United States. Like Medicare, Social Security and unemployment insurance receive their funding from payroll taxes on employed individuals. Unlike the taxes that cover Social Security and unemployment insurance, however, there is no limit on income to which the Medicare tax can be applied. As a consequence, higher-income American workers pay substantial taxes to support the program. Medicare is the most expensive public health care program in the United States. In 2008, the Medicare program cost U.S. taxpayers over $430 billion.[33]

Medicaid pays for care received by poor people. People eligible for Medicaid include, first, beneficiaries of the Temporary Assistance to Needy Families (TANF) program. TANF is a version of America's traditional public assistance programs, which have typically provided financial assistance to single mothers. Recipients of Supplemental Security Income (SSI), a program providing income support to the disabled, may be eligible for Medicaid. In 1997, Medicaid expanded to cover children whose families were not poor, but earned limited income (up to three times the federal poverty limit in some states). This program is known as the State Children's Health

Insurance Program (SCHIP). The Patient Protection and Affordable Care Act contained provisions aimed at expanding Medicaid eligibility to include childless, low income individuals.

Medicaid more closely resembles a welfare program than an insurance setup. All U.S. residents may qualify for Medicaid, regardless of work history. But unlike Medicare, Medicaid is *means tested*—to become beneficiaries, applicants for Medicaid must pass stringent income tests.

Medicaid is funded jointly by the federal and state governments. States have latitude to fine-tune their programs' benefit and eligibility structure; hence, there are individualized state programs with names like *Tenncare* and *Medi-Cal*. Federal funds are allocated according to a formula that provides higher subsidies for states with lower per capita incomes. Medicaid programs in states with the highest per capita incomes receive 50 percent of their funds from the federal government. States with the lowest incomes may receive over 80 percent. The costs associated with Medicaid in 2007 were $333.2 billion, with $190.6 billion coming from the federal government and $142.6 billion from state governments. Medicaid funding has become increasingly burdensome for states, precipitating fiscal alarm in jurisdictions as requirements for the program approach one-third of some state budgets.

What Is Social Insurance?

Earlier in this chapter it was stated that government financing for health services resembles insurance in some respects. Metaphorically, one may speak of Medicaid as insurance against becoming poor and Medicare as insurance against getting old. But neither Medicare nor Medicaid is an insurance program in the traditional sense.

Rather, both Medicare and Medicaid are funded through social insurance mechanisms. Social insurance is a government-operated hybrid of traditional insurance and public welfare. As is typical of social insurance plans, payment (though not eventual participation) is mandatory.

Funding for Medicaid is generated by federal and state taxation. Nonpoor individuals pay a disproportionately high share of these taxes. Few higher-income taxpayers will eventually become Medicaid beneficiaries. Funding for Medicaid, then, represents not insurance but a transfer of funds from the relatively well-off to the indigent.

In contrast, many working people whose payroll taxes fund Medicare will eventually become beneficiaries. But the monies these individuals contribute are unlikely to cover their needs as Medicare beneficiaries. Since the program's inception, Medicare expenditures have been funded not by prior contributions of beneficiaries themselves but by younger individuals who are still in the labor force. Medicare benefits, then, represent a transfer of resources from younger to older individuals.

(Continued)

(Continued)

Social insurance programs are open to the entire public, another feature that distinguishes them from private insurance. As noted earlier, private insurance companies expend much effort to limit adverse selection into their plans. No such restrictions can be applied to Medicare and Medicaid. This feature exposes both programs to financial risk that would be unacceptable to private plans.

All private insurance entities are obliged to maintain an ability to pay claims. Insurance companies have contractual obligations to beneficiaries for coverage of specific services and associated financial loss for the life of a policy. State laws mandate that companies maintain adequate reserve levels to meet potential claims. Social insurance programs, however, are based on laws and regulations that can be changed.[34] Government decision makers have the liberty to increase taxation, tighten eligibility requirements, or restrict benefits at any time.

Maintaining sufficient reserves to pay claims is a key challenge of both private and social insurance programs. The Medicare Trust Fund's adequacy for the baby boom generation's needs is a topic of considerable public concern. Maintaining the fund's solvency into the twenty-first century will remain a policy concern far into the future.

Both Medicare and Medicaid emerged from intense debates during the 1950s and 1960s. During that era, many Americans were becoming concerned with the burden that health care costs were beginning to exact on the elderly. Just as today, most Americans obtained private health insurance through their jobs. Although some advantaged workers received health care coverage as a retirement benefit, many did not. The switch of Blue Cross from community to experience rating, moreover, made indemnity insurance prohibitively expensive for many elders.

Many elders feared poverty. "Medical care for the aged" became a key issue in the 1960 presidential campaign and was championed by John F. Kennedy, the eventual victor. Under President Lyndon B. Johnson, who succeeded Kennedy after his assassination, Medicare and Medicaid were tacked onto an extension of the Social Security Act renewal in 1965. Title XVIII of the act, health care for the aged and disabled, became known as Medicare; Title XIX, a health plan for the poor, was later called Medicaid.

Several smaller programs to cover health care for specific segments of the United States population followed in subsequent decades. Some of these, such as the Indian Health Service and the Veterans Administration, have been mentioned earlier. Another is the Ryan White Comprehensive AIDS Resources Emergency Act. The Ryan-White Act established a program intended to be the "payer of last resort" for people with AIDS. The program supports treatment for people with AIDS when no other resources are available to them.

Table 7.2 shows the impact of Medicare and Medicaid on patterns of United States health care spending. Unlike Table 7.1, which covers only individuals

TABLE 7.2   **Percentage contributions to health care funding by form of insurance, all U.S. residents**

Source of Funds (%)	Year			
	1960	1980	2000	2005
Consumer out of pocket	55.2	27.2	16.9	15.0
Private health insurance	21.4	28.4	35.4	35.9
Other private funds	2.0	4.3	5.0	4.1
Government	21.4	40.0	42.7	45.0
Federal government	8.7	28.9	32.5	34.2
Local and state government	12.7	11.1	10.2	10.7

Source: National Center for Health Statistics. *Health, United States, 2007.* Table 125. Hyattsville, MD: National Center for Health Statistics; 2007.

under sixty-five, Table 7.2 presents data on the entire U.S. population. In 1960, consumer out-of-pocket payments comprised the majority of dollars spent on health care in the United States. By 2005, individual out-of-pocket payments covered only 15 percent of the bill. Between 1960 and 2005, however, private insurance increased its share by over 50 percent. The percentage of payment supplied by federal programs, chiefly driven by Medicaid and Medicare, saw a fourfold percentage increase.

Managed Care as Insurance. Chapter Five introduces the concept of managed care as an arrangement under which an administrative entity—a scheduling bureaucracy, case manager, or utilization review agency, for example—intervenes between the consumer and the provider. Supporters of managed care characterize such arrangements as means that simultaneously ensure optimal care and control costs. According to supporters, these dual purposes are achieved through (1) avoiding unnecessary care and (2) substituting expensive interventions or medications with cheaper ones when these are presumed equally effective. Critics have contended that managed care functions largely as a rationing device, a deliberate barrier to care for the purpose of saving money for the plan sponsor.

Large managed care organizations such as the Health Insurance Plan of Greater New York, Group Health Cooperative, and Kaiser Permanente emerged at midcentury, serving a restricted but stable market. In the 1970s, federal and state legislation established conditions under which many more consumers received services under some form of managed care. HMOs proved too restrictive for consumer tastes. However, plans such as PPOs, a form of managed care allowing greater consumer choice, flourished.

It is important to understand that managed care operations are insurance operations as well as delivery systems. Traditionally, HMOs have provided a *service benefit* to insured consumers. The consumer or his sponsor pays a premium. In exchange, the HMO provides services as needed. Under plans now operated by Blue Cross or commercial carriers, consumers receive benefits on an indemnity basis. Physicians, hospitals, and other service providers receive cash payments from the insurance company. Alternatively, the patient pays a bill and receives cash back. In the PPO situation, providers bill on a fee-for-service basis. But they are restricted to the delivery of services allowed by the PPO for specific conditions or patient histories. The utilization review process regulates the services the patient may receive. Physicians who are found to practice in a manner exceeding the PPO's financial restrictions may be dropped.

Like all companies with health insurance products, managed care operations enter a competitive process to obtain contracts from employers and government agencies. In doing so, they take financial risks. A managed entity examines data on past claims, demographics, and health characteristics of prospective groups to establish rates that it believes will be profitable. At they same time, competition may force all competitors to reduce the rates they offer dangerously close to break-even.

Government agencies have looked to managed care as a way to provide alternatives, promote prevention, and control costs. In the 1980s, Medicare began an experimental program to enroll beneficiaries in HMOs. The program was extended to other types of managed care plans in the ensuing decade. The *Medicare Advantage* plan was enacted in 2003, with the intention of making more plans available to beneficiaries and increasing payments to the plans. Enrollment in Medicare Advantage plans reached ten million in 2008, approximately 23 percent of the Medicare population.[35]

Enrollment of Medicaid beneficiaries in managed care plans has increased even more rapidly. In the late twentieth century, all states implemented policies encouraging or requiring Medicaid beneficiaries to join managed care plans.[36] Between 1994 and 2004, enrollment in Medicaid-funded managed care plans grew from 7.9 million to 27 million. During that period, the proportion of Medicaid beneficiaries in managed care plans increased from 23 percent to 60 percent.[37] Many, if not most, of these plans enroll only Medicaid beneficiaries.

ADDITIONAL INSURANCE CONCEPTS AND TERMINOLOGY

The historical sketch presented earlier provides an overview of how insurance helps pay for health care in the United States. The sketch also covers concepts and nomenclature essential to understanding and communicating about health insurance. The following concepts and terms provide additional perspectives and vocabulary relevant to public and private health insurance.

Underwriting. Underwriting is the process by which an insurer determines whether to accept a client, the premium the client is to be charged, and exclusions and caps on claims in an ensuing policy. In health care, the underwriting process takes account of the claims history of an employer or the health status of an individual. Through the underwriting process, an insurer attempts to identify profitable risks and screen out individuals or groups likely to result in high individual claims or significant claims by numerous individuals. A team involved in health insurance underwriting may include specialists such as actuaries, epidemiologists, and health economists.

Loss Ratios. Insurance companies compute a series of ratios as indices of their performance. These ratios are useful for both business and policy purposes. They enable seekers of insurance as well as potential investors to assess the efficiency of a company. They enable policy makers and analysts to track the profitability of insurers.

The most fundamental type is known simply as the *loss ratio,* computed by dividing claims paid by premiums received in a given year. This chapter has so far discussed insurance as a process by which premiums are established on the basis of expected claims. In reality, premiums need to reflect other expenses involved in operating an insurance entity. In addition to paying claims, insurance companies must cover expenses such as brokers' commissions, claims adjuster salaries, administrative services, and legal fees. The *total ratio* reflects these expenditures and is computed by dividing the sum of claims and other expenses by premiums received in a given year. Achievement of a total ratio of less than 1.0 signifies an insurer with superior underwriting and administrative capabilities. A total ratio that is too low, however, may reflect excessive profits.

Reinsurance. Insurance companies and managed care organizations themselves buy insurance. They buy policies from *reinsurance* companies to protect themselves against extraordinary losses. A large risk pool generally protects an insurance company against extraordinary risk. But events such as natural disaster, terrorism, or public health emergencies such as epidemics may increase the company's losses catastrophically.

Self-Insurance. Although most employers buy health insurance policies from insurance companies to cover their workers, some choose to *self-insure.* Under such an arrangement, a company assumes the financial risk typically assumed by an insurance company. Only large companies with sufficient cash may opt for self-insurance. They choose the self-insurance option because they wish to avoid charges made by insurance companies for managing the money they pay in premiums. Companies that self-insure believe they can manage the expenses and risks of covering their employees as well as an insurance company can by budgeting for predictable losses due to health care utilization by their own employees. Insurance companies may in fact provide specialized services to a company such as underwriting, processing claims, and issuing payments to health care providers.

Fiscal Intermediaries. As indicated earlier in this chapter, some of the most important insurance programs today are operated by the public sector. The most visible is Medicare, which most closely resembles insurance in the private sector. Working Americans are required to pay a tax to support the Medicare Trust Fund. Upon retirement or other eligibility portals, the beneficiary draws on the Medicare Trust Fund, whose assets are invested in U.S. government securities. Medicare operates in collaboration with the private sector. The *Center for Medicare and Medicaid* (CMS), which administers these programs, does not make payments directly to providers. Rather, it contracts with private sector *fiscal intermediaries,* which manage the accounts and write the checks. In California, for example, Blue Cross has often held fiscal intermediary contracts.

Entitlements. Public programs such as Medicare are often known as *entitlements.* This label reflects the fact that an individual is entitled to benefits under the program when he meets specific standards of employment history, age, and disability status. Entitlement programs have become an object of concern, since demographic trends project massive increases in the number of people legally entitled to benefits.

MEDICARE SPECIFICS AND ISSUES

Because Medicare is the single largest payer for health services in the United States, it is important to understand the program in detail. Table 7.3 lists major parts of the program, including benefits and costs to the participant. Dollar figures in the table represent costs to beneficiaries in the mid-2000s. Medicare as a whole must be viewed as an extremely generous program, but specific features of the program have raised significant policy issues.

The program summarized in Table 7.3 may appear complicated to people unfamiliar with Medicare. Actually, the program is even more complex. Certain disabled individuals are eligible for benefits even if they are under age sixty-five. People below certain income levels can seek relief from some premiums and deductibles. Under some conditions, individuals may receive benefits under both Medicare and Medicaid. Elders must often make choices among multiple options that even experts find difficult to understand.

Medicare does not cover all the services a beneficiary may require, and fees that providers charge might not be covered under the program. To cover associated expenses, beneficiaries often purchase "Medigap" insurance to pay for unexpected deductibles, copayments, and nonallowed expenses. Numerous and varied Medigap policies are available to elders. It is not uncommon for elders to purchase several policies whose benefits overlap.

Medicare Parts A and B have existed since the program's inception. Medicare Parts C and D are of relatively recent vintage. Under Medicare Part C, beneficiaries may enroll in managed care plans. Plans covered by Medicare Part C include HMOs, PPOs, and fee-for-service plans with elements of managed care. Those who opt for Part C obtain more complete coverage in areas such as hospitalization and have fewer out-of-pocket expenses. The need to purchase Medigap insurance is minimal.

TABLE 7.3   **Medicare parts A through D: benefits and costs to consumer**

Program	Year Enacted	Benefits	Costs	Comment
Part A	1965	Hospital: 60 days without charge after deductible; additional charges after 60 days	No premium; $952 deductible	Coverage of nursing homes includes only skilled nursing facilities
Part B	1965	Physician and other health professions services	Premium required: $88.50/month in 2006; $124 deductible	Not all services covered; physician charges may exceed Medicare allowable
Part C	1997	Medicare Advantage, requiring coverage by managed care plan, with extra benefits	Premium varies	Consumer must enroll in plan in her residential locality
Part D	2006	Pharmaceutical benefit	Premium approx. $32/month in 2006; $250 deductible	75% of drug costs from $250 to $2,000; 0% next $2,850; 95% above $5,100

Medicare Part D was added in 2006 as part of the Medicare Modernization Act. This legislation aimed primarily to provide elders with coverage for pharmaceuticals, an area of rapidly increasing importance and cost in the early twenty-first century. A highly contentious debate preceded passage of the legislation. Policy makers realized that the cost of Medicare Part D would be extremely high. To reach a compromise, legislators created a gap in funding. Under the compromise, relatively low costs and relatively high costs were covered. Beneficiaries whose pharmaceutical consumption fell into midrange (between $2,000 and $5,100 in 2006) received no coverage. This coverage gap was dubbed the *donut hole.*

Long-term care has never been covered under Medicare. Medicare pays for limited care in a skilled nursing facility (SNF). Hospitalized patients are often discharged to SNFs for services to prepare them to resume life in the community, such as training and rehabilitation. But Medicare does not pay for residence in a *long-term care facility,* as nursing homes are called in the health care industry. Insurance policies are sold to cover long-term care facility stays. These, however, are unpopular among the young and expensive for the elderly. Long-term care expenses are covered under Medicaid. But to become eligible for Medicaid, a consumer must divest his assets and become, in effect, poor. Self-induced poverty of this kind greatly diminishes the elder's independence and the degree of control he may exercise over care and conditions of life.

Medicare Parts A and B are strongly institutionalized in American society. Fundamental criticism of these program elements is infrequent. In the years following their enactment, however, Medicare Parts C and D have been subject to controversy. Some observers believe that Medicare Advantage plans are overpaid by the government and cuts to the program may be in the offing. The original Medicare Part D legislation prohibited Medicare authorities from negotiating prices directly with pharmaceutical companies. It is reasoned that the volume of pharmaceuticals paid for by Medicare would give Medicare authorities immense bargaining power and lead to huge savings. Others have raised the possibility and cited supporting data that elders whose expenditures fall in the donut hole are likely to stop taking needed medications.[38]

Other policy issues associated with Medicare concern the fairness of the program. U.S. elders are not the most disadvantaged members of society. Children and single mothers generally have fewer material advantages. It has been argued that children, single mothers, and others who are clearly disadvantaged should enjoy the relatively rich benefits provided to elders. In addition, some have argued that Medicare, like Medicaid, should be means tested. Wealthy elders, then, would either become ineligible or be charged premiums for Part A and be charged higher premiums for Part D than their less affluent counterparts. Public policy has begun to move in this direction. The Medicare Modernization Act of 2007 mandated that high-income elders pay a Medicare Part B premium twice as high as that of beneficiaries in the lowest-income categories.[39]

If There Were No Health Insurance . . .

It is tempting to speculate how health care in the United States might be different if health insurance had never been invented.

According to one perspective, health insurance is an unfavorable method for financing health care. Evidence suggests, for example, that health insurance creates inflation in the health care sector. This is because the market supports out-of-pocket payment at a particular level for each unit of health care. People will pay the same amount for that unit of care whether or not the amount represents payment in full or merely a small share of costs. For this reason, it has been reported that a pre-Medicare elder paid about the same out-of-pocket amount for a doctor visit as the Medicare beneficiary paid in cost sharing twenty years later. The additional amount paid by Medicare, then, represents inflation.

However, people living in countries that have no system of health insurance or a very weak system are likely to be denied vital health services. China at the start of the twenty-first century furnishes an example. Collective farms and government-owned factories once provided basic health care to most Chinese. But many of these institutions had been disbanded or sold to the private sector by the beginning of the new century. Health care became a personal fiscal burden for most Chinese. By 2002, out-of-pocket payment covered 60 percent of health care expenditures, compared with 16 percent in the United States.

Often Chinese are required to pay in advance for the care they or their family members require, and treatment stops when the money runs out. Journalists have reported grisly stories about the results of this practice. Doctors threatened to stop treating a child with curable leukemia when his father could raise no more money from family and neighbors. According to another report, a woman who had just delivered her baby was bleeding profusely and needed an emergency blood transfusion. A witness heard nurses screaming at the woman's husband, "If you don't have any money, we don't operate!"

Lack of a health insurance system may place limits on China's economic development. Fear of financial burden due to illness causes many Chinese to save money that would otherwise be spent in the consumer economy. Officials have expressed fear that widespread financial ruin caused by health care expenses may produce social unrest.[40]

THE PROBLEM OF UNINSURANCE

Lack of health insurance—sometimes referred to as **uninsurance**—has been a key issue in U.S. health care for generations. In the early 2000s, the percentage of Americans under age sixty-five without health insurance varied between 16 and 17 percent. In 2005, individuals who lacked health insurance at any time in the preceding year comprised approximately 20 percent of U.S. residents under age sixty-five.[41]

As indicated in preceding chapters, people without health insurance often have access to sources of health care. People without health insurance may receive care at community clinics, free clinics, and hospital emergency departments (see Chapter Five). Individuals with sufficient funds may pay out of pocket for care at doctor's offices, urgent care facilities, and hospitals. For those without sufficient financial means, however, options for care are limited.

Even when they are able to obtain health care, the uninsured often find it chaotic and unpleasant.[42] Continuity of care cannot be counted upon. Wait times are often long.

Ironically, the costs for which people without health insurance may become responsible are often very high. In the event of hospitalization, costs can be astounding. Third-party payers today negotiate with hospitals for favorable fee scales. But hospitals are free to charge uninsured individuals whatever they deem appropriate. In 2008, a young, employed woman without health insurance was charged nearly $9,000 for a twelve-hour stay in an emergency room.[43] Patients receive bills for several times this amount for a few days in the hospital. A Johns Hopkins University professor has reported that in 2004 "the rates charged to many uninsured and other 'self-pay' patients for hospital services were often 2.5 times what most health insurers actually paid and more than three time the hospital's Medicare-allowable rates."[44]

It is tempting to think of the uninsured as primarily the poor. However, the problem is considerably more complex. The behavioral model of health service utilization (see Chapter Four) provides clues to the likelihood of "uninsurance" among different demographic groups. Ethnicity, immigration, and lifestyle influence whether an individual may have access to health insurance and when, if offered, the option of purchasing insurance will be accepted. Many poor people in the United States are in fact insured under public programs such as Medicaid and Medicare.

Economist Victor Fuchs highlights the importance of factors other than simple poverty. According to Fuchs, people who hold jobs or are dependents of job holders constitute many of the uninsured. Others may have access to plans or are able to purchase them individually, but do not. Fuchs divides the uninsured in the United States into the following six categories:

- *The poor.* This is the largest group of uninsured people in the United States. A majority of the poor and uninsured individuals in the United States hold jobs or are members of families in which there is one or more job holder. Nearly 80 percent of individuals in this category are employed or are the dependents of employed persons. The incomes of these individuals and families, however, are too low to enable then to acquire insurance. They hold jobs in firms that do not offer insurance and may not have enough money to pay for insurance even when it is offered on the job.

- *The sick and disabled.* Many men and women who are not poor are still unable to afford health insurance because they have "preexisting" health problems. These individuals face very high premiums or are excluded from some coverage entirely.

- *The "difficult."* Some people are neither poor nor sick, but have difficulty in obtaining insurance at average premiums. They may be self-employed or out of the labor force entirely. In order to reach and service such individuals, insurance companies incur abnormally high sales and administrative costs.

- *Low users.* Some people do not expect to use much medical care. They may be in particularly good health; they may be Christian Scientists. For them, health insurance is a bad buy unless they can acquire it at below-average premiums.

- *Gamblers.* Most people buy health insurance in part because they are risk-averse. They would rather pay a fixed, known premium than run the risk of a huge expense in the event of a serious illness. But not everyone is risk-averse. The gambler says, "I'd rather save the premium and take my chances."

■ *Free riders.* The final category consists of individuals who remain uninsured because they believe that if they do get sick, they will get care anyway, with somebody else paying the bill.[45]

Table 7.4 highlights the most and least likely individuals in the United States to lack health insurance. Lack of insurance varies not only by demographics but by location.

TABLE 7.4 Selected categories of high uninsurance, 2003

Category	Percentage Uninsured
Ages 18–24	30.1
Ages 25–34	25.4
Native Americans or Alaska Natives	35.0
Latinos	34.7
Below 100% poverty	31.1
100–149% poverty	31.9
150–159% poverty	27.6
Texas residents	27.7
New Mexico residents	24.4
Oklahoma residents	22.5
Noncitizens	45.7
Total U.S.	**17.6**

Sources: Demographics: *Health, United States 2005*, Tables 134 and 138.

States: Employee Benefit Research Institute estimates of the Current Population Survey, March 2002, 2003 and 2004 Supplements.

Citizenship: Employee Benefit Research Institute estimates of the Current Population Survey, March 2005 Supplement.

As the table indicates, Texas, New Mexico, and Oklahoma led the nation in uninsurance, at 27.7, 24.2, and 22.5 percent, respectively, between 2002 and 2004. During this time period, Minnesota, Hawaii, and Iowa had the lowest percentages of uninsured, at 9.5, 11.6, and 11.7. Of all categories displayed in Table 7.4, citizenship status is the strongest predictor of not having insurance. In 2004, the uninsurance rate among noncitizens was 45.7 percent. Among citizens, uninsured individuals comprised 15.4 percent.[46]

A close examination of a group with an extraordinarily high rate of uninsurance helps identify the numerous and complex factors associated with not having health insurance in the United States. Rates of uninsurance are quite high among Mexican Americans. In the first decade of the twenty-first century, approximately 38 percent of this group had no health insurance. A survey of working Latinos in California asked those who were not insured their reasons for not having insurance.[47] The main reasons given by these individuals are presented in Table 7.5.

It is apparent from Table 7.5 that economic factors predominate as explanations of uninsurance among California's working Latinos. Costs were cited as the most important reason for lack of insurance more often than any other reason. A strong majority of the uninsured cited costs as *one* of the reasons they did not have insurance. Lack of access to a plan at work was also an important factor.

However, pocketbook issues did not tell the whole story. Almost a third of the uninsured cited trouble understanding plans or associated forms as a reason for their

TABLE 7.5   **Reasons for not having health insurance among working Latinos in California**

Reason	Gave as main reason (%)	Mentioned as reason (%)
Cost of premiums, deductibles, or copayments too high	31.8	64.8
Insurance not offered by employer or ineligible because of part-time status	23.7	45.8
Insurance not necessary due to good health, ability to pay without insurance, or access to free or inexpensive care	13.9	36.0
Too much trouble to understand plans and forms	6.3	30.7
Other or no response	23.0	—

status. Personal and cultural factors played a role as well. Among people offered a health plan at work, those who felt that they could affect what might happen tomorrow by what they did today were more likely to enroll. Working Latinos born in the United States or living in the United States twenty years or longer were as likely to have health insurance as non-Latinos with similar levels of income and education.

Cases of working Latinos who choose not to have insurance even when it is offered provide clues to why uninsurance exists in other population segments. On the personal or family level, health insurance is often not a good buy. Young, healthy individuals are relatively unlikely to need health services—as is true for many working Latinos. People of this description who are placed in risk pools with less healthy individuals in effect subsidize the requirements of others. Public policy must address this issue in a far broader perspective than that relevant to only Latino workers.

CONTINUING ISSUES

Financing constitutes the core of management and policy challenges in U.S. health care. Issues cited in this chapter have included controlling overall costs, the viability of insurance as a funding mechanism, covering the uninsured, and the solvency of public insurance programs. Several additional issues are likely to remain of concern over the coming decades.

The role of employers. As suggested in Table 7.1, the role of employer-spon- sored health insurance appears to be in decline. Employers often cite health care costs as a major barrier to making profits and staying in business. Employers have begun offering high-deductible plans and opting for self-insurance as expedients. Some employers now offer *cafeteria plans.* These plans provide employees with a fixed amount of money for all employee benefits. The employee is allowed to select an inexpensive health plan with high deductibles if she prefers to allocate more of the benefit amount to other purposes, such as retirement. Under such arrangements, it is unclear how reliably employees can make appropriate choices.

Equality of care. A great deal of headway could be made in establishing insurance coverage for all Americans if such a system did not have to assure that all would receive equal health care quality. A second-tier system might be established as a basic insurance payer of last resort. Medicaid managed care arrangements may in fact comprise such a system. The value placed on meritocracy supports a dual system, but Americans have been reluctant to acknowledge the possibility that some individuals will receive inferior care.

Fairness of public programs. There is reason to ask whether the funding and distribution of benefits under Medicare and Medicaid are fair. Medicare, the largest single health insurance plan in the United States, requires only that beneficiaries be over sixty-five years of age and have a qualifying work history. Analysts have asked whether the public should pay for the health care of wealthy elders. Perhaps the income differential applied to Medicare Part B premiums should be extended to the program as a whole. Medicare, furthermore, provides benefits to people under sixty-five with end-stage renal disease and end-stage liver disease. Is it fair that only younger individuals with these diseases receive Medicare benefits? Would it not be justifiable to include people with multiple sclerosis, schizophrenia, and many other serious, expensive diseases under the plan?

Insurance pooling and income transfers. Participation in insurance schemes is a concern at the core of health care financing. As heath care in the United States has evolved, risk pools have successively subdivided to accommodate people with similar levels of risk. This process makes it very expensive to cover people at high risk, such as those with chronic illnesses and the elderly. Only by including the healthy with the potentially ill can a risk pool function over the long run. Medicare is at particular risk of insolvency because it contains only elders.

Mandating that people at low risk join insurance pools, a provision of the Patient Protection and Affordable Care Act would provide a solution. However, such a requirement imposes costs on people at low risk who might choose not to buy insurance or would have cheaper insurance available to them in a free market. A mandate of this kind would institute yet another *income transfer* mechanism, taking resources from low-risk people and giving them to people at higher risk.

At present, the Medicare tax system has just such an effect. Working people pay for the current expenses of elders. This amounts to an *intergenerational income transfer.* Medicare costs are projected to rise significantly in the coming decades. If taxes on working people rise proportionally, serious political opposition may develop to the continuation of Medicare and other public programs.

Acceptance of responsibility. A skeptical observer of the United States might see the heath care system as a paradox. A great many benefit from the system. Most Americans receive high-quality services. The system provides stable, well-paid employment to millions more. Yet almost everyone appears eager to minimize his financial contribution. Direct or indirect cost shifting prevails. Insurance companies and Medicare negotiate for reduced rates from hospitals and push for lower fees for health professionals. Individual consumers often evade payment to hospitals, clinics, and emergency departments. Economically advantaged elders fight against higher Medicare premiums. Advocates for victims of individual diseases lobby for special programs. The U.S. health care finance system can be said to resemble a shell game of grand proportions.

The spiral of public expectations. The most basic of U.S. health policy dilemmas may be characterized as an upward spiral of expectations. The rising incomes and improving life conditions of the late twentieth century have encouraged the public to expect progress in all sectors. Accordingly, every generation expects to be healthier than its predecessor. Rising expectations create desire for new technology, including medical interventions and pharmaceuticals. Actual development of new technology allows public expectations to be, to some degree, fulfilled. The deployment of new technology depends on health insurance. Without health insurance, few people could pay for the new technology. It would be deployed much more sparingly and perhaps not be developed at all. Expectations, technology, and health insurance, then, mutually reinforce each other in increasing health expenditures. Control of costs, then, must involve one of these three actions: (1) dampening of expectations, (2) upstream control of technology, or (3) limitation of health insurance. Each of these would require a serious exercise in public choice.

Trade-offs between health care and other uses of funds. Ultimately, the United States will have to decide on a limit to spending for health care. The level at which this limit is established will be a difficult public choice. Health care enables Americans to live longer and more functional lives. It contributes to the economy without necessitating inconvenient foreign alliances or damaging the global environment. Some argue that high expenditures for health care represent not excess but a highly favorable investment in social well-being. Even so, a favored status for health care among public priorities may reduce resources for other necessities such as education, public infrastructure, and business investment.

Issues regarding health insurance are most challenging in the public sector. Some critics contend that a single payer plan, under which the government would pay all providers, would be superior to the current system of benefits and subsidies. These critics have argued that a simple, universal plan would be cheaper to administer and more comprehensive for the population as a whole. Americans, however, have rejected such initiatives in the past. Some innovators have experimented with low-fee clinics for the uninsured. Bargain service of this kind would abandon the insurance concept in favor of discounting with or without public subsidies. The matter of how much subsidy some groups should receive, and how much other groups should contribute, remains unsettled.

Could the United States Become Another China?

The United States has a far better system of health care and health insurance than China. Situations similar to those described earlier in this chapter, however, are occurring in the United States. They underscore the need to develop a system that is both affordable to Americans and capable of covering their needs. A growing tendency of U.S. cancer facilities to require prepayment for services indicates that even people with health insurance today face financial barriers to care.

In 2008, the *Wall Street Journal* reported that 14 percent of nonprofit hospitals questioned in an Internal Revenue Service survey "required patients to pay or make an arrangement to pay" before being admitted. Two of the largest U.S. for-profit systems, Tenet Healthcare and HCA, have adopted similar policies. Consequences for people seeking treatment for cancer resemble the anguish of Chinese patients and

(Continued)

(Continued)

their families. Experiences of individual cancer patients captured in the news story included the following:[48]

In 2006, Lisa Kelly, a leukemia patient, sought urgent treatment at a nonprofit and world-renowned facility in Texas, the M.D. Anderson Cancer Center. According to the *Wall Street Journal,* "the nonprofit hospital refused to accept [her] limited insurance. It asked for $105,000 in cash before it would admit her." The patient, accompanied by her husband, had brought with her a check for $45,000. The *Wall Street Journal* article further reported:

> The hospital demanded an additional $60,000 on the spot. It told her the $45,000 had paid for the lab tests, and it needed the additional cash as a down payment for her actual treatment. . . . Hospital representatives explained that M.D. Anderson would not accept her insurance "because the payout, a maximum of $37,000 a year, would be less than 30 percent of the estimated costs of her care. . . . In the hospital business office, she was crying, exhausted, and confused.

> The hospital eventually lowered its demand to $30,000. Mr. Kelly lost his cool. "What part don't you understand?" he recalls saying. "We don't have any more money today. Are you going to admit her or not?"

Ms. Kelly was eventually admitted for an eight-day course of chemotherapy. She needed periodic treatment over the subsequent year, for which advance payment was also required. The story continues:

> At times, she arrived at the hospital and learned her appointment was "blocked." That meant she needed to go to the business office first and make a payment.

> One day, Ms. Kelly says, nurses wouldn't change the chemotherapy bag in her pump until her husband made a new payment. She says she sat for an hour hooked up to a pump that beeped that it was out of medicine until he returned with proof of payment.

Critics of the U.S. health care system suggest that advance payment for vital health care is socially undesirable, if not simply cruel. Hospitals as prominent and prosperous as M.D. Anderson seem to be attractive targets for such comments. M.D. Anderson is one of the most profitable hospitals in the United States. In 2007, the hospital had net income of $310 million; its total value in cash, investments, and endowment was $1.88 billion.[49] Yet M.D. Anderson's prosperity, if not its survival, may depend on advance payment for treatment. Prior to initiation of the system in 2005, the hospital had millions in unpaid patient bills on its books.

KEY TERMS

Third-party payers
Upstream resources allocation
Insurance
Indemnity policies

Cost sharing
Deductible
Copayments
Uninsurance

SUMMARY

This chapter specifies how health care is paid for in the United States and the purposes for which health care funds are spent.

Private health insurance and government programs cover the majority of health care expenses today. However, direct consumer payments still amount to a considerable sum. Private insurance has become less readily available to Americans because of its increasing costs. Many people who formerly had health plans at work have become beneficiaries of public programs.

Health insurance increases the cost of health care by promoting demand. Insurance enables individuals to buy more health care services than they could if they had only ready cash or its equivalent. Despite the importance of health insurance, a large number of Americans lack coverage.

To control costs, managers and policy makers have made a variety of innovations in health finance since the 1980s. Both public programs and private plans have looked to managed care and competition among suppliers to control costs. Private insurers have developed new products such as high-deductible and limited coverage policies designed to attract a wider variety of customers.

DISCUSSION QUESTIONS

1. Should a system of upstream control be instituted to help control U.S. health care costs? What kind of upstream control mechanism would be most practical and beneficial? What negative consequences might such upstream control have for Americans?

2. Of all U.S. residents, noncitizens are among the most likely to be uninsured. What factors might contribute to their high rate of uninsurance and what solutions would you recommend?

3. How likely is it that Medicaid beneficiaries receive care inferior to that of privately insured people? Would such a situation be acceptable to Americans?

4. Medicare taxation results in transfer of wealth from younger to older individuals. Is this arrangement fair? Is it viable for the long term?

5. Might Medicare serve as a model for reform of the U.S. health care financing system?

CHAPTER

BIOMEDICAL RESEARCH AND PROGRAM EVALUATION

LEARNING OBJECTIVES

- To appreciate the importance of research in the health care industry
- To comprehend the choices available to researchers in assessing interventions
- To assess the adequacy of research as a tool for decision making
- To realize the limitations of research
- To recognize the social and ethical issues in biomedical science

THE IMPORTANCE OF RESEARCH

Systematic research in biomedical and related sciences deserves credit for the explosion of new treatments and technologies evident today. Research techniques whose fundamentals originated in the days of research pioneers such as Koch and Pasteur have made this progress possible. Biomedical research today is a multibillion-dollar industry that employs hundreds of thousands of people worldwide. Individual research projects may cost many millions of dollars, involve hundreds of thousands of subjects, and take decades to complete.

An ever-greater proportion of medical techniques in use today have been subject to evaluation via scientific research. This development is sometimes referred to as the *evidence-based medicine* movement. Even so, much that occurs in health care today has never been systematically tested or evaluated.

An indicator of the scale on which biomedical research takes place today is illustrated in Figure 8.1. This figure presents the number of patents awarded by the U.S. Patent and Trademark Office during the twenty-one-year period of 1988 through 2008 for drugs, related chemical compounds, and specific molecules of potential therapeutic benefit. Over sixty thousand patents for such substances were awarded during this period. Considerable research effort was required for each patent application. Additional research of a considerable scale followed award of many of these patents.

FIGURE 8.1   *Patents awarded for "drug, bioaffecting, and body-treating compounds," 1988–2008*

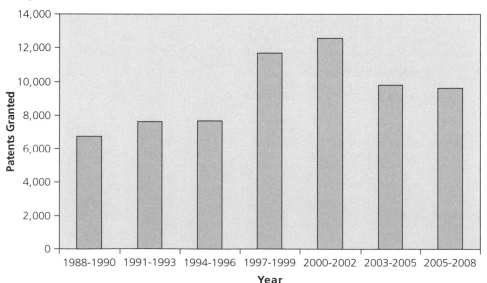

Irrespective of a patent award, significant clinical research is required to establish efficacy and safety in administration to humans.

Figure 8.1, it should be noted, reflects only a fraction of the health-related innovation resulting from and necessitating further research. During the period referenced in Figure 8.1, thousands of additional patents were awarded for medical devices, imaging technology, patient handling and transportation, and numerous other applications. Although uneven, the trend in technological innovation, whether widely adopted or eventually abandoned, is clearly up.

Beyond the importance for improved patient care, research is crucial for decision making in management and policy. Solutions for the rising cost of care and uninsurance, for example (covered in Chapter Seven), have become the subject of intense research efforts. To assess the potential value of proposed solutions, decision makers require a basic understanding of the techniques that researchers employ and the limitations inherent in these techniques. Equally important, decision makers require an understanding of the professional and economic pressures under which the research community works. These pressures materially influence the results presented to clinicians and reported to decision makers.

PRINCIPLES OF EXPERIMENTAL DESIGN

Use of valid research methods by honest scientists has given health care providers a number of effective tools. Research has also helped medical practice dispose of time-honored yet ineffective treatments and set to rest contentions by zealots and mountebanks. Sophistication and breadth of research methods in the biomedical sciences have steadily increased over the past century. However, the fundamental logic of inquiry has remained the same.

Pasteur's 1881 demonstration of his anthrax vaccine at Pouilly-le-Fort, France, illustrates classic biomedical research procedure. In collaboration with a local agricultural society, Pasteur selected 60 farm animals. He vaccinated 31 of these with a weakened strain of anthrax bacilli and left the remaining 29 untreated. About a month later, Pasteur inoculated all 60 beasts with a highly virulent anthrax strain. After another two days, hundreds of people—including government officials, journalists, farmers, and veterinarians—assembled to view the results. None of the vaccinated animals developed anthrax. All 29 untreated animals developed the disease; 25 of these had died by the end of the day.[1]

The Pasteur demonstration included basic elements of modern **experimental design:** (1) random assignment of subjects to distinct intervention options (in this case vaccination versus no vaccination); (2) specification of one or more outcome measures (here, illness and death); (3) comparison of outcome measures applied to individuals in each study condition. Informing this process, of course, would be a hypothesis stating the researcher's expectations. Pasteur stated his hypothesis in this way: "All [animals] that were not vaccinated will perish; all . . . that were vaccinated will resist infection, and we will [return] to a normal state."

A graphic presentation summarizing the experiment and numerical findings such as the one presented in Table 8.1 facilitates evaluation of the hypothesis. This table is a four-cell (or four-fold) table comparing survival numbers and percentages among individuals subjected to each intervention option. In most science, statistical tests would be applied to determine whether outcomes differed across intervention options.

Inspection alone would seem to suffice in assessing the results of Pasteur's experiment. Formally, however, the relationship between vaccination and vital status is quite strong. According to a statistic known as *gamma*, near-perfect association (gamma = .99) exists. A *chi square* test indicates that the results presented in Table 8.1 could have occurred by chance less than one time per thousand repetitions of the experiment (p < .001).

Experimental logic when applied to human beings acquires pathos far greater than did Pasteur's anthrax demonstration. A fictional description illustrates a clash between the interests of individual subjects and a greater good to be served by scientific validity. In his Nobel Prize–winning 1925 novel, *Arrowsmith,* Sinclair Lewis describes an experiment intended to test the value of an agent called *phage* against bubonic plague on a Caribbean island:

> [In his experiment, Dr. Arrowsmith] divided the population into two equal parts. One of them . . . was injected with plague phage, the other half was left without.
>
> The pest attacked the unphaged half of the parish much more heavily than those who had been treated. There did appear a case or two among those who had the phage, but among the others there were ten, then twenty, then thirty daily victims.[2]

Unlike Pasteur's creatures, experimenter Arrowsmith's subjects were human. But Arrowsmith believed that a far greater good justified the sacrifice of the Caribbean Islanders: he saw far-off India, with its annual four hundred thousand deaths from plague, saved by his efforts.

TABLE 8.1   Pasteur's 1881 anthrax experiment as a fourfold table

Outcome (Vital Status):	Intervention (Vaccination):	
	Yes	No
Alive	30 (97%)	4 (14%)
Dead	1 (3%)[a]	25 (86%)
N (100%) =	31	29

Note: Gamma = .99; chi square = 42.0 (p < .001).

[a]The single death among vaccinated subjects was attributed to a cause other than anthrax.

More is expected today of scientists than in Pasteur's era or the fictionalized plague experiment. Modern experiments produce more information than a simple yes-or-no answer to an intervention's effectiveness. Human subjects receive far better protection. But basic objectives, methods, and concerns have remained constant.

MODERN RESEARCH DESIGNS

Scientists working in health care–related fields use a wide variety of methods. The designs in widest use retain key features in common with the classic examples described earlier. Such designs still focus on testing of hypotheses, although today's researchers often specify *null hypotheses,* which they then attempt to reject based on their observations. In a drug trial, for example, scientists might attempt to reject a null hypothesis that states: "There is no statistically significant difference between outcomes observed across separate interventions." Outcome measures are likely to be multiple, comprising, for example, mortality risk, side effects of interventions, function, quality of life, and economic benefit.

Randomized Controlled Trials

The most direct descendent of classical biomedical science is the **randomized controlled trial (RCT).** Under the RCT method as traditionally applied, individuals participating in the experiment, or *subjects,* are randomly assigned to one of two groups. Some are assigned to a treatment group, receiving a drug or other intervention believed to be effective. Others are assigned to a control group, whose members receive no treatment or an intervention known to be biologically inert. The biologically inert substance sometimes given to control subjects is called a *placebo.*

RCTs with simple assignment to a potentially effective agent or a placebo are in fact unusual today. Modern legal and ethical standards dictate that every subject receive the best known treatment for her condition. Control subjects, then, are given a standard treatment of known, though limited, efficacy. Today's RCTs, moreover, are likely to omit the classic control group. Instead, subjects are assigned to one of several *arms* of a study, each calling for a different intervention to be administered. According to the current state of science, interventions under each arm are presumed to be equally effective.

The gold standard for research is achieved in the double-blinded RCT. Under such a procedure, both experimenters and subjects are *blinded,* in the sense that they are not told (and cannot otherwise determine) which subjects have been assigned to any specific arm. Double blinding reduces the possibility that the **placebo effect**—a tendency among subjects assigned to any intervention to experience health improvement due solely to expectations engendered by being in an experiment—will confound the study findings. It also reduces the likelihood that the experimenter's hopes, expectations, or material interests contaminate his observations.

The RCT produces the highest possible level of design *validity.* As long as the number of subjects is sufficiently large, random assignment ensures that subjects assigned to different study arms will have, on average, the same characteristics. Thus, only the experimental interventions can explain subsequent differences—in health status or mortality, for example—among subjects assigned to each arm. **Validity**—the degree to which a research design allows a scientist to reject all but one explanation of the results she obtains—is the primary criterion according to which research methodology should be judged. A highly valid research design allows the experimenter to definitively attribute changes observed to the intervention applied.

It is important to understand that RCTs, as attractive as they may seem, are not applicable to some of the most important research questions being asked today. Examples include determination of health risks, assessment of health trends, delivery of health services, and reduction of health disparities. RCTs are also less useful in some strictly biomedical research concerns. RCTs require sufficient control over subjects for randomization. In real life, subjects may attempt to influence the intervention to which they are assigned. They are free at any time to leave the trial. RCT design requires procedures that adjust for self-selection and loss to follow up. Finally, people cannot be randomized into different lifestyles, communities, and socioeconomic groups, some of the factors that have the strongest impact on health.

A study of a drug for treatment of generalized anxiety disorder illustrates application of the RCT. The drug under investigation was paroxetine—a selective serotonin reuptake inhibitor, or SSRI, marketed under the name Paxil.[3] A widespread condition, generalized anxiety disorder is characterized by worry, restlessness, fatigue, irritability, muscle tension, and difficulty concentrating and sleeping. The condition impairs social and occupational function.

In the study, 566 patients from 50 medical centers were randomly assigned to three interventions: one group received only a placebo; the second received 20 milligrams of paroxetine per day; the third received 40 milligrams of paroxetine per day. The investigators assessed patient responses according to several standard scales, primarily the Hamilton Rating Scale for Anxiety, which measures a variety of dimensions such as anxious mood, general tension, and somatic manifestations.

Patients were followed for eight weeks. At the eight-week time point, the investigators found that anxiety had declined within all three groups. Responses defined as meaningful reduction in Hamilton Rating Scale scores were observed in 62 percent of the 20-milligram paroxetine group and 68 percent of the 40-milligram paroxetine group; responses were observed in 46 percent of those receiving placebo. Despite a considerable placebo effect, responses to the medication at either dosage exceeded those of the placebo by margins unlikely to have occurred purely by chance. The investigators concluded that their study offered strong evidence for the efficacy of paroxetine for treatment of generalized anxiety disorder.

Case-Control Studies

In the **case-control method**, scientists match cases of individuals with a particular disease or health risk with others who, though similar according to known dimensions, are disease-free and outside the risk category. This comparison may promote understanding of how a suspected risk factor actually affects health, the degree to a particular characteristic may have given rise to illness, or to what degree a disease affects function. Case-control studies can be done on either a prospective or retrospective basis.

Studies of this kind identify individuals who have the disease, health risk, or functional deficit of interest as *cases*. Individuals who are presumably the same except that they lack the disease or deficit are known in this context as *controls*. In the case-control method there is no random assignment of subjects to interventions. Rather, controls are selected according to actions they have taken on their own or diseases they have developed spontaneously. RCTs cannot be used to address questions such as responses to risk and disease; it is unthinkable today to induce disease among subjects in order to compare them with others allowed to remain healthy.

A study of the effect of helmet use by skiers and snowboarders provides an illustration of the case-control method. To obtain definitive information on the benefits and potential detriments of helmet use, the investigators obtained data on 578 skiers and snowboarders who had sustained head injuries. They looked at the nature and severity of the injuries, the demographics of the individuals injured, their skiing or snowboarding skills and styles (cautious versus aggressive), and their use or nonuse of helmets. They compared the injured skier and snowboarder sample with a sample of 2,992 noninjured skiers and snowboarders, obtained by questioning one of every tenth person waiting at selected ski lift lines. Noninjured skiers and snowboarders were more likely to wear helmets than their injured counterparts. The authors concluded that "helmet use is associated with reduced risk of head injury among snowboarders and alpine skiers."[4]

Lacking random assignment to interventions, case-control studies have a lower level of validity than RCTs. It is important to remember that randomization ensures that subjects assigned to each intervention arm will be on average identical. No unobserved variable can then be suspected of explaining outcomes. In the case-control method, an infinite range of unobserved (and unsuspected) factors might explain the differences between cases and controls. Researchers in the ski helmet study acknowledge that their case and control samples may ski different average distances and that accident history may be reported in a faulty manner.

Surveys

Surveys are widely used as tools to assess the prevalence of known risk factors or the incidence of specific diseases. Multivariate statistical techniques allow scientists to analyze survey data in a manner that compensates for the kinds of bias always possible in surveys, such as self-selection. Survey data may also be used to simulate experiments through various statistical procedures.

A great deal of the basic health data used in the United States and throughout the world is obtained via surveys. Surveys are used to determine health and illness facts about Americans, behavioral and lifestyle practices that affect health, and health care utilization. The National Center for Health Statistics (NCHS), an agency of the federal government, conducts a number of major surveys on a continuous basis. One program, the Health Interview Survey, randomly contacts about 43,000 households, asking individuals about the family's health status, health problems, and access to and utilization of care. In this fashion, the survey obtains data on over 100,000 individuals. Another continuous program is the National Health and Nutrition Examination Survey, which visits and physically examines a representative sample of 5,000 individuals per year. This survey has been crucial in identifying health issues such as overweight and obesity. NCHS also obtains and merges data collected by individual states on births, deaths, and health behavior obtained through standardized questions used in state-level surveys on health behavior known as the Behavioral Risk Factor Survey.

An important report entitled Declining Disability Among the Elderly illustrates the use of survey data as applied to health.[5] The report draws in part on the National Long Term Care Survey (NLTCS). Funded by the federal Administration on Aging, this program has conducted periodic surveys of individuals ages sixty-five and over since 1982. By 2004, a database of over 35,000 individuals had been accumulated. Disability, the outcome of interest, is measured as difficulty with basic activities of daily living such as eating, bathing, dressing, and getting around, or difficulty with instrumental activities of daily living, such as light housework, shopping, and preparing meals. NLTCS surveys conducted between 1984 and 1999 have revealed a steady decline in disability according to these indices. The researchers attribute declining disability to factors such as new treatments for diseases of the elderly, better public accommodation for people with physical dysfunctions, and a rising level of education.

Survey research encounters several key challenges. Most basic is its inability to explain observed phenomena in a definitive fashion. Any number of unobserved variables could explain declining disability instead of those cited by the investigators. Survey research is also subject to many sources of bias. These include omission of key population segments from samples, faulty recall of past events by subjects, and a tendency for subjects to respond to survey questions in a socially desirable manner.

Disease Surveillance

Disease surveillance is methodologically similar to surveys. Surveillance data are obtained from individuals and organizations linked to *disease registries*. Disease registries accumulate information and make it available for purposes ranging from academic to vitally practical. The geographic areas monitored by these registries range from local to worldwide. The value of surveillance systems depends on methods capable of reasonably complete reporting and standardized categorization of diagnoses, tissues, and, increasingly, genetic markers.

Surveillance today plays a crucial role in research on disease incidence and prevalence. The National Cancer Institute–funded Cancer Surveillance System illustrates surveillance techniques. This system contacts pathology laboratories and cancer-oriented physician practices to rapidly identify new cases of cancer that occur in selected geographical areas. Diabetes and asthma registries have been instituted in various localities. On the international level, the UN World Health Organization conducts surveillance of influenza and other contagious diseases, alerting public health and medical care systems across the globe to the possibility of large-scale health risks.

Registries such as these have been useful for identifying geographical risk factors and tracking incidence trends. Of importance to clinical practice and management, registries are used to monitor interventions and outcomes within health care organizations. Registries are important resources for advancement of quality control and evidence-based medicine. Accumulation of records for specific diseases enables organizational leadership to determine whether protocols are being followed and whether these protocols are effective. Increased use of registries has led to the establishment of very large databases known as *data warehouses,* either proprietary or shared among a number of organizations.

Case Studies

Case studies are fundamental to all professional practice. The term *case study* captures a wide range of procedures for observing and organizing data. The case study is distinguishable from other approaches in its presumption that each case (or set of cases) may be unique. Case studies, of course, provide information applicable to a broader universe of cases. But the researcher cannot assume that the combination of features in a case she observes is duplicated in any other laboratory, community, or patient.

The most fundamental types of case studies are known as *descriptive* or *interpretive.* A **descriptive case study** simply provides facts about a particular disease or intervention. The *interpretive* case study applies principles and tests to descriptive material in order to formulate an explanation or diagnosis. In a *logic model case study,*[6] researchers compare sequences of observed events with those theorized to explain phenomena such as development of a disease or impact of a public health program.

A widely followed feature in the *New England Journal of Medicine* presents case studies in the form of clinical puzzles. One such case involved a nineteen-year-old college student.[7] The student presented with what appeared to be mononucleosis, but with complaints not readily explainable by this disease, including severe joint and aural pain. Application of a complex of laboratory and tests and cultures led to diagnosis that included mononucleosis. The student, however, also had gonorrhea sufficiently disseminated to affect several areas of her biological functioning.

Table 8.2 summarizes key features of each research design described here, along with the challenges and limitations faced by each. Variations within each study design are also shown. Sources more specialized than this textbook need to be consulted for details on these variations. The table suggests that although high levels of validity are not assured outside the RCT, non-RCT methodologies are necessary for addressing a wide range of issues.

Measures of Outcomes

High-quality research requires accurate and practical measures of both interventions and outcomes. Measures in biomedical research are usually quantifiable metrics reflecting degree or intensity of independent and dependent variables. Metrics

TABLE 8.2   Types of research methodology, applications, and validity

Research Method	Variations	Applications	Validity
Randomized controlled trial	Blinded (single or double); cross-over; prerandomization	Drug trials	High
Case-control study	Prospective; retrospective; cohort	Natural history of disease; treatment effects; late sequelae; risk factor identification	Moderate
Survey	Random sampling or stratified sampling; quasi-experimental	Health services research; epidemiology; risk factor identification	Moderate
Case study	Clinical; exploratory; interpretive; logic model	Disease description; drug safety; natural history of disease; hypothesis generation; program evaluation	Low

used as independent variables in some of the preceding examples include assignment to a treatment or placebo group and variations in medication dosage. Outcome measures include tumor size and vital status. Metrics such as these are straightforward. Reflecting the ever-widening application of health care and medicine, more complex and problematical measures have come into widespread use.

Many measures used today are known as multi-item indicators. These instruments contain multiple items (such as survey questions or clinician-assessed symptoms), each of which is believed to measure a central dimension (such as morbidity) using different verbal or written cues. Such instruments measure complex outcomes such as physical function, emotional well-being, and total impact of an illness. Multi-item indicators include *indices,* sets of items that are summed (sometimes differentially weighted) to produce a total score, and *scales,* sets of ranked items indicating successively higher magnitudes.

The value of a research design is no better than the validity and reliability of the measures it uses. For a measure to be valid, it must actually measure what the researcher thinks it measures. Before using *intelligence quotient* (IQ) metrics in a study explaining human intellectual capability, for example, the researcher must possess evidence that this measure actually reflects the diffuse and variable phenomenon of human reasoning acuity.

For a measure to have a high level of **reliability**—whether it is a laboratory test or the volume of a tumor—it must yield the same value when administered by different observers or repeatedly observed in the same subject. The tendency of individual human beings to view the world differently makes it necessary to develop instruments that will ideally yield identical findings, no matter who administers them. Questions eliciting a subject's report on her condition must be sufficiently meaningful and clear to ensure uniform responses on repeated administrations.

Table 8.3 illustrates the range of indicators used by biomedical scientists, epidemiologists, and program evaluation researchers to assess outcomes. In some instances measures have been validated through direct experimentation. For example, the visual analogue scale of pain was validated by subject responses on the instrument to laboratory procedures intended to produce pain at varying levels. Pain was administered to the subjects by having them immerse extremities into cold water or the tightening of bands around their limbs to produce ischemia.

TABLE 8.3 Outcome indicators widely used in biomedical research

Name of Instrument	Description	Purpose
Laboratory protocol	Laboratory values such as blood pressure, PSA; Pap and other screening tests; imaging output	Assessment of medical condition; extent and progress of disease
Quality-adjusted life years	Years of survival adjusted for function and comfort	Health services and pharmaceutical research
Visual analogue scale	Printed lines to represent degrees of pain	Pain assessment for clinical or research purposes
MOS-36	36-item questionnaire assessing physical and mental health	Outcomes of medical interventions and health service experiments
Karnofsky scale	Observer rating scheme	Level of function and alertness

(Continued)

TABLE 8.3 *(Continued)*

Name of Instrument	Description	Purpose
Profile of Mood States	Self-administered questionnaire	Assessment of individual mood dimensions such as depression and anxiety
Gleason Coma Scale	Observer-administered protocol	Depth of coma
CARES	Self-administered questionnaire	Impact of gynecological conditions on relationships and sexuality
International Index of Erectile Function	Self-administered questionnaire	Male sexual function

PROGRAM EVALUATION

Program evaluation focuses not on medical agents or procedures but on practices, policies, and organizational arrangements to deliver services and prevent illness. Investigations of such interventions are also called *evaluation research* or *action research.* Public agencies initiate evaluation research to assess the impact of the programs to which they allocate funds. In 1999, for example, Congress appropriated $10 million for evaluation of the multibillion-dollar State Children's Health Insurance Program.[8] Many private-sector sponsors allocate a percentage of the budget of an intervention to evaluation.

Technically, evaluation research has drawn on many of the same procedures used by more traditional biomedical research. Evaluation of an intervention outside the laboratory or physician's office, though, is necessarily more than traditional science. For this reason, evaluation researchers have employed an eclectic mix of methodologies. The most frequently used evaluation techniques are described next.

Traditional Experiment

Several widely cited evaluation efforts have mimicked RCTs. Group Health Co-operative of Puget Sound, for example, used a randomized experimental procedure to assess a program of preventive services for elders.[9] Elders consenting to participate received health risk assessments and were randomly assigned to an intervention or a

control group. Those exposed to the intervention were invited to attend health educa-
tion sessions and participate in activities that addressed their individual health risks.
Individuals in the control group received normal preventive services available at the
HMO, but were not invited to health education sessions or risk-related interventions.
Data were collected on health status, components of care, and costs at twenty-four and
forty-eight months postrandomization.

Survey Methods

Survey techniques have also been widely used for evaluation purposes. This approach
was applied, for example, to evaluate a foundation-funded effort to educate California
legislators and others capable of influencing state health policy on the importance of
health promotion and disease prevention.[10] The evaluation team conducted a telephone
survey of legislators, lobbyists, staff, and executive branch officials. Items on survey
instruments asked about respondents' familiarity with the education program, the
importance they attributed to prevention, and the degree to which their policy making
may have been influenced by the foundation's efforts.

Case Studies

Attempts by evaluation researchers to utilize techniques of traditional biomedical science have often met with frustration. This is particularly true of efforts to conduct randomized experiments. Human beings tend to resist control over their behavior. When
a subject is randomized into a control group, there is no assurance that the person will
not simply opt to behave as those in the intervention do, or obtain the same resources
as those in the intervention have received. As noted earlier, surveys often suffer from
bias and inaccuracy due to subject recall or self-report.

Frustrated by these difficulties, the evaluation field has developed some of its
own approaches. A very popular evaluation approach is the logic model case study,
as described earlier. When guided by a well-thought-out theory of how an intervention should work, the logic model case study can provide plausible evidence for the
intervention's efficacy. Less methodologically sophisticated case study procedures
have also proven useful to evaluators. Strictly descriptive case studies, for example,
can serve as important means for recording and interpreting complex and far-reaching
events in an extended intervention. Descriptive case studies are likely to be more
meaningful to some stakeholders than more abstract forms of data recording, analysis,
or presentation.

Quasi-Experimental Design

Evaluation researchers have also embraced the so-called quasi-experimental design
as an alternative to the RCT or straightforward survey methodology. Campbell and
Stanley, pioneering exponents of quasi-experimental design, conceive of it as a category of procedures intended "to achieve some degree of control where random
assignment to equivalent groups is not possible."[11] Such control is achievable via mechanisms such as schedule and differential exposure of subjects to interventions short

of randomization. Quasi-experimental design admits multiple methods of observation and analysis. It is most valid when the researcher is aware of the variables he has not been able to control or measure.

A study by investigators at Kaiser Permanente in Portland, Oregon, illustrates one type of quasi-experimental procedure called an *interrupted time series design*.[12] This study assessed the efficacy of medical record alerts in reducing prescription of warfarin along with potentially adverse interacting (contraindicated) medication. Warfarin is a widely prescribed medication for preventing blood clots and embolisms. Originally developed as a rat poison, warfarin exposes patients to the possibility of internal bleeding. This risk increases when the drug is used at the same time as certain other medications. Alerts in the electronic medical record system at Kaiser Permanente regarding drugs that should not be used alongside warfarin constituted an intervention intended to reduce this risk. A physician prescribing both warfarin and a contraindicated medication via the Kaiser Permanente's electronic medical record system would receive an alert on her computer screen.

An interrupted time series experiment was conducted with physicians in fifteen primary care clinics. All physicians in the clinics were exposed to the intervention. The hoped-for outcome was a decrease in prescription of contraindicated medications among patients taking warfarin. Physician prescribing behavior was followed for thirty months prior to the intervention and eighteen months afterward.

A modest decline in prescription of contraindicated medication occurred immediately following introduction of the intervention. The decrease was sustained throughout the subsequent followup period. Such results would appear to substantiate the intervention's efficacy. However, this conclusion must remain tentative. The quasi-experimental approach cannot rule out alternative explanations.

Empowerment Evaluation

It is important to note that high-quality evaluation research requires cooperation among several parties with traditionally different interests and concerns. The evaluator depends on subjects of the evaluation (including managers, providers, and clients) to furnish data. Evaluation, however, is seldom a primary concern for operations personnel. These individuals tend to focus strongly on making sure that action is initiated and clients are served. Evaluation, moreover, can be scary for those being evaluated. One method for creating the necessary collaboration is called *participatory* or *empowerment evaluation*. This approach allows people normally considered objects of study to help specify evaluation questions and share in the interpretation of data.[13]

Empowerment or participatory evaluation makes sense. In addition to promoting collaboration, this approach enables people normally considered subjects of research—health professionals, managers, and clients—to pose evaluation questions that will help them improve the intervention while it is still ongoing. Possible payoff of this kind can motivate strong and constructive collaboration.

Alternatively, however, participatory evaluation can have a negative effect on the evaluation process. This occurs when program personnel use the mandate for participation in a defensive manner. In this respect, they may try to keep difficult but crucial questions—those that address program performance and outcomes—off the evaluation agenda. Evaluation professionals face the task of demonstrating to operations personnel and clients that high-quality evaluation is in everyone's interests.

COST-EFFECTIVENESS AND COST-BENEFIT ANALYSIS

Cost-effectiveness and cost-benefit analysis, both techniques in widespread use, may be applied in the context of both traditional biomedical research and program evaluation. **Cost-effectiveness analysis** determines the financial cost of a desired health or health-related outcome. Formally, cost-effectiveness comprises a ratio of dollars to number of successful outcomes achieved. Analysis yields the dollar cost of a unit of output such as deaths avoided in a particular year, days of continued ability to work, years of physical function preserved, or number of teen pregnancies avoided.

Cost-effectiveness analysis can be applied to indicators that capture multiple dimensions of health outcomes. Quality-adjusted life years (QALYs), for example, reflect both lives saved and quality of life experienced during each year. Applying cost-effectiveness analysis to QALYs is particularly valuable in deciding whether to add a new treatment to the array of services covered by an insurance plan.

Two studies of cancer therapy illustrate this application. An investigation headed by economist Louis P. Garrison assessed the cost-effectiveness of adding a new and expensive chemotherapeutic agent (trastuzumab) to standard breast cancer therapy. Other research had already determined that adding trastuzumab to standard treatment extends life expectancy. Assuming that treatment would take place over a period of twenty years, the research team found the cost-benefit ratio of adding trastuzumab to be $34,201 per QALY gained.[14] Another research team compared alternative treatments for prostate cancer. For a sixty-year old man, the cost of relatively conventional radiation treatment was $39,355; the cost of newer, potentially more effective proton beam therapy $64,989. The incremental cost-effectiveness ratio for proton beam therapy was $55,726 per QALY.[15]

Cost-benefit analysis yields the magnitude of dollars lost or gained as a result of a health intervention. To perform cost-benefit analysis, dollar values must be computed for the outcomes achieved. In this fashion, the monetary value of an additional year of life or an unwanted pregnancy avoided must be ascertained. The complexity of computing money values for health outcomes has discouraged some investigators from engaging in cost-benefit analysis, although the research literature contains examples of great importance.

THE SOCIAL AND ECONOMIC CONTEXT
OF RESEARCH

This chapter has so far addressed research and evaluation largely as technical matters. While important for a critical understanding of the implications of research for management and policy, a technical overview is necessarily limited. Of greater importance in some instances is the broader array of constraints, motivations, and institutions that govern science. These factors materially influence the quality and applicability of both biomedical research and program evaluation. Managers and policy makers require as full an understanding of this context as of the technicalities themselves.

Research Funding

Funding drives both biomedical and evaluation research. Research of any importance today requires sponsorship. Even a small project requires laboratory space, equipment, and technical personnel costing far more than an individual scientist can pay through personal resources. Payers for research include government agencies, nonprofit organizations, and private firms. These entities provide funds via grants and contracts to universities and free-standing research organizations, both profit-seeking and nonprofit.

At the extreme, large-scale clinical trials or observational studies cost many millions of dollars. Availability of generous funding draws talent from all quarters of the research community, while reduced funding drives people out. Financial support for biomedical research, the manner in which it is obtained, and the way in which it is used constitute key concerns for everyone involved in health care.

Biomedical research today should be viewed as an industry in its own right. Like other industries, biomedical research carries out training and recruitment functions, establishes organizational structures, and maintains hierarchies. The industry supports significant numbers of personnel who do no actual research but play support, administrative, and executive roles. Thus, research operations require funding not only to cover the pay of scientists and maintenance of laboratories but also for indirect costs to meet the broader needs of the organizations.

The support requirements of research add significantly to the cost of sponsorship. Typically, organizations that apply for grants or contracts compute a percentage of the direct cost of the proposed research and add it to their total request for funding. This percentage is known as the *indirect rate.* For grants received in 2008, Stanford University negotiated an indirect rate with the federal government of 58 percent.[16] This meant that on a grant awarding $1 million to a biomedical scientist to cover his research, Stanford received an additional $580,000 for maintenance of facilities, research support salaries, and the like. Critics have commented that payment of indirect expenses by funding agencies unjustly escalates the cost of science. But universities and other research organizations contend that they do not fully recover their indirect expenses, even with such payment.

In 2003, nearly all funds for biomedical research came from seven sources. Total revenue from these sources approximated $94 billion. Amounts and percentages allocated by source included the following:

Pharmaceutical firms	$27.0 billion (29 percent)
National Institutes of Health	$26.4 billion (28 percent)
Biotechnology firms	$17.9 billion (19 percent)
Medical device firms	$9.2 billion (10 percent)
Other federal agencies	$6.9 billion (7 percent)
State and local government	$4.3 billion (5 percent)
Private sources (including individuals and foundations)	$2.5 billion (3 percent)

In summary, government agencies at all levels provided $37.6 billion (40 percent), profit-seeking firms $ 54.1 billion (58 percent), and noncommercial private sources $2.5 billion (3 percent).[17]

Important changes in sources of research funding occurred between 1994 and 2003. Government-allocated dollars approximately doubled during this time period. But the percentage allocated by private, profit-seeking firms including pharmacy, biotech, and medical device companies outstripped the government-funded growth. Resources contributed by private individuals and firms increased in dollars, but declined as a percentage of the total. A longer historical look would reveal an even more strongly declining role for noncommercial private dollars in biomedical research.

Each potential source of funding for biomedical and related fields of research has its own objectives, procedures, and challenges. Although obtaining funds from any source is difficult and uncertain, each of the sources described next has its own risks, rewards, and challenges.

For-Profit Companies. Decisions by commercial entities to fund research must depend on the estimated likelihood of business success. A new drug or device must be approved by the FDA in order to recover the huge expenses of research. Once the decision to fund has been made, research may take place in-house or under contract to outside organizations, often to universities. Research on new interventions always represents a gamble for the private firm. For this reason, funding typically favors interventions for highly prevalent conditions, ensuring high sales volume should the new drug or device prove effective.

Public Agencies. Public agencies provide most of the funding for research unrelated to near-term commercial opportunity. Basic science research and clinical investigations, as well as studies relevant to health care delivery and policy, are funded predominantly by the U.S. Public Health Service (PHS), itself part of the Department of Health and Human Services. Relevant units of the PHS include the National Institutes of Health (NIH), the Centers for Disease Control and Prevention, and the Agency for Healthcare Research and Quality. These and several other PHS units provide grant funding to outside scientists through extramural research programs. The process of obtaining funds from these agencies is complex and highly competitive. In 2006, for example, only about 20 percent of the applications to NIH received funding.

Private Foundations and Individuals. A private foundation is a nongovernmental, nonprofit organization with funds from a permanent portfolio of investments known as an *endowment*. Typically, an endowment originates from a single source, such as an individual, a family, or a corporation. Legally, foundations are chartered to maintain or aid social, educational, religious, or other charitable activities serving the common good. They are owned by trustees who hold the foundation's assets in trust for the people of the jurisdiction in which they are chartered. Governance is carried out by a board of directors. Trustees usually sit on boards of directors, but directors are not always trustees. Foundations of significant size employ staff to recommend policy, evaluate applications for funding, and perform day-to-day administrative tasks.

Like federal agencies, private foundations identify areas of interest and disseminate this information to the grant-seeking community. New interests and areas of emphasis emerge periodically through initiation by staff or discussion among directors and trustees. Large foundations such as Robert Wood Johnson and W. K. Kellogg seem to change their areas of emphasis approximately every decade or upon accession of a new president. Foundations often develop initiatives articulating interests focused on specific concerns, and issue program announcements and RFAs in these areas.

The process of evaluating grant requests is less formal in private foundations than in government. Still, funding is highly competitive. In 1999, for example, the Robert Wood Johnson Foundation's Web site advised potential applicants that their chances of success were one in twenty. In the 1990s, this foundation operated an investigator program in health policy. Each year, this program received over four hundred letters of inquiry and awarded no more than ten grants.

Research Advocacy and Politics

Closely associated with the struggle for funding is the political atmosphere that inevitably surrounds biomedical research. Large-scale issues in the politics of research sometimes come into the view of the general public. Early twenty-first-century examples included prohibitions in federal policy against funding research involving fetal stem cells and recombinant DNA. Earlier epochs saw controversy over use of public funds for research on agents believed by some to be effective against cancer. These included vitamin C, advocated by Nobel Prize–winner Linus Pauling, and Laetrile, an agent derived from apricot pits. Mainstream scientists saw no evidence to suggest that either agent merited a definitive RCT. Yet prominence in the press and widespread public interest eventually compelled NIH to fund RCTs for both vitamin C and Laetril, neither of which proved effective.[18, 19]

Public Agitation. Breast cancer provides perhaps the best example of a successful political effort to move a particular focus of research into prominence and public support. During the late twentieth century, advocates of breast cancer awareness and intervention did much to promote public awareness. First Ladies Betty Ford and Nancy Reagan and events such as the Race for the Cure helped give the disease visibility. Breast cancer advocates championed increased research into the disease. During the 1990s federal funding for breast cancer research increased from $81 million to more than $400 million.[20]

The Politics of Program Evaluation. Evaluation researchers face challenges in some ways akin to those of traditional biomedical science. Sometimes multiple responses to evaluation RFPs are assessed by committees of technically qualified personnel in a manner similar to the NIH selection process. This is particularly true in government agencies. Private agencies have greater liberty to seek a bid from only one vendor (a process called *sole sourcing*) for evaluation services. By negotiating a sole source contract, the agency seeks to work with an evaluator in which it has confidence due to earlier association or public reputation.

In practice, evaluation researchers face pressure to report positive results. Funding agencies often have ambitious expectations regarding operating units and grantees, and a strong interest in their success. Whether public or private, funding agencies value evidence of success in order to please stakeholders. Foundation staff would rather bring encouraging messages to their boards, just as executive branch officials would prefer to report positive results to congressional committees.

Program operations staff or external grantees have a more direct motivation to press for positive evaluation. Government agencies prefer to see their programs positively evaluated in part because favorable evaluation increases the likelihood of steady or increased resource allocations. Many foundation grantee organizations are small, community-based nonprofits. Like biomedical researchers, they occupy an intensely competitive and uncertain funding environment. Grantees tend to view evaluators with suspicion. Findings by evaluators that goals have not been achieved may jeopardize future funding. Many of the problems tackled by grant-funded nonprofits are in fact quite difficult to achieve, such as adverse health behavior, urban blight, racism, lack of economic opportunity, and crime.

Evaluators need to work collaboratively with both funding agencies and grantees. Evaluation professionals require favorable relations with funding agencies for future business. Evaluators also need to work cooperatively with program operating units and grantees. The goodwill of operating units and grantees is crucial, because evaluators depend on them for data. Cooperation is advanced by expectations of favorable findings among those being evaluated. An empowerment evaluation approach helps forge ties between evaluation professionals and program personnel. This dynamic may result in omission of the most difficult evaluation questions, spinning of marginal achievements into allegedly important lessons, and presentation of indefinite or ambiguous conclusions.

Striking Back at Science: Threatened Interests Shoot the Messenger

The findings of biomedical and evaluation research today can have immense financial, policy, and public health impact. Interests threatened by the results of research do not stand idly by. Rather, they protect themselves by challenging scientific findings, discrediting scientists, and depriving investigators of resources necessary for scientific inquiry.

A striking example of opposition by financial interests to potentially damaging research findings occurred in response to a series of studies led by Dr. Richard A. Deyo. According to these studies, a widely used procedure for chronic back pain called spinal-fusion surgery was found to have "few scientifically validated indications" and to be "associated with higher costs and more complications than other back operations."[21] Deyo's research team recommended nonsurgical approaches instead.

The team's findings drew a sharp reaction from orthopedic surgeons involved in spinal fusion work. Members the North American Spine Society launched a letter-writing campaign to their congress members alleging that Deyo's research team had been biased and inept. The surgeons lobbied for a total defunding of the Agency for Health Care Policy and Research (AHCPR), which had awarded grants to Deyo and whose mandate from Congress included research on outcomes of medical interventions.

The lobbyists' efforts were successful. In the following year, the House of Representatives passed a budget with no funds for AHCPR. Although the Senate restored some funding, AHCPR's scope was substantially reduced.

SCIENCE GONE WRONG: ERROR, DISTORTION, AND FRAUD

History suggests that the products of science must be viewed with skepticism. Even the best-conducted science is subject to error, sometimes avoidable and sometimes not. Human ethical lapses, moreover, have led to intentional corruption of science, famously illustrated in scandals ranging from Charles Dawson's faked Piltdown Man of 1912 to Hwang Woo Suk's bogus patient-derived embryonic stem cell colonies of 2005. The social and economic context of science today—notably competition, careerism, and the profit motive—has raised the odds of scientific error and misconduct.

Scientific Error

Error is endemic and necessary in science. Scientific progress may be said to proceed via detection and correction of error. Experiments and less systematic observations build the literature of a scientific field. This literature in turn generates hypotheses regarding matters such as disease prevention and cure. When further experimentation and observations indicate that such hypotheses are erroneous, the literature behind them must be rethought. Individual researchers also fall into less forgivable types of error as well.

Erroneous Leads from the Scientific Literature. The field of cancer prevention illustrates how initially exciting theories may give rise to disappointment. The rise and fall of *cancer chemoprevention* provides an example.

Prominent biomedical scientists in the 1980s looked at diet as a way to prevent certain cancers. Epidemiological studies and experiments with animals had suggested that ingestion of substances such as vitamins A and E could prevent cancers of the lung and breast. A series of randomized clinical trials gave high dosages of these vitamins (or their chemical precursors) to people at high risk of these diseases.

The trials were large and long term. In one study, 29,133 subjects were randomly divided into groups receiving vitamin E (tocopherol), a vitamin A precursor (beta carotene), or a placebo.[22] These individuals were followed for five to eight years. In another study, over 18,000 individuals were randomized into groups receiving both beta carotene and vitamin A or a placebo.[23] To the disappointment of chemoprevention advocates, individuals given the presumably preventive substances had higher rates of cancer incidence than those given placebos. One of the trials had to be terminated early to avoid further health risks to the subjects.

Similarly disappointing results have emerged from theory related to the prevention of smoking among adolescents. In a landmark randomized trial involving 8,388 children and youths, researchers tested an intervention based on the most widely accepted principles of health education at the time. Expertly designed and conducted, the study lasted from 1984 through 1999. The report concluded, however, that there was no evidence from this trial that the intervention was effective.[24]

Investigator and System Bias. Often unaware, researchers themselves can introduce error into their experiments, analysis of data, and reporting of results. The desire to find positive results, for example, can contribute to the publication of erroneous findings. Positive findings consistent with expectations in the investigator's field are most easily published in widely read journals. Resulting publications promote successful careers.

John Ioannidis, a widely published analyst of biomedical research, defines *bias* as "the combination of various design, data, analysis, and presentation factors that tend to produce research findings when they should not be produced."[25] He cites manipulation in the analysis or reporting of findings and selective or distorted reporting as examples of bias. Bias, he writes, "should not be confused with chance variability that causes some findings to be false by chance even though the study design, data, analysis, and presentation are perfect." Bias in favor of results that are positive and consistent with current scientific literature, however, pushes investigators to use a variety of means to produce such results. Such means include *data dredging*, or seeking the hoped-for results within selected groups of subjects, rather than within the entire study population. According to Ioannidis, such bias has introduced error into biomedical literature on a huge scale.[26]

Distortion of Findings

As opposed to literature-driven and other unconscious bias, findings from research may be distorted intentionally. Investigators with commercial objectives provide examples. It is important to remember that drug trials have crucial financial implications for the pharmaceutical firms that sponsor them.

RCTs of Iamin, a medication otherwise known as Blue Goo used for diabetic foot lesions, illustrate a process leading to distortion of research findings.[27] After an early round of trials, Blue Goo manufacturer ProCyte reported that the medication seemed effective in healing wounds on the feet of diabetic patients who otherwise faced amputation. But after conducting more advanced tests, ProCyte announced that the drug failed to outperform a placebo. Within minutes of the announcement, ProCyte's stock fell 68 percent.

It became apparent that ProCyte scientists had used biased methodology to make Blue Goo appear a successful product in the early trials. These scientists engaged in data dredging by dismissing negative overall results and focusing on apparent success among intentionally selected patients.

In one study, eighty-one patients were randomly assigned to receive treatment with Blue Goo or a placebo. After the trial ended, company scientists examined the data for the distinguishing characteristic of those who responded consistently well to Blue Goo. They found that the medication worked consistently well within a highly specific group of patients—individuals with diabetic ulcer wounds on the soles of their feet (excluding those with leg wounds) and whose wounds had started out bigger than four inches square.

Reactions to medication by individuals within a specific population segment can be a legitimate focus of research. However, the motivation of ProCyte seems to have been retaining the interest of its investors and keeping its stock from losing value. To do this, the firm made a special effort to identify a small group of patients who seemed to do well on Blue Goo. In such a situation, however, it cannot be concluded that members of this group responded favorably because of a shared feature of their illness. These patients may have escaped deterioration of their foot wounds purely by chance.

Fraudulent Science

The frequency of outright fraud in biomedical science is unknown. Journals and review panels do not normally check tables and narrative against a scientist's raw data. Although readers may criticize logic and inference, they generally accept the observations reported as having been actually made.

However, scientific fraud certainly occurs. Fraud may take the form of outright fabrication of data, lying about how the data were obtained, or intentionally misleading readers about what a sample represents. Motivation for fraudulent science arises from diverse sources. University-based scientists may compromise their standards due to pressure for high-volume publication and grant getting. Among industry scientists, the desire to obtain regulatory approval for a new intervention or promote public confidence in it may lead some to fraudulence. The wish to support a concept or theory that does not quite fit the data obtained from an experiment may tempt a researcher to fabricate, distort, or misrepresent observations. Ironically, people who merely wish to be thought of as members of the scientific community—for reasons of self-esteem and prestige—may use fraudulent science to obtain the desired status.

A famous case involving fraud concerned heart researcher John R. Darsee, who was reported to have fabricated data for more than one hundred papers he wrote while at Harvard and Emory Universities. There was no controversy regarding Darsee's misdeeds. However, rancorous disagreement arose over whether the Darsee fabrications reflected merely the deeds of an isolated rogue or flaws in the operation of modern science itself. NIH investigators, for example, implied that large numbers of Darsee's colleagues and coauthors shirked their responsibility to examine his work for inconsistency and evidence of fraud.[28]

KEY TERMS

Experimental design	Descriptive case study
Randomized controlled trial (RCT)	Reliability
Placebo effect	Program evaluation
Validity	Cost-effectiveness analysis
Case-control method	Cost-benefit analysis

SUMMARY

This chapter summarizes methods of research used in the biomedical sciences and health services delivery and suggests standards for acceptability of research for making management and policy decisions.

Research is a major component of the U.S. health care industry. Funds expended within this sector approximated $100 billion in 2008. The importance of research extends well beyond this funding level, because research helps determine the service delivered by the system as a whole.

The randomized controlled trial (RCT) constitutes the gold standard of traditional biomedical research. But the RCT is unable to address many concerns that arise in the prevention, treatment, and cost of illness. Widely used alternative research designs include case-control studies, surveys, and quasi-experimental procedures. For definitive findings, all research techniques require standardized measures of outcomes such as disease parameters, patient-reported symptoms, and quality-of-life indices. A critical component of this research concerns the degree to which added cost of new technology may be justified by benefit to the consumer.

Challenges to research today extend beyond scientific methodology. These include potential exclusion from RCTs of minorities, scarcity and attrition of research subjects, and increasingly stringent ethical and legal concerns. The majority of biomedical research dollars today come from profit-seeking industry, raising the possibility of conflict with scientific and consumer interests. Error, distortion, and fraud are always possible in science.

DISCUSSION QUESTIONS

1. How much confidence should the public have in findings published in leading medical journals today?

2. Observational research designs involving case studies and surveys have clearly lower levels of validity than RCTs. To what extent can observational methods have genuine value in (a) biomedical science and (b) evaluation research?

3. To what degree should advocacy—including agitation for attention to particular diseases—play a role in research funding decisions by public agencies?

4. It has been asserted in this chapter that the degree of competition that prevails in science today promotes fraud and corruption. To what degree is this true? What remedies might be feasible and effective?

5. Is the balance that exists today between public and private biomedical research funding favorable or unfavorable to the public interest? If not, what remedies might be considered?

PART

PATHS FORWARD

Despite the stability of some essential elements, the U.S. health care system has undergone significant change in recent decades. A variety of innovations has been formulated and implemented. Some of these innovations have been sustained, others abandoned, and still others are evolving in unforeseen ways. Changes now in the process of implementation and soon to be implemented will determine access to and quality of health care that the United States will experience for generations to come.

The late twentieth and early twenty-first centuries saw fundamental changes in the ways U.S. health care was financed and delivered. Examples included selective contracting, cost sharing, and managed care. These innovations have unquestionably saved money for some payers over the short run. But their ability to promote sustained control over costs is in doubt. Quality of care, moreover, may have begun to suffer as a consequence of cost-control interventions.

Many professionals and members of the public have looked to prevention as a means of controlling health care costs and maintaining the public's health. The health care system can do much to prevent illness through immunization and early detection of diseases. In addition, research has demonstrated that certain dietary and exercise practices can help maintain individual health. However, Americans do not consistently practice healthy lifestyles. Economic and neighborhood factors reduce opportunity for health promotion among the disadvantaged. Cost-effectiveness analysis, moreover, suggests that health promotion and disease prevention will not reduce health care costs in the United States.

Government and public policy makers must participate as drivers of change in U.S. health care. Despite the private character of the U.S. health care system, government today plays an increasingly important role. Health care professionals and organizations operate in an environment crowded with government requirements and regulations. Analysts have disputed the degree to which the consumer benefits from government participation in health care. Since the 1940s, a series of major legislative mandates have helped make the U.S. health care system what it is today. Some have clearly benefitted the public; others have had unanticipated, adverse consequences; still others have been implemented, found impracticable, and abandoned. Public action in the United States takes place through the building of coalitions, an activity whose difficulty should not be underestimated.

The future of U.S. health care will depend on how Americans resolve several long-standing issues. Concrete solutions to some of these were presented to Americans in the Patient Protection and Affordable Care Act. But controversy surrounding the associated legislation underscores the challenges long prominent in U.S. health care. Responsibility for payment remains the master controversy, raising, in turn, dilemmas regarding how much care individuals may expect to receive, how the disadvantaged are to be treated, and how much of the system's direction will be handled by the private versus public sector. Although policy makers have looked to other countries for models, few if any of these are directly applicable to the U.S health care system. In making changes that will be required, Americans will have to reconcile seemingly incompatible values, such as meritocracy versus equality. Age-old features of health care, including the mystery of its application and emotional involvement of its recipients, suggest that associated management and policy issues will never be fully resolved.

CHAPTER

IMPACT OF INNOVATION

Utilization, Cost, and Quality of Care

LEARNING OBJECTIVES

- To review historic innovations in health service delivery
- To understand the quality of care
- To grasp the impact of selective contracting, cost sharing, and managed care on utilization, cost, and quality
- To anticipate the outcomes of evidence-based medicine, pay for performance, and public dissemination of cost and quality information
- To apply a critical approach to innovations

HEALTH SERVICE INNOVATIONS: STRATEGIC AND TACTICAL

Although fundamentally stable, the U.S. health care system has continually evolved through successive innovations. These innovations may be thought of as both strategic and tactical. Innovations classifiable as strategic influence actions across most, if not all, segments of the health care industry. Other initiatives, because of their selective and often discretionary adoption, may be thought of as *tactical* or *limited.*

Key strategic innovations have included selective contracting, cost sharing, and managed care. To review earlier chapters, *selective contracting* emerged from a desire among public officials to control Medicaid costs and was rapidly adopted by the private sector. Legislation and regulatory decisions enabled hospitals and physician groups to bid against each other for contracts to serve health plan enrollees. Resulting contracts often featured price discounts or prospective payment provisions. *Cost sharing* requires consumers to make out-of-pocket payments for care in the form of deductibles and copayments at the point of purchase. *Managed care* involves the placement of an organizational mechanism between the patient and the provider to regulate utilization.

Many less comprehensive but potentially quite important interventions have been developed for the purpose of controlling costs, improving quality, or both. Only three examples will be addressed in this chapter to illustrate widely discussed and deployed interventions in the early twenty-first century. These include evidence-based medicine, pay for performance, and public dissemination of price and quality information.

Evidence-based medicine may be thought of as using systematic, high-quality research as the basis of medical education and decision making. The goal of evidence-based medicine is ultimately to develop standards of care validated through both new research and synthesis of existing studies. Strong scientific evidence is lacking for the efficacy of many medical interventions in widespread use today. As a consequence, great variability has been reported in both the cost and content of medical care across geographical areas.

Evidence-based medicine represents a break with past practice by de-emphasizing unsystematic clinical observation and the authority of teachers, superiors, and tradition. The evidence-based medicine concept, though, continues to recognize the validity of judgment in individual cases and the importance of patient preferences.[1]

Closely tied to the development of evidence-based medicine is *pay for performance* applied to hospitals, health plans, and individual clinicians. Availability of research-based treatment guidelines enables managers and physician leaders to develop templates for patient care. Under pay-for-performance schemes, physicians who practice according to these guidelines receive monetary rewards. Key U.S. health care institutions such as the Institute of Medicine and the Centers for Medicare and Medicaid Services (CMS) have promoted the concept of pay for performance. Commercial insurance companies have implemented the concept by creating scorecards to reflect quality of care by providers.[2]

In turn, firms and agencies concerned with health care have developed mechanisms for *dissemination of price and quality information to consumers.* CMS, for example, has instituted Hospital Compare, a publicly available web site displaying hospital-level quality measures.[3] A near majority of U.S. states make quality measures for individual Medicaid health plans available on the web.[4] HEDIS has instituted a consumer-accessible database allowing comparison of health plans. *Value-based insurance* designs are a related concept. Insurance designs of this kind maintain cost sharing for interventions of uncertain value, but reduce cost sharing for interventions known to be effective.[5] Other proposed approaches include deployment of information technology throughout the health care industry and expansion of high risk insurance pools at the state level.

Proposals for comprehensive health care reform have periodically emerged in the U.S. policy arena. Such proposals are of much larger scale than those covered in this chapter. But these proposals require assessment according to the same criteria as smaller-scale innovations.

INNOVATIONS AND HEALTH SERVICE OBJECTIVES

Before examining the impact of the innovations outlined above, it is important to review the objectives of the U.S. health care system—or systems providing health services anywhere in the world. A health care system's fundamental objectives today should be to increase life expectancy and to preserve physical and mental functioning. Objectives widely considered creditable include enhancement of quality of life, even in the absence of readily observable disease. Thus, people in the United States and other affluent countries expect that services such as cosmetic dentistry and surgery, psychotherapy, and fertility enhancement will be available to them. Americans look to the health care system for information and guidance for preventing illness through exercise, nutrition, and overcoming alcohol and tobacco abuse.

Assessment of innovations in health service delivery, then, cannot focus exclusively on potential cost savings. Too great an emphasis on this objective ignores the fact that health services benefit the public. Assessment of innovation needs to include impact on availability and affordability of services, appropriate utilization by consumers, and the quality of care.

Assessing Innovations

Considerable research has taken place on the impact of the strategic and tactical innovations outlined earlier. This research has used many of the principles detailed in Chapter Eight. A brief description of the approaches taken by researchers to assess these innovations is important for a critical understanding of their findings. In researchers' terminology, appearance of innovations such as selective contracting, cost sharing, and managed care constitute *independent variables.* Key *dependent variables* include cost, utilization, and quality of care.

The Concept of Quality

Of the effects hoped for from an innovation, quality is the most difficult to define and measure. This is true in part because the ultimate effect of a medical intervention is often difficult to observe. People remain sick or get well for multiple reasons. The effect of a medical intervention may not be immediate and may address only some of the causes or consequences of an illness. This is particularly true of *modern disease* as defined in Chapter Three. For generations, clinicians and scientists have worked toward developing widely accepted quality measures and means of applying these measures throughout the health care system.

The work of Dr. Adevis Donabedian, a pioneer in research on the quality of health care, has contributed significantly to this objective. As early as the 1960s, Donabedian proposed that quality be assessed according to three dimensions: structure, process, and outcome. His formulation continues to help define how quality is measured.

According to Donabedian, **structure** involves qualifications of staff, adequacy of financial and administrative arrangements, and availability of resources such as equipment and infrastructure in a practice, facility, or community. **Process** addresses the question, in Donabedian's words, of "whether medicine is properly practiced." From the vantage point of process, quality is signified by consistency of practice with applicable standards of diagnosis and treatment. In today's language, standards of care for specific clinical issues and evidence-based medicine constitute criteria for quality on the process dimension. Donabedian conceives of **outcomes** according to such familiar health status objectives as recovery, function, survival, and "social restoration of patients discharged from psychiatric hospitals."[6]

In summary, the process dimension of quality of care may be thought of as "what is done to the patient." The outcome dimension might be considered "what ultimately happens to the patient." While some may contend that concern with outcomes should predominate, favorable outcomes depend on the presence of quality in structure and process. Process measures are particularly important in view of the fact that outcomes may not become apparent for many years or may be difficult to observe for other reasons.

Assessment of quality has become an important function within individual health care organizations. For many years hospitals, managed care operations, and other health care organizations have maintained data systems on quality of care. These systems have played an important role in quality assurance, cost control, and accountability. They have served as a resource for discussion among clinicians for the purposes of recognizing errors and taking steps to avoid them in the future. Research on quality measurement has accelerated as the health care system has become more competitive and transparent. Many of the same measures used for the internal purposes of health care organizations are important as well in assessing the impact of innovation within the system as a whole.

Levels of Analysis

The impact of innovation must be assessed on two levels. First, innovation may be expected to affect an entire *community, city,* or *region.* Analysis at this level is important

Dr. Codman and the Origin of Quality Assessment

The origin of quality assessment is sometimes traced to a publication by Ernest Amory Codman—*A Study in Hospital Efficiency,* sometimes called the **Codman Report**. Published in 1917, it has been reprinted by The Joint Commission as late as the 1990s.

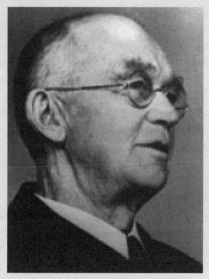

Ernest Amory Codman (1869–1940)

A prominent Boston surgeon, Codman made a lifelong practice of tracking patients for years after treatment to assess the outcomes of his care. He recorded his surgical errors and assessed their relationship to ultimate patient outcomes for the purpose of improving surgical practice. This process would today be called *continuous quality improvement.* In order to pursue this course, Codman resigned from a prestigious post at Massachusetts General Hospital and started his own facility, which he named End Result Hospital. There, Codman worked with some of the most talented surgeons of his day. Nevertheless, his team reported diagnostic or surgical error in one of every three patients.

Codman made the facts about his hospital's performance public in annual reports. Sending these reports to hospitals throughout the United States, he urged others to conduct similar record keeping and reporting. Antagonizing the Boston medical establishment with his campaign, Codman saw his income decline and his professional reputation maligned.

The Codman story serves as a reminder that calls for quality assurance and accountability are not always well received. Reviewing his own work, Codman commented that assessment and criticism of results were rare in the hospitals of his time. Memorably, he wrote: "It is the duty of no one and for the interest of no one—except for the patients and for the community."[7]

for assessment of the impact of competition among health care providers. Impact assessment of policies favorable to competitive contracting, for example, must determine whether they produce the hoped-for reduction in costs. Relevant information must be collected from hospitals and health plans. Prices and service offerings must be compared across market areas with varying levels of competition.

The effects of other innovations are best determined by observing *individual consumers.* Analysts, for example, have conducted numerous studies on the impact of cost sharing and managed care on consumer behavior. Elements of consumer behavior that have been studied include the volume and types of health services consumers utilize. Impact of an innovation on quality of care may be assessed according to the criterion of appropriateness of utilization. An innovation that reduced utilization of low value—unnecessary services, for example—would be considered favorable in terms of the system's objectives. An innovation that reduced utilization of high value—such as important services—would be considered unfavorable.

Equally important is assessment of the quality of services that consumers are offered. Researchers have assessed care that patients receive through standardized measures. In some instances, researchers have used *process* measures, comparing the care that individuals receive to standards developed by expert clinicians and evidence-based criteria. In other instances, researchers have assessed impact on care through patient *outcomes* such as health, function, and longevity.

Types of Studies

To assess prices, service availability, utilization, and quality, health services researchers have typically used *observational studies.* As noted in Chapter Eight, this term designates research methods other than the randomized controlled trial (RCT) typical of biomedical experimentation. Rather than randomly assigning individuals to experimental and control groups, health service researchers obtain data from patient records, conduct surveys, or use administrative databases containing information on utilization and costs. Such procedures are less clearly able to assess actual impact of an intervention than more traditional scientific methods. But they are often the only means practically available.

Among studies of the impact of innovation in health service delivery, the **Rand Health Insurance Experiment (Rand HIE)** stands out in importance. The Rand HIE represents a rare use of the RCT in health services research. Although the study took place in the 1970s, it is still widely referenced and serves as the basis for continuing research. As indicated in Chapter Eight, the RCT has greater validity than observational studies of any kind. Just as the RCT represents the gold standard for research in general, the Rand HIE is often called the gold standard for research on health insurance and outcomes.

In the Rand HIE, researchers randomly assigned U.S. families to insurance plans with differing characteristics.[8] Among the plans to which subjects were assigned, five produced the clearest and most widely cited results. Four of these plans were of the indemnity type, in which consumers received care on a fee-for-service basis in their communities. Each of the four indemnity plans differed in the amount of cost sharing required of the consumer. A "free care" plan made the consumer responsible for neither deductibles nor copayments. Other indemnity plans required payment of 25, 50, or 95 percent of medical expenses. People responsible for 95 percent of their costs received full coverage after they had expended an out-of-pocket maximum based on their income. A fifth plan was an HMO and, like the free care plan, required no cost sharing. After three to five years, the researchers began comparing utilization of services and health outcomes among approximately six thousand individuals who participated in the study. Analysis of the large and complex data set that resulted continued for the remaining years of the twentieth century.

A number of limitations in the Rand HIE should be recognized. The study selected subjects randomly from the population and followed them for only a few years. Most initially healthy people are unlikely to contract serious or chronic illnesses during this time frame. Thus, the Rand HIE followed people who were usually well. The effects of cost sharing or managed care may be most relevant to individuals with established health problems. Among such people, access to a broad range of services and specialists unimpeded by cost or organizational mediation may be most important. Longer-range studies of people with definite health problems have been needed to supplement the Rand HIE.

Measures of Impact

Chapter Eight introduced the topic of measurement in biomedical research. These measures are generally quantitative, many expressing a dimension of individual health status and well-being as a number on a scale (see Table 8.3). Researchers have applied some of these measures in assessing the impact of innovations such as those discussed in this chapter. Development of new indicators on a very large scale began in the late twentieth century as concern increased over achieving an appropriate balance between cost control, utilization, and quality.

At the community or area level, assessing innovation has concerned mainly structural variables. Structure in this sense includes costs and availability of services. Data for such assessments are obtained from administrative sources such as CMS and state health agencies and private sources such as the American Hospital Association (AHA).

Process and outcome assessments are more readily done when data on individual consumers are available. These data have been obtained from patient charts, logs kept by clinicians, interviews of health care consumers, and surveys of community residents. Indicators of utilization are straightforward. Development of indicators of other potential effects of innovation, however, has been the subject of significant research in its own right. Table 9.1 presents a sample of measures that have been used or proposed to evaluate the quality of health services.

Table 9.1 presents types of measures and illustrative examples arranged by (a) dimension (structure, process, or outcome), and (b) the level of analysis at which each may be applied. Availability of services is a key structural variable on the community level. Concrete indices of availability include the time the average consumer must wait for an appointment with a primary care physician or specialist. Indices of this kind have been used to assess the potential impact of supply of providers and facilities on service availability.[9] The availability of sufficient emergency facilities to meet a community's needs, measurable by the average amount of ambulance diversion, constitutes another structural variable.

Structural indices applicable to individual facilities may address the adequacy of laboratory or medical records functioning, or the presence or availability of specific

TABLE 9.1   Structure, process, and outcome measures of health care: selected examples

Dimension	Level	Measure	Examples
Structure	Community	Availability of services	Wait time for appointment
		Price of services	Price stability and acceptability
	Facility	Availability of equipment	Diagnostic or treatment, such as angiography
			Support, such as computerized medical record or clinical decision support
		Availability of personnel	Perinatologist available to obstetric service; neurosurgeon on call in emergency department
		Quality assurance systems in place	Systems to record adherence to protocols and trends in quality measures and patient well-being
Process	Facility	Diagnostic procedures	Enzyme test for myocardial infarction
		Treatment interventions	Beta-blocker for acute myocardial infarction
			Prophylactic antibiotic one hour prior to surgery
		Followup procedure	Regular followup visits for patients taking steroids
		Timeliness	Anti-embolism therapy for acute heart attack
			Diagnosis of cancer following detection of symptoms

TABLE 9.1

Dimension	Level	Measure	Examples
Outcome	Consumer	Consumer satisfaction	Communication with providers
			Responsiveness of staff
		Health perceptions	Self-reported health
			Anxiety or worry
		Health behavior	Smokers who quit smoking
			Hypertensives who adopt low-salt diets
		Mental health	Self-reported anxiety or depression
		Level of functioning	Lack of activity restriction
			Zero or few bed disability days
		Physiologic measures	Diabetic blood sugar lower than 200 mg/dl
			Hypertensives' blood pressure reduced to normal
			Vision corrected to 20/40 or better
		Stage of disease	Cancer detected in early stage
		Patient safety	Adverse events and injuries
		Risk of dying	Age- and risk-adjusted death rate

personnel. For example, a perinatologist—an obstetrical subspecialist concerned with high-risk deliveries—enhances quality by safeguarding newborns and providing alternatives to emergency hysterectomy. However, these specialists are not available in all birthing facilities (in-house or on call).

In Table 9.1, process indicators address components of care and the efficiency with which a patient is scheduled or otherwise moved through the system. Often process measures of quality are complaint- or disease-specific. Table 9.1, for example, includes beta-blocker and prompt therapy to dissolve embolisms among individuals presenting with acute myocardial infarction (heart attack). Many similar process indicators have been developed by CMS (available at www.cms.hhs.gov/hospitalqualityinits). Regular followup visits for patients taking steroids, specifically among patients with chronic obstructive pulmonary disease, have been used as a process indicator in the Rand HIE.[10] Prompt follow-up and diagnosis of patient symptoms or screening results potentially indicating malignancies is a process measure of obvious importance.

Outcome measures are usually confined to individual consumers. CMS recommendations and the Rand HIE both include measures of consumer satisfaction. Self-described health status is captured by multi-item indicators such as the MOS-36 (see Chapter Eight). Physiologic measures expressed as lab values for specific health risks or illnesses are widely used in both quality assurance and in research; they appear, for example, in Rand HIE reports. Mental health is an important outcome of health care, and many multi-item indices have been developed for its measurement. For use in the Rand HIE, the Rand Corporation developed the Mental Health Inventory. This multi-item index assesses mental health according to questionnaire items reflecting various types of psychological distress (such as anxiety and depression), counterbalanced by items reflecting psychological well-being.[11]

Stage of disease and risk of dying are outcomes of clear importance. Cancer is the most familiar example of the importance of early-stage detection. Early-stage detection is often associated with longer life expectancy. Early detection of other illnesses such as heart disease and diabetes also promotes effective treatment and survival. Risk of dying can be computed from patient-level data indicating the presence of life-threatening disease or disease precursors, such as high cholesterol and high blood pressure. For comparative purposes, it is important to adjust health risk for background factors such as age, gender, and race, which often affect likelihood of survival through a variety of mechanisms.

OUTCOMES OF STRATEGIC INNOVATION I: SELECTIVE CONTRACTING

Selective contracting has played an important part in U.S. health care since the 1980s. Initiated in response to fiscal issues in California's Medicaid program, legalization of selective contracting gave rise to the preferred provider organization (PPO) movement and other competition-driven forms of contracting. As the years went by, a large amount of data became available to answer the question of whether selective contracting has actually saved money within the industry as a whole.

It is unquestionable that large purchasers of health services initially saved money by awarding contracts to provider organizations on a selective basis. The state of California, for example, reduced the costs of its Medicaid program through selective contracting. For the health care system as a whole, however, the financial benefits of the innovation are less certain.

Economists Zwanziger, Melnick, and Bamezai compared California hospital costs and revenues over time in the years following enactment of selective contracting (1983 through 1997). They found that hospital costs and revenues increased less rapidly in areas where competition was more intense in comparison with areas where there was weaker competition.[12] The study did not directly address charges to insurance plans, but the economists' findings on costs suggest that a measure of control on expenditures was achieved. It is important to note, however, that costs rose substantially during the period covered by the study. Any impact that may have occurred was confined to reduction of the rate of increase.

The manner in which hospitals achieved their cost savings remains at issue. Achievement of savings at the expense of quality of care would constitute an adverse impact. Some evidence has surfaced that the reduction in hospital cost increases found between 1983 and 1997 did occur at the expense of quality. According to a study covering hospital care in the 1980s, reduced hospital expenditures were accompanied by increases in death rates among patients.[13]

Returning to the issue of cost control, other studies suggest that moderation of expenditure increases may have been short-lived. A study extending into the early 2000s found that in areas where strong competition prevailed, hospitals tended to duplicate each other's service offerings.[14] In an atmosphere of intense competition, hospitals sought to achieve and maintain a full line of services. Comprehensive service offerings are attractive to health plans because they simplify the process of concluding and managing contracts. Maintaining comprehensive services amounts to a form of nonprice competition. This strategy may benefit individual hospitals, but it does not lower costs. Optimal cost control requires operating hospital services at high volume. Duplication among hospitals lowers the volume and potentially the quality of a given service.

A late twentieth-century study of HMO penetration and cost containment casts further doubt on the long-term benefit of selective contracting. Most HMOs do not operate their own hospitals, but contract out for the services their members require. Early in this history of selective contracting, the presence of competing HMOs in a given market area seemed to reduce hospital costs. As major purchasers of services, HMOs were well positioned to obtain discounts. However, as the public became discontent with the restrictions involved in HMOs, the ability of HMOs to obtain hospital services at reduced rates declined. The authors of the study conclude: "High managed care penetration is no longer associated with lower-cost growth—and may even be associated with higher-cost growth—in the most competitive markets, indicating that the synergistic effect between managed care penetration and hospital competition to hold down hospital cost inflation no longer exists."[15]

Finally, it is important to remember that competition eventually results in failure of some of the players. Less competitively successful hospitals either close or are acquired by the hospitals that survive. In the extreme case, a single hospital may be left in a given market area. Absence of competition allows such hospitals to charge monopoly prices.

OUTCOMES OF STRATEGIC INNOVATION II: COST SHARING

Cost sharing affects a larger number of Americans than any of the other innovations identified in this chapter. Increased cost sharing has taken the form of copayments and deductibles, as well as enrollment in high-deductible health plans associated with health savings accounts. Thus, the impact of cost sharing on utilization, quality, and outcomes is of key importance.

The Rand HIE produced especially important results in analyzing the impact of cost sharing. Findings addressed both impact on service utilization and on consumer health status. Scores of articles and reports emerged from the Rand HIE. The findings summarized in the next section originally appeared in a 1993 book presenting comprehensive study results titled *Free for All: Lessons from the Rand Health Insurance Experiment.*[16]

Effect on Utilization

The most widely influential findings from the Rand HIE concerned reduction in service utilization as an effect of cost sharing. Following are some of the key findings.

■ *Strong impact on service utilization.* In one of its most important findings, the Rand HIE determined that cost sharing markedly reduced utilization of health services. When consumers were required to pay for 95 percent of their care, they reduced their use of services by about 30 percent in comparison with those in a plan requiring no cost sharing. Lower levels of cost sharing corresponded to smaller reductions, but utilization was found to be smaller whatever the level of cost sharing imposed. Imputed annual expenditures for individuals in the no-cost-sharing plan were (in 1991 dollars) $833; expenditures in the 95-percent-cost-sharing plan were $628. Notably, emergency department visits for urinary tract infections declined by about 50 percent and for asthma by over 60 percent under the cost sharing plans.

■ *Highly comprehensive impact.* The impact of cost sharing found in the Rand HIE was striking in comprehensiveness. As the investigators commented, "Cost sharing markedly decreased all types of services among all types of people." The effect of cost sharing on relatively high- and low-income adults was about equal. However, the dampening effect of cost sharing on service utilization was much stronger among poor than nonpoor children.

■ *Lack of differentiation between high- and low-value services.* Of particular importance was the finding that consumers were no more likely to reduce utilization of high-value, appropriate, or vital health services than low-value or unnecessary services.

This was true even for hospitalization, a decision seldom, if ever, made independently by the consumer but by physicians in consultation with consumers. The Rand investigators concluded that "our analysis suggests that cost sharing has a nonspecific effect on the use of services. In particular, it reduces appropriate and inappropriate services by the same proportion."

Health Savings Accounts and High-Deductible Plans

As discussed in Chapter Seven, use of health savings accounts (HSAs) has gained widespread visibility as an insurance innovation. HSAs are tax-free accounts provided as an employee benefit. Typically, HSAs combine high-deductible health plans with a financial account to which the employer contributes. The beneficiary enjoys the privilege of accumulating funds earmarked for health insurance cost sharing from year to year. HSAs, then, provide strong incentives for consumers to think seriously about the health care they consume and shop for value. Findings from the Rand HIE suggest that health care consumption should drop for both necessary and unnecessary services under these plans.

Research on the behavior of consumers with high-deductible policies and HSAs has not borne this out as strongly as the Rand HIE. A study of manufacturing company employees compared those enrolled in a high-deductible plan and a traditional PPO. Few consumers in either plan were found to forgo diagnostic or therapeutic services they thought they needed, delay medical treatment, or take lower than prescribed doses of medications. People enrolled in the high-deductible plan were initially more likely to engage in these adverse behaviors than those in the PPO. However, most differences between the high-deductible plan and PPO members disappeared one year later. None of the hoped-for behaviors of a favorable nature—including use of generic drugs and seeking cheaper diagnostic procedures—differed between the two plans.[17]

Another study of employed individuals yielded similar results regarding preventive health care. Employees in a high-deductible plan were compared with those in a PPO. No differences were detected in utilization of cancer screening or diabetic monitoring services.[18]

Adverse effects of high-deductible plans are yet to be demonstrated.

Effect on Quality of Care

For the average consumer, the Rand HIE reported minimal or no adverse health consequences associated with higher cost sharing. Two adverse effects were noted, however. People with poor vision were more likely to have their vision corrected in the no-cost-sharing plan. Of potentially greater importance, low-income people with high blood pressure were more likely to improve in the no-cost-sharing plan than in the cost sharing plan. This difference resulted in a lower risk of dying among low-income people in the no-cost-sharing plan. No differences were detected on other quality-of-care and patient outcome indices, including cholesterol level, self-reported health status, and health behavior.

Since completion of the Rand HIE, significant additional research has investigated the impact of cost sharing on quality of care and health status. Summaries of illustrative studies (along with the HIE results) are presented in Table 9.2. Both the Rand HIE

TABLE 9.2   Impact of cost sharing on quality of care and patient outcomes

Subjects	Utilization	Outcomes	Study Authors
Consumers in Rand HIE	Reduced use of services of all kinds	Reduced control of high blood pressure among low-income patients Reduced correction of poor vision	Brook RH, Ware JE Jr, Rogers WH, et al.[19]
Cancer patients	Delay in diagnosis	No effect on stage at detection or survival	Greenwald HP[20]
Medicare beneficiaries	Reduced use of pharmaceuticals	Increased emergency department visits and hospitalization Reduced control of hypertension, hyperlipidemia, and diabetes	Hsu J, Price M, Huang J, et al.[21]
Medicare beneficiaries	Reduced mammography screening	—	Trivedi AN, Rakowski W, Ayanian JZ[22]
Retired public employees	Reduced pharmaceutical use and doctor visits Increased hospitalization	—	Chandra A, Gruber J, McKnight R[23]

and a study of Medicare beneficiaries under plans with capped pharmaceutical benefits indicate poorer health status as a result of cost sharing in at least some populations. People at highest risk appear to be low-income earners with chronic diseases. Other studies of cost sharing among cancer patients and elders summarized in Table 9.2 either do not present findings on outcomes or failed to detect adverse outcomes. But delay in diagnosis, reduced mammography screening, and presumably avoidable hospitalization may reflect poor quality of care or foreshadow adverse health outcomes.

OUTCOMES OF STRATEGIC INNOVATION III: MANAGED CARE

As with the preceding sections on strategic innovation, it is important here to start with the results of the Rand HIE. This research reported that individuals randomly assigned to the Group Health Cooperative of Puget Sound HMO had about the same likelihood of ambulatory care visits as persons assigned to indemnity (fee-for-service) plans. In a finding of key importance, the Rand HIE reported that the HMO patients were hospitalized about 40 percent less often than those in the indemnity group. Largely because of less frequent hospitalization, the total expenditure rate for services in the HMO was about 25 percent less than in the indemnity groups. Individuals in the HMO were more likely to visit doctors for preventive purposes than those in indemnity plans. However, preventive services did not explain the lower rate of hospitalization among the HMO patients.[24]

The Rand HIE, then, suggests that managed care saves money. But even if managed care organizations do operate more economically, they may not save much money for actual consumers, employers, or government programs. Evidence suggests that managed care organizations may not pass on the savings they achieve to purchasers of health care. A Minnesota study, for example, suggests that managed care plans typically engage in *shadow pricing*—charging for its services at rates just below those of indemnity plans.[25] A review of research conducted following the Rand HIE suggests that managed care operations deliver services no more efficiently than indemnity plans. This review concludes: "It is fair to say that the jury has yet to return a verdict on whether 'managed care' is more efficient than the old [fee-for-service] system."[26]

Turning to quality and outcomes, the Rand HIE researchers found that consumer satisfaction was lower in the HMO. But as in findings regarding cost sharing, they did not find evidence that assignment to the HMO had generally affected consumer health in an adverse manner. Health effects were found, however, for people who began the study with health problems of specific kinds. These effects were confined to low- and high-income groups. The low-income initially sick group assigned to the HMO reported significantly more bed-days per year due to poor health and more serious symptoms than those assigned to no-cost-sharing indemnity care. The low-income, initially sick people in the HMO also had a greater risk of dying. For the high-income initially sick group, the HMO produced significant improvements in cholesterol levels and in general health ratings by comparison with indemnity care.

It is important to remember that the Rand HIE selected participants randomly from the population and followed them for only a limited time. In addition, the Rand sample included neither children under fourteen nor elders. For these reasons, the experiment was conducted on people in less need of, and potentially less responsive to, health care than others in the U.S. population. The study, moreover, looked at only one managed care organization, an HMO that operated in a restricted geographical area. Table 9.3 summarizes, in addition to the Rand HIE results, findings from a number of later studies. Although these studies lacked the RCT design of the Rand HIE, together they include a broader range of patients and providers.

TABLE 9.3   Impact of HMO membership on quality of care and patient outcomes

Subjects	Utilization	Outcomes	Study Authors
Consumers in Rand HIE	Increased preventive visits Decreased hospitalization	Generally lower satisfaction Poorer health status among initially ill low-income consumers	Ware JE, Brook RH, Rogers WH, et al.[27]
Child Medicaid beneficiaries in managed care	Increased outpatient visits, reduced ED visits, and less hospitalization	Greater frequency of delayed care Lower consumer satisfaction	Baker LC, Afendulis C[28]
Cancer patients (prostate)	Less surgery and more radiation treatment	Low-income patients have significantly greater likelihood of survival	Greenwald HP, Henke CJ[29]
Heart attack patients in Medicare	Reduced use of angiography	—	Guadagnoli E, Landrum MB, Peterson EA, et al.[30]
Adults with asthma	More likely to have primary care physician and use inhaled steroids	HMO and indemnity patients similar	Ferris TG, Blumenthal D, Woodruff PG, et al.[31]

Years after completion of the HIE, a group of researchers studied the impact of managed care on children funded under Medicaid in seven states. Managed care tended to result in lower rates of emergency department use and hospitalization, which, along with higher rates of outpatient visits, may be considered a favorable sign. But managed care was found to be associated with more delay in care and, as reported by the Rand HIE, lower consumer satisfaction.[32]

Three other investigations summarized in Table 9.3 focus on patients who, unlike most of those in the Rand HIE, had established illnesses and definite health service needs. A study in Seattle compared treatment received by cancer patients and their subsequent survival in an HMO versus an indemnity plan. The HMO in this study was the same as the one used in the Rand HIE. The strongest results were found in prostate cancer, for which surgery or radiation (though not both) are usual forms of care. Patients in the HMO were less likely to receive surgery and more likely to receive radiation. This finding was consistent with that of the Rand HIE's observation of less hospital-intensive care in the HMO. Radiation is usually an outpatient procedure, whereas surgery for prostate cancer is typically done in a hospital. But the Seattle study found that low-income people in the HMO had much better survival chances than those in indemnity plans.[33]

A study with similar aims compared Medicare beneficiaries in managed care and indemnity plans. Subjects in this study had had heart attacks and were initially treated in hospitals. The investigators applied an appropriate care criterion for quality: receiving angiography in cases where, according to American College of Cardiology and American Heart Association guidelines, the procedure would likely provide benefit. Among patients who were considered appropriate candidates for angiography, those in managed care were less likely to receive the procedure than those covered by indemnity arrangements.[34]

Finally, a study of asthma patients produced findings seemingly favoring managed care. In comparison with indemnity plan patients, those in managed care were more likely to indicate that they had a primary care physician and to appropriately use inhaled steroids. Outcomes in measurable pulmonary function did not differ across the groups.[35]

As with the case of costs, research findings on quality and outcomes in managed care do not provide clear guidelines about whether quality of managed care is better or worse than that obtained under traditional indemnity. Generally, services in managed care seem to be more subject to delay than in indemnity plans. Consumer satisfaction seems lower under managed care, an observation confirmed by the managed care "backlash" that has fueled the popularity of PPOs and point-of-service plans. The Rand HIE reported worse health outcomes for low-income people with established health problems treated in an HMO. But a study of cancer patients in the same HMO found that low-income individuals had a much better chance of surviving the disease.

It appears that some patients may obtain better services from a managed care organization than they would under indemnity. This would be most true of an assertive, medically literate, low-income consumer. Other people, such as the low-income sick in the Rand HIE, may lack sufficient education or assertiveness needed to obtain the best care of which an HMO is capable.

In interpreting the research on managed care, it is important to remember that the "managed care" label includes a wide variety of actual insurance arrangements and organizations. Although the Rand HIE focused on an HMO, most managed care organizations today are PPOs. These organizations present consumers with fewer restrictions than traditional HMOs.

Major differences appear likely even among managed care organizations of the same type. Group Health Cooperative, on which both the Rand HIE and prostate cancer findings presented earlier are based, is a case in point. Group Health Cooperative, a nonprofit and consumer-governed organization, originated in response to a community-level initiative in the 1950s. Most managed care organizations today have origins and governance structures of a very different nature. Thus, they may have organizational and professional cultures quite different from those of Group Health Cooperative. Differences of equal importance appear likely among many of the managed care organizations now operating across the United States.

For many reasons, concluding that managed care is superior or inferior to traditional indemnity fee-for-service care is difficult, if not impossible, on the basis of facts available today.

OUTCOMES OF TACTICAL INNOVATIONS

As indicated earlier, selective contracting, cost sharing, and managed care constitute examples of strategic innovation in the U.S. health care system. Less revolutionary seeming and pervasive, a number of innovations that may be characterized as tactical have also taken place. Some of the best-known examples are evidence-based medicine, pay for performance, and public dissemination of data on quality.

Evidence-Based Medicine

The health care industry has widely implemented the concept of evidence-based medicine. The concept is receiving increased attention in medical schools and continuing medical education programs. Hospitals and integrated delivery systems have internally disseminated evidence-based practice guidelines. Computerized decision support systems to promote application of research in clinical practice have been developed. Systems transmitting e-mail reminders of practice guidelines to clinicians have been implemented. Evidence has been reported of the efficacy of such systems in changing the behavior of clinicians.[36]

Research has supported the economic potential of evidence-based medicine. Adherence to evidence-based guidelines in medication, for example, has been cited as a major money saver. According to one study, adherence to such guidelines can reduce the cost of medication by 40 percent.[37]

However, the principle of evidence-based medicine must still overcome resistance by clinicians. Traditionally, clinicians have been taught to focus on the unique features of each patient. This approach contradicts the reliance on protocols and templates that characterizes some mechanisms for applying the principles of evidence-based medicine.

Pay for Performance

Pay for performance represents an application of guidelines developed or adopted by health care systems for clinical practice. These guidelines may be formulated according to evidence-based medicine. They may also reflect attempts of health care systems to control costs.

The concept of pay for performance has spread throughout the health care industry. The impact of pay for performance on health care outcomes, however, is uncertain at this time. A comparison of hospital care following heart attacks at hospitals with and without pay-for-performance systems, for example, found no difference in outcomes.[38]

Assessing the impact of pay for performance is hampered by differences in methods from organization to organization. Some pay-for-performance systems are focused on hospitals, others on individual physicians or other clinicians. It has also been suggested that the size of the incentives currently being offered are too small to affect physician behavior.[39]

Just as some physicians are uncomfortable with evidence-based medicine, many appear to reject the validity of pay-for-performance. Among the challenges to more widespread and efficacious implementation of the concept are objections by physicians. Physicians raise questions about the number and inconsistency of quality metrics according to which they are rewarded. Suspicion has arisen about whether these metrics truly reflect evidenced-based medicine versus schemes by insurance companies to save money. In this connection, one physician has commented:

> I can't help suspecting that underneath all these quality improvement and pay-for-performance initiatives lies yet another scheme that will work out well for insurers and very badly for providers and patients. The tens of thousands of dollars I'm going to lose out on for failing to achieve my electronic prescribing or obesity management goals have certainly caught my attention, but it's not the big prize. The big prize will come from creating a multitude of grading systems that rate doctors against one another, making them increasingly dependent on quality-improvement goals and payments while distracting them from patient care and making reimbursement more complicated than ever.[40]

Public Dissemination of Quality Findings

A revolution has taken place in public availability of health information of all kinds. As noted earlier in this chapter, both private firms and public agencies have developed significant resources for the public on interventions, quality, and price. The development of the web has greatly facilitated public access to these resources. A key social development has played as important a role in the appearance of these resources as the technical surroundings. In the past few generations, the educational level of the U.S. public has increased markedly. Along with rising levels of education has come increased medical literacy in the general population. More educated, confident patients would seem likelier to question their health care providers and independently explore health care alternatives.

The twenty-first century has indeed spawned a wide variety of user-friendly, web-based information sources on health care options, costs, and quality. The *Wall Street Journal* reports that in 2008 there were two hundred health care–related sites online. In that year, 72 million people visited sites with names like RevolutionHealth, EveryDayHealth, and WebMD Health. WhyNotTheBest.org, a site developed by the nonprofit Commonwealth Fund, compares 4,500 hospitals nationwide on quality measures such as safety and disease-specific clinical criteria. Through these and other web sites, consumers can obtain not only comparative information on treatments and facilities but personalized feedback on their illnesses and concerns. A web site operated by the Cleveland Clinic allowed consumers to seek second opinions on medical questions.[41]

Many health-related web sites are operated by for-profit organizations, and consumers should use these with discretion. Drug companies directly fund some of the sites. Sites not tied directly to manufacturers are often laced with advertisements. Privacy is also of concern, as consumers often reveal personal information to obtain the feedback they desire. The open access provided by the web creates tremendous opportunity for free public discussion. But this same feature bypasses processes of scientific and editorial review that have traditionally promoted validity and accuracy and minimized bias.

Whether disseminated through the web or other media, widespread use of quality information for decision making by consumers or clinicians presents challenges. Commentators, for example, have raised questions about the validity of quality measures—specifically, whether all such indices in widespread use actually measure quality. Many measures that are routinely reported lack firm connections to outcomes. Second, reporting of quality indicators is subject to error and self-interested manipulation. Individual hospitals may selectively report or exaggerate the importance of measures upon which they perform well. A group of physicians at Johns Hopkins and the University of California has advocated the establishment of standards for reporting on quality akin to the "generally accepted accounting principles" formulated by the Financial Accounting Standards Board.[42]

The ultimate question regarding public dissemination of quality indicators is whether the process will affect consumer behavior. Concepts such as market-based and consumer-driven health care assume that the public will respond to such information by selecting higher-quality and lower-cost plans and services. Research findings, however, suggest that public response, at least in the near future, is likely to be small. Consistent with reports extending back into the 1980s, a 2009 synthesis of the highest-quality research on public dissemination of quality indices concluded that "there is limited evidence about the effectiveness of quality information on consumer choice."[43]

This is true in part because most consumers do not enjoy complete freedom to exercise choice. They are constrained by the range of health plans offered by employers and government agencies, as well as the cost of care outside these plans. Finally, the ability of disadvantaged consumers to use information on health care quality is often limited. Barriers to use of such information seem to be most common among low-income, minority, and elderly consumers.[44]

The Big Picture: Outcomes of Uninsurance

No one has formally proposed uninsurance as a method for controlling health care costs. In the past, however, both employers and government agencies have made changes in the insurance they offer, which have had the effect, if not the intent, of reducing the number of people covered. Employers have discontinued health insurance or passed increased costs on to employees in the form of higher premiums. Government programs have tightened eligibility requirements for programs such as Medicaid.

Higher premiums cause consumers to forgo insurance even if they qualify for a plan. A team of health economists in 2004 reported that a 20 percent cost increase in premiums caused 10 percent of employees to drop family coverage and 20 percent to drop individual coverage.[45] As noted in Chapter Seven, cost rather than availability causes many Latino workers to forgo insurance.

Research clearly indicates that uninsurance results in adverse health outcomes. Representative study results include the following:

When uninsured, the near-elderly (ages fifty-five through sixty-four) with established chronic diseases—diabetes, hypertension, and heart disease, for example—face higher mortality risks than similarly aged and afflicted individuals with insurance. A study of the near-elderly concluded that over 100,000 people ages fifty-five through sixty-four die each year due to lack of health insurance that might allow life-threatening yet treatable diseases to be controlled or cured.[46] As might be expected, low-income elders are more likely to experience adverse effects of uninsurance than their more affluent peers.

A study of adults with asthma found that those without insurance received poorer-quality care than their counterparts with insurance. The uninsured experienced worse clinical outcomes in terms of peak expiratory flow. Type of health plan made little difference in this study, with both HMO and indemnity patients enjoying better outcomes than the uninsured.[47]

KEY TERMS

Structure

Process

Outcomes

Codman Report

Rand Health Insurance Experiment
(Rand HIE)

SUMMARY

This chapter summarizes the impact of significant attempts by managers and policy makers to control costs and maintain quality in health care. Key innovations for these purposes have included selective contracting, cost sharing, and managed care.

Selective contracting has reduced hospital costs under programs such as Medicaid. But the atmosphere of competition promoted by selective contracting has produced some adverse consequences. To place themselves in competition for contracts with health plans, hospitals duplicate each other's services. Costs are reported to have increased in areas where competition has enabled one hospital to become predominant.

Research has consistently reported that cost sharing reduces the consumer's tendency to utilize services. But in reducing utilization, consumers do not discriminate between vital, high-value services and unnecessary, low-value ones. Special concern has arisen over adverse effects of cost sharing among the disadvantaged.

Early studies identified savings achieved through managed care. HMOs have been found to practice a less hospital-intensive style of medicine. Savings through reduced hospitalization have produced significant reductions in costs for some HMOs. But studies on quality in managed care versus indemnity plans (under which providers are paid on a fee-for-service basis) have not produced consistent results.

DISCUSSION QUESTIONS

1. Dr. Ernest Codman encountered fierce resistance from the medical profession of his day to publicly open assessment of end results. To what degree has the outlook of the health care industry changed in this matter?

2. Cosmetic dentistry and surgery are widely valued and utilized by the public. Should availability and affordability of such services be considered a structural measure of quality provided by the system?

3. How concerned should we be about the decline in health service utilization reported by researchers due to cost sharing by consumers?

4. Research has found that selective contracting, cost sharing, and managed care all have limited ability to produce their hoped-for effects, and sometimes they produce adverse results. In view of these findings, can constructive use still be made of these innovations? What illustrative examples can be cited?

5. Early research on selective contracting found that this innovation resulted in a slowing of the increase in hospital costs. Do you believe that selective contracting is having this effect at present?

6. What, if any, innovations might produce a *decline* in health care costs?

CHAPTER

10

HEALTH PROMOTION AND DISEASE PREVENTION

LEARNING OBJECTIVES

- To appreciate the importance of prevention
- To review the scientific basis of prevention
- To understand how public health, medical care, and individual behavior can contribute to prevention
- To identify challenges in prevention
- To assess the cost-effectiveness of preventive interventions
- To anticipate the role that prevention may play in the future

THE APPEAL OF PREVENTION

The idea of prevention has natural appeal. No one wants to get sick. Avoidance of illness, with its physical discomfort, impairment of function, and potential threat to survival is a natural feature of human behavior. Clearly, prevention should play an important part in efforts to promote quality of life and longevity among Americans. But detailed examination is necessary to identify the most effective means of prevention. In addition, it is important to critically examine claims that prevention can help solve the problem of high and increasing health care costs in the United States.

Throughout the ages people have placed great importance on avoiding disease. Ancient civilizations favored building sites in breezy places away from swamps because these venues seemed more healthful. Chronicling a great plague in Athens, the Greek historian Thucydides observed a connection between human crowding and the risk of epidemic.[1] Physicians through the ages have recommended a moderate lifestyle and regular exercise as practices effective in the prevention of illness.

Magic and myth have played important roles in prevention. Aboriginal tribes wear amulets and beads to ward off disease and other forms of evil. As recently as the early twentieth century, Americans in congested immigrant neighborhoods hung pouches of garlic around the necks of their children to protect them from contagious diseases. Today, Americans spend billions of dollars on vitamins and food supplements of unproven efficacy in preventing disease. According to a 2008 report, for example, Americans were spending $100 million per year on gingko supplements. Although widely believed to prevent Alzheimer's disease, these preparations have demonstrated no clinical efficacy.[2]

Humankind, however, has effectively practiced prevention for thousands of years. The ancient Romans established basic public health facilities for their populous cities in the form of water and sewage systems and public baths.[3] In medieval Europe, lepers were subjected to ritual isolation, ordered to wander with hood and bell, and prohibited from eating or drinking in the company of nonlepers.[4] During fourteenth-century epidemics of Black Death, thousands fled from urban centers. Cities active in international trade during the Renaissance established the practice of quarantine, ordering that ships lie at anchor for a period of four weeks before being permitted to dock, and then only if no disease had become evident on board.[5]

People concerned with health understood several risks associated with human behavior that were later confirmed by modern science. Commenting on the premodern physician's understanding of the risk that obesity represented to elders, medical historian Daniel Schafer writes that "although a modern understanding of hormones and molecular genetics was obviously lacking, basic knowledge of the influence of nutrition in old age was prevalent."[6] As early as the nineteenth century, insurance underwriters identified certain trades, such as those involving asbestos, as hazardous to health. These observations were later confirmed in the 1960s by Dr. Irving Selikoff, whose studies of asbestos and lung disease led to stringent controls over use of the mineral.[7]

Underscoring the significance of prevention, U.S. policy makers have also embraced the principle. Politicians of both major parties cite prevention as a means of addressing the seemingly implacable increase in prevalence of premorbid conditions such as childhood obesity. Statesmen also look to prevention as a means of controlling health care costs.[8,9]

Although subject to exaggeration by enthusiasts, the importance of prevention cannot be ignored. Writing in the *Journal of the American Medical Association,* physician Steven H. Woolf cites key statistics. According to Woolf, "exercise can lower the incidence of diabetes by 50 percent. Four health behaviors (smoking, diet, physical inactivity, and alcohol use) account for 38 percent of all U.S. deaths. Other forms of . . . prevention can intervene more dramatically, as when vaccines all but eradicate infectious diseases. [Screening] can reduce colorectal and breast cancer mortality by 15 percent to 20 percent."[10] Earlier, a highly influential report in the same medical journal asserted that about 50 percent of all deaths that occur in the United States are attributable to factors such as tobacco use, unfavorable dietary practices, lack of exercise, unsafe sex, traffic accidents, and exposure to toxic agents.[11]

Three Types of Prevention

Health professionals today refer to three types of prevention. **Primary prevention**, the most familiar, includes activities intended to prevent an individual's contracting a disease. Polio immunization and tobacco cessation are both forms of primary prevention; immunization prevents the individual from ever developing polio, while quitting tobacco use reduces the individual's risk of cancer, heart disease, and chronic obstructive pulmonary disease. **Secondary prevention** refers to early detection and prompt treatment of disease. Many screening techniques today are effective in helping detect disease at an early stage when it is often more readily treatable. Early detection of cancer and HIV infection are both considered forms of secondary prevention. **Tertiary prevention** comprises procedures intended to prevent a disease already present from producing avoidable limitations on function and quality of life. Hospice services and control of otherwise debilitating pain from arthritis both fall within the definition of tertiary prevention. Measures taken to promote a patient's ability to maintain activities of daily life such as self-care and employment also are considered tertiary prevention.

THE SCIENTIFIC RATIONALE FOR PREVENTION

Prevention of illness through public health and medicine has contributed significantly to the increase in life expectancy cited in earlier chapters of this book. The impact of prevention is perhaps clearest in the decline of mortality among mothers, infants, and children during the twentieth century. Pathogen-free milk and drinking water have markedly reduced the risk of tuberculosis and diarrhea among children. Immunization has minimized the risk of death in children aged five years or less from a wide variety of infant and childhood diseases. Skilled birth assistance and antisepsis have transformed maternal mortality from a frequent to rare event. Prevention of maternal, infant, and child mortality helps explain the population explosion of the late twentieth century. During that period, global population increased from 3 billion to over 6.5 billion.

A vast body of scientific research supports the value of preventive interventions. When applied by clinicians, public health officials, health education specialists, and individuals in their daily lives, the resulting information preserves function and extends lives. Due to resource limitations, a failure to apply known science to prevention explains in large part the high mortality rates that prevail in the world's poorest countries today.[12]

Efficacy of Public Health and Medicine

Commentators have often contrasted the contributions of clinicians and public health officials to human health. Such a separation, however, cannot be clearly made with respect to prevention. Preventive practices of both modern medicine and public health rest on the same scientific basis. They may also involve identical techniques. Public health agencies, for example, may operate early detection facilities and mass immunization programs. But the same early detection procedures and inoculations may be delivered in the offices of private doctors.

The evidence supporting the efficacy of prevention as practiced by modern medicine and public health is too voluminous to be covered here. But two areas illustrate its scope. Immunization is a good example of primary prevention. Screening constitutes a well-known application of secondary prevention. Vaccines and screening technology represent applications of basic science, whose principles are confirmed by the outcomes achieved through their use.

Immunization. Both science and practice experience have demonstrated the value of immunization against many diseases. Some of the strongest evidence for these benefits is visible among young people and elders. The vast majority of nineteen- to thirty-five-month-old children in the United States now receive inoculations against nine diseases: diphtheria, tetanus, pertussis (whooping cough), polio, meningitis-causing Haemophilus influenzae (HIB), measles, mumps, rubella, and hepatitis B.[13] For decades, vaccination against influenza has been a routine procedure for elders in the United States and Europe.

As a consequence of immunization, diseases that once threatened the lives and health of children in the United States are now rare. The history of pertussis illustrates the benefit of immunization. Between 1934 and 1943, annual incidence of the disease averaged over 200,000, including over 4,000 deaths. After introduction of childhood pertussis vaccination during the 1940s, reported cases declined dramatically, reaching a low of just over 1,000 in 1976.[14]

A report from the Netherlands has demonstrated clear benefits from annual influenza vaccination among people ages sixty-five and over. The study observed elders over a six-year period. Those who received annual vaccination experienced a reduced mortality risk of 24 percent. Influenza vaccination was estimated to prevent one death for every 302 people vaccinated. Notably, the vaccination program was conducted as a mass public health intervention effected by the country's general practitioners. Annual vaccination days were scheduled in October and November, during which elders were invited to receive the shots in their doctors' offices. Data on vaccination were recorded in an electronic patient record, which facilitated their availability to researchers.[15]

Screening. The term **screening** refers to a process by which evidence of possible disease is detected prior to the appearance of signs and symptoms. Positive findings from screening do not constitute diagnosis. Rather, they constitute indications that the clinician should look for further evidence. Findings from screening often initiate more thorough diagnostic procedures, including detailed imaging, biopsy, or exploratory surgery.

From the perspective of management and policy, only some conditions are appropriate for screening. Screening is most worthwhile when

■ The disease involved is highly prevalent

■ An inexpensive, convenient, and reliable procedure is available for screening

■ Patients can benefit from early detection of the disease

Unless these conditions are met, few cases of actual disease will be identified within the population. Among the cases identified in this scenario, few, if any, will be cured, and costs associated with each life saved will be high.

Screening has proven particularly effective in early detection of some cancers. Research on colorectal cancer screening has demonstrated the effectiveness of associated techniques for reducing both incidence and mortality from the disease. A recent review of the evidence indicates that many procedures used for detecting colorectal cancer are effective, including fecal occult blood testing (FOBT). FOBT detects small amounts of blood in the stool that may be produced by bowel tumors. Studies of biannually administered FOBT indicate that the procedure (along with medical and surgical follow-up) reduces mortality from colorectal cancer by 15 to 21 percent.[16] The value of FOBT is easier to demonstrate for the population as a whole than for the individual patient. The authors of another study comment that "screening with FOBT . . . may require offering annual testing to 500 to 1,000 people for 10 years to prevent one death from colorectal cancer."[17] The Papanicolaou (Pap) test for early cervical cancer most closely approaches the ideal. Between the early 1970s and 2000, widespread use of the Pap test decreased incidence and mortality from invasive cervical cancer by 40 percent in the United States.[18] The test is inexpensive, convenient, and effective at detecting precancerous as well as actual malignancies. Cervical cancer, moreover, is highly curable when detected early.

Evidence-Based Recommendations. Since the 1980s, the U.S. government has sponsored a body of physicians, scientists, and others to determine the most important steps clinicians can take to prevent their patients from contracting illness. Known as the U.S. Preventive Services Task Force (USPSTF), it studies research findings related to prevention and develops priorities for clinicians. The USPSTF ranks services according to the strength of evidence regarding efficacy and the net benefits it believes patients may obtain.

The USPSTF ranking classifies preventive interventions from grade A to D, plus grade I where evidence is inconclusive:

A. *Strongly recommended:* good evidence that the service improves health outcomes and that benefits substantially outweigh harms.

B. *Recommended:* at least fair evidence of benefits in health outcomes and that benefits outweigh harms.

C. *No recommendation for or against:* at least fair evidence that the service can improve health outcomes, but the balance of benefits and harms is too close to justify recommendation.

D. *Recommended against:* at least fair evidence that the service is ineffective or that harms outweigh benefits.

E. *Insufficient evidence:* evidence is insufficient to recommend for or against routinely providing the service.

A sampling of the services classified into each of these categories by the USPSTF appears in Table 10.1. It is important to note that USPSTF has classified some interventions as B or C for the general population, but as A for individuals at elevated risk. Evidence for prevention carried out by clinicians is complex because of the variability of the people likely to be seen in a given practice.[19]

Lifestyle and Risk Reduction

Important as public health and medicine have been, popular attention today has focused on environment and lifestyle. Research on prevention in the twentieth and twenty-first centuries has produced striking findings in these areas. Most important for the average individual have been findings in four areas: tobacco, body weight, diet, and exercise. An accumulation of research on prevention of cancer added sun exposure to the widely known dangers of tobacco and asbestos exposure.[20] A search for the causes of AIDS after the disease was first identified in the 1980s alerted people to the dangers of unprotected sex. Risk of HIV infection was added to the many health hazards already recognized in intravenous drug use.[21]

Several scientific investigations of very high quality in the latter half of the twentieth century underlie much of today's thinking about prevention. The most important of these studies have followed thousands of individuals for decades to assess the impact of biological factors and lifestyle on health and survival. These include two studies

TABLE 10.1 Clinical prevention services according to USPSTF grade (adults), 2008

Intervention	Applicable Population
A. Strongly recommended	
Screening for cervical cancer	Women who have been sexually active and have a cervix
Screening for colorectal cancer	Men and women 50 years of age or older
Aspirin for prevention of coronary heart disease	Adults who are at increased risk
Screening for high blood pressure	Adults aged 18 and older
Screening for chlamydia infection	Sexually active nonpregnant women aged 24 and younger and older women at increased risk
Screening and cessation interventions for tobacco use	All adults
Annual influenza vaccination	All patients 50 years of age or older
Pneumococcal vaccine	All patients 65 years of age or older
B. Recommended	
Genetic counseling regarding breast cancer risk	Family history associated with increased risk for mutations predisposing to breast cancer
Chemoprevention for breast cancer (such as tamoxifen therapy)	Women at high risk who are able to tolerate chemoprevention
Screening for breast cancer via mammography every one to two years	Women aged 40 and older

(Continued)

TABLE 10.1 *(Continued)*

Intervention	Applicable Population
Dietary counseling	Adults with high cholesterol levels and other risk factors for cardiovascular and diet-related disease
Counseling and behavioral interventions for weight loss	Obese adults
C. No recommendation for or against	
Screening for HIV	Persons not at increased risk for HIV
Screening for osteoporosis	Postmenopausal women younger than 60 who are not at increased risk for osteoporotic fractures
D. Recommended against	
Screening for testicular cancer	Asymptomatic adolescent and adult males
Screening for coronary conditions with resting electrocardiogram, treadmill, and CT scan	Adults at low risk for coronary heart disease events
Combined estrogen and progestin for prevention of osteoporosis, high blood pressure, lipid disorders, and cancer	Postmenopausal women
I. Insufficient evidence	
Screening for dementia	Older adults
Behavioral counseling to promote physical activity	Inactive adults

named after the localities in which they took place: Framingham in Massachusetts and Alameda County in California. Long-term studies of Harvard alumni, female nurses, and women from the general population have been of great value as well. Also of note is a landmark study by English epidemiologists Doll and Peto on the causes of cancer.

The **Framingham Heart Study** has been a definitive source of information about the individual characteristics that lead to cardiovascular disease (including heart attacks, heart failure, and stroke). The study was begun in 1948 on 5,209 men and women, who were given physical examinations. These individuals were followed continuously well into the twenty-first century, receiving additional physical examinations every two years. In 1971, the study was expanded to include children of the people initially examined to help identify familial risk factors.

Key findings from the Framingham study began to appear in the 1970s, enabling researchers to develop a "portrait of the potential candidate for coronary heart disease."[22] These early findings identified smoking, high blood pressure, and metabolic variables such as serum cholesterol and glucose intolerance (a feature of diabetes) as risk factors for heart disease. Prior to the Framingham study, heart disease was considered by many to be unpredictable.

More recent research based on the Framingham subjects has refined initial discoveries. Low-density lipoprotein cholesterol, rather than cholesterol itself, was found to predict heart disease. High-density lipoprotein cholesterol turned out to be a protective factor. By the 1990s, researchers had developed a scoring system that allowed physicians to accurately estimate the risk of coronary heart disease in middle-aged patients.[23] The fact that many of the risk factors were amenable to identification and reduction by physicians led a key researcher to comment that "most [heart attacks] represent medical failures; the conditions should have been detected years earlier for preventive management."[24]

The Framingham study had major implications for lifestyle. Low-density lipoprotein cholesterol and diabetes are less common, and higher levels of high-density lipoprotein cholesterol more common among those who are physically active. The Framingham study did not find that overweight in itself contributed strongly to heart disease. But overweight is associated with definite risk factors such as lower levels of high-density lipoprotein cholesterol, high blood pressure, and diabetes. The importance of cholesterol as a predictor of heart disease and related ailments has obvious implications for dietary practices.

More direct evidence for health benefits from exercise was found by Stanford's Ralph S. Paffenbarger in the Harvard Alumni Health Study, which followed thousands of men who matriculated as undergraduates at Harvard University between 1916 and 1950. As do many elite universities, Harvard maintains continuously updated records on its alumni for fundraising purposes, facilitating continual contact. Paffenbarger evaluated the efficacy of exercise by seeing whether men who had been college athletes had greater longevity than their relatively sedentary classmates. This hypothesis was substantiated. Even more convincing was a later finding that sedentary men who began an exercise program in middle age tended to outlive their contemporaries who remained sedentary.[25] Even occasional exercisers who expended a minimum amount of energy experienced a survival benefit.[26]

A study of women found similar results. Meir Stampfer of Harvard used data from the Nurses' Health Study to investigate the effects of diet and lifestyle on cardiovascular disease. Since 1976, the Nurses' Health Study has followed several thousand nurses who, serving as volunteers in a number of investigations regarding lifestyle-related causes of disease. Stampfer's study found that nurses who did not exercise regularly experienced a significantly higher risk of death from heart disease and stroke than those who did. Women who were overweight, consumed a high-calorie diet, or used tobacco also had a higher risk of death from heart disease and stroke. Part of this study's importance derived from its power to set aside the widespread belief that heart disease was a "male" illness from which women were relatively free.[27]

Exercise Isn't Only for the Young and Able

The Framingham Heart Study and several other investigations have demonstrated the benefits of exercise for a wide range of age groups. Young athletes may strive for steadily increasing performance, but the true benefits of lifelong exercise may become most apparent in old age. Following is the story of a one-time Olympic swimmer:

> After turning ninety on Friday, Adolph Kiefer will rise early this morning and swim. That has been his routine since childhood, since before the 1936 race in Berlin that earned him an Olympic gold medal. He doesn't plan to stop.
>
> . . . Once a medal winner at the trials, Mr. Kiefer now owns a company that furnishes the event with stopwatches, whistles, pace clocks and other equipment.
>
> . . . For twelve years, Mr. Kiefer dominated international races in the backstroke as well as the individual medley. In a career that spanned more than 2,000 races, he lost only twice. One of his world records stood for twelve years.
>
> A condition called idiopathic peripheral neuropathy has stiffened Mr. Kiefer's hands and robbed him of the balance needed to walk without assistance. One recent morning, he used a walker to travel from his bedroom to the natatorium on the far side of his house.
>
> In the water, his long backward strokes offer a hint of the power he once wielded. But he no longer swims like an Olympian. His is the routine of a ninety-year-old seeking to limit the effects of an incurable disease, and he is succeeding. His chest and legs remain muscular, giving him the strength to use a walker, to pull himself out of chairs, to remain self-sufficient more than two decades after his neuropathy first struck.
>
> "Anybody else with his level of neuropathy would be getting pushed around in a wheelchair," says Gail Lucks [a physician and Mr. Kiefer's daughter].

Source: K. Helliker. Swimming the distance: as the Olympic trials begin, a 90-year-old medalist is watching the water. *Wall Street Journal.* June 28, 2008:W1.

Diet is perhaps the most familiar concern regarding health risks. Scientists have paid special attention to trans fats—semisolid substances for use in margarines, commercial cooking, and food manufacturing to enhance consumer convenience and shelf life. Randomized controlled trials have demonstrated that consumption of trans fatty acids raises levels of low-density lipoprotein cholesterol, reduces levels of high-density lipoprotein (HDL) cholesterol, and increases the ratio of total cholesterol to HDL cholesterol, all powerful predictors of heart disease.[28] A 1996 review of nearly 150 medical journal articles concluded that a diet rich in non–trans fats, whole grains, abundant fruits and vegetables, and adequate in omega-3 fatty acids offered significant protection against heart disease.[29] Other studies have linked historically high life expectancy in Japan, and especially Okinawa, with diets rich in vegetables and low in fat.[30] A variety of studies supports the potential benefits of omega-3 fatty acids, particularly in the form of fish oil, for prevention of heart disease.[31]

The **Alameda County Study**, a large-scale longitudinal investigation like several already discussed, provides a different perspective. Studies such as Framingham sought to explain heart disease risk on the basis of metabolic variables. The Alameda County investigation focused specifically on behavioral and social correlates of mortality. The study began in 1965 by collecting lifestyle data via questionnaire from 6,928 randomly selected adults. Nine years later, the researchers determined the vital status (alive versus dead) of these individuals and sought statistical relationships between various health-related practices and survival. Five factors were determined to have helped the study participants remain alive: never having smoked, regular physical activity, low alcohol consumption, average weight status, and sleeping seven to eight hours per night.[32]

Later work by the Alameda County researchers produced important findings on the importance of social relations and surroundings for staying alive. In a finding replicated in many other communities (see Chapter Three), the Alameda County researchers reported that frequent and intimate social contact correlated with increased longevity.[33]

Still other findings from the Alameda County Study indicated that people who resided in poor neighborhoods had a 50 percent greater chance of dying than those in nonpoor neighborhoods. This was true even after individual health-related characteristics had been accounted for.[34] Other research has suggested that lack of opportunity for physical exercise helps account for increased mortality risk in poor neighborhoods.[35] But an actual mechanism that may promote survival among the socially connected has not yet been demonstrated.

Cancer presents a more complicated challenge for prevention than cardiovascular disease. Malignancies may occur in any body tissue and may involve a variety of cell types, even within the same organ. Behavior predisposing individuals to cancer ranges from familiar practices such as tobacco use to rare occupational exposure to specialty chemicals.

The work of epidemiologists Doll and Peto has long served as a resource for advocates of cancer prevention. Their classic publication, *The Causes of Cancer: Quantitative Estimates of Avoidable Risks of Cancer in the United States Today,*[36] asserts that 35 percent of U.S. cancer deaths are caused by diet, 30 percent by tobacco, and 7 percent by reproductive and sexual behavior. Notably, Doll and Peto attribute few cancer deaths to pollution (2 percent), food additives (less than 1 percent), and industrial products (less than 1 percent). Doll and Peto pay considerably more attention to consumption of fat, lack of dietary fiber, and general overeating. Later generations of researchers have maintained this emphasis, reporting evidence that fat and overweight may promote breast cancer[37] and that diets low in fruits and vegetables may be conducive to some forms of colon cancer.[38]

Doll and Peto's comments on reproductive and sexual behavior are provocative. They observe that women who begin menstruating early and do not have children are more susceptible to cancers of the endometrium, ovaries, and breast. They speculate that greater numbers of menstrual cycles correlate with increased likelihood of contracting cancer. They consider the possibility that young women who exercise may help prevent cancer by delaying the onset of menstruation. Later research on reproductive and sexual behavior has concentrated on cervical cancer. As noted above, mortality from this disease is declining, due in large part to early diagnosis via the Pap test. Considerable interest remains in a possible relationship between exercise and breast cancer. A second cycle of the Nurses' Health Study has found women who have regularly engaged in "high amounts of physical activity" to be at lower risk.[39]

PREVENTION IN PRACTICE

Disease prevention is usually associated with medical and public health activity. Thus, immunization and other forms of prevention carried out by physicians conform to the guidelines of disease prevention. The same would be true of traditional public health measures. **Health promotion**, on the other hand, connotes behavior ultimately under the control of individuals themselves. Exercise, healthy eating, weight control, and avoidance of tobacco, excessive alcohol use, and high-risk sex fall under the rubric of health promotion. Collectively, such activities may generally be considered dimensions of individual lifestyle.

Public Health and Medicine

The preceding section on the scientific basis of prevention covers the principal contributions of public health and medicine. Traditional distinctions between medicine and public health become less clear in the context of prevention. Principal contributions of medicine to primary prevention include immunization and counseling about health behaviors such as diet, exercise, and smoking. Public health and medicine both conduct screening, a fundamental secondary prevention procedure.

Many mainstream medical interventions may be classified as tertiary prevention, in that they retard the progression of disease and reduce its impact. Musculoskeletal surgery, it may be argued, helps prevent heart attacks: by enabling people with back, neck, and limb discomfort to remain active, these interventions promote cardiovascular conditioning. The same is true of coronary artery bypass graft (CABG). By removing coronary artery occlusions, CABG prevents the occurrence of heart attacks.

Relatively new interventions in chronic disease management (CDM) may be regarded as secondary prevention. Within primary care settings, CDM systems combine and coordinate resources required for optimal treatment of diseases such as asthma, diabetes, hypertension, and congestive heart failure. Under such systems patients receive instruction and support in self-care. Resources made available to primary care physicians include ready access to specialists for consultation.[40] Electronic data facilities may promote periodic patient contact procedures to ensure regular checkups and medication adjustment. Through routine management, it is hoped that patients will avoid acute episodes necessitating emergency care or hospitalization.

In view of the importance of lifestyle and behavior in prevention, it would seem important for clinicians to promote favorable behavior by informing and counseling their patients. Today influencing individual behavior remains the method of choice for preventing heart disease, some cancers, and AIDS. Health systems such as Kaiser Permanente have undertaken large-scale efforts to encourage their clinicians to deliver relevant information and counseling. But physicians in high-volume practice may have limited opportunity for such action. Individuals most in need of such intervention, moreover, may seldom see a doctor. Other mechanisms for promoting favorable health behavior have begun to receive emphasis.

Behavior and Community

Most attempts to promote healthy behavior have taken place outside formal health care settings such as doctors' office and hospitals. Rather, such efforts have been undertaken principally by government agencies, schools, and health-oriented nonprofits such as the American Cancer Society or American Lung Association. Community-based organizations—including community improvement associations, health-oriented community coalitions, and religious congregations—have begun to assume an important place in prevention. Initiatives intended to improve human behavior have employed a variety of approaches. Following are some of the major ones:

- *Information dissemination:* concentrating on simultaneous delivery of information to mass audiences

- *Instruction and counseling:* conducted in small-group or classroom settings and designed to affect the way people think about health risks, deal with adverse social influences, and process information received from others

- *Community partnerships:* focused on alerting people in a given neighborhood about the health risks they face and building the social capital needed to reduce these risks

- *Policy change:* utilizing laws and ordinances at all levels of government to reduce threats to health and increase opportunities for prevention

Efforts to improve behavior related to health have focused on a broad range of health concerns. They have utilized methods ranging from posters and public service announcements to intensive individual counseling. Some of the longest-standing efforts have sought to promote avoidance or cessation of tobacco use. Since the emergence of AIDS in the 1980s, safe sex has occupied a significant part of the prevention agenda. More recently, diet and exercise have achieved increasing prominence.

Information Dissemination. Simple dissemination of information is the most familiar of all mechanisms employed in hopes of changing health behavior. This approach assumes that people engage in risky health practices because of an information deficit. Associated interventions have focused on providing information about the dangers of adverse practices such as tobacco use and the benefit of favorable actions such as immunization and cancer screening.

Most traditional health education and hygiene classes fall into the category of information dissemination. Prevention-related information is also widely disseminated in the mass media. Among key participants in such interventions is the Advertising Council. The Ad Council, as it is better known, is a nonprofit organization supported by the advertising industry that has produced numerous broadcast messages on health matters such as safe driving and colon cancer screening. Health messages today appear on product packaging, the most familiar being those on packages of cigarettes sold in the United States.

Informational messages have sometimes included content intended to arouse fear among target persons. Messages on tobacco products sold in Canada are apply this thinking. Graphics on tobacco product packaging in Canada include images of diseased lung tissue and people breathing through tracheotomy tubes. A polio immunization campaign on U.S. television in the 1950s included footage of a woman in a wheelchair chillingly implying that she had taken a chance, rather than taking her polio shot.

A program to discourage the use of methamphetamine by young people continued the information deficit approach into the twenty-first century. Sponsored by the Siebel Foundation, a campaign known as the Meth Project has featured expertly produced, powerful, and grim television images to demonstrate the consequences of using the drug. The prevention mechanism envisaged by the program was to promote balanced information regarding perceived benefits and costs of methamphetamine use. According to an official statement, "Many perceive benefits in using the drug, but little to no risk. This is the root of the problem. The goal of the Meth Project is to arm teens and young adults with the facts about methamphetamine so that they can make well-informed decisions when presented with the opportunity to try it."[41]

Instruction and Counseling. Individual and small-group counseling and support have found widespread use in prevention. Nutrition and fitness counselors aid individuals in losing weight and planning cardiovascular conditioning programs. Classes in exercise and relaxation techniques, along with popular Eastern practices such as yoga, address important dimensions of counseling. Instruction and counseling involve health

promotion mechanisms different from information dissemination. Information dissemination provides people with facts about one particular kind of behavior. Instruction
and counseling in the sense used here are intended to change people's assumptions
about themselves and the world around them and also the *process* by which they
think, assess options, and make choices.

Many intensive programs utilizing one-on-one counseling have been formulated
to help people stop using tobacco. Such interventions have, among many others, utilized *aversion therapy* techniques intended to reduce the appeal of smoking to people
wishing to quit. Aversion-based interventions have included requiring that clients who
have relapsed into tobacco use smoke multiple cigarettes in rapid succession. The
associated toxicity and discomfort, it is believed, makes smokers associate a cigarette
not with pleasure but with a repulsive experience.

Innovators in prevention have utilized sophisticated psychological approaches to
advance prevention objectives. Two such approaches are the *social influence model*[42]
and the *cognitive-affective model*.[43] The social influence model asserts that people can
be taught how to resist social and media pressure to engage in unhealthy practices.
Techniques based on this model emphasize informing individuals of the actual behavior of peers, often incorrectly portrayed by media as accepting of risk. The cognitive-
affective model emphasizes improving generic personal and social skills as an aid to
resisting adverse influences.

Psychological approaches such as these have been widely applied as classroom,
telephone, and Internet-based interventions for health risks such as tobacco and overeating. Tobacco Quitlines, or systems of telephone-based counseling and coaching for
tobacco cessation, represent an increasingly popular example.[44] Quitline counseling
is typically provided by paraprofessionals following a semistructured protocol. The protocol may include setting a quit date, removing smoking paraphernalia from their home
and car, striving for total abstinence, and anticipating future triggers or challenges.
Clients may receive training in problem solving and other skills. Such procedures combine elements of several counseling approaches such as the cognitive-behavioral model.
Quitlines often provide coaching to friends and relatives. Quitline services may include
written materials to reinforce telephone counseling and pharmaceutical adjuncts such
as nicotine patches. A number of commercial quitlines market their services to employers, unions, and health care systems throughout the United States.

Community Partnerships. The terms *community partnership* and *community coalition* may be used interchangeably. This approach to prevention relies on neighborhood-
based collaboration of institutions, organizations, and individuals to promote health
and prevent illness. Objectives of these coalitions sometimes emphasize changes
in individual behavior. But generally, their perspective is communitywide, seeking
change in factors that simultaneously affect large numbers of people. Accordingly,
community coalitions usually focus their efforts on issues such as public safety, access
to health care, employment opportunity, education, and housing. Matters such as these
are sometimes characterized as *upstream determinants of health*. Achievements in

these areas might not immediately improve the health of a given individual, but in the long run may have significant impact on the health of thousands.

Potentially, a community partnership can serve as a powerful asset for prevention. A successful partnership combines the resources, expertise, and creativity of numerous parts of a community. Membership of a coalition may include one or more churches, synagogues, or mosques; a public health department; a school system; a police department; one or more hospitals, clinics, or health systems; and a chamber of commerce or business roundtable. Each of these community sectors can help ensure involvement of a different segment of the community's population, transmitting information to individuals and obtaining their services as volunteers or financial contributors. Community partnerships may arise spontaneously or develop in response to availability of funding from philanthropic foundations or government agencies.

Community partnerships also depart from traditional prevention approaches by promoting the community's capacity to organize itself and advocate for change conducive to health. From a social scientist's point of view, the community coalition's characteristic focus is the building of *social capital*—that is, the presence of local networks that link individuals and facilitate working relationships among organizations and institutions. Social capital defined in this manner is invaluable in bringing about communitywide change.

Advocates of community organization argue that networks of individuals, organizations, and institutions alone can have substantial impact on the environmental conditions that fundamentally determine health risks. One example is the built environment. The term *built environment* denotes the pattern of housing, roads, sidewalks, and commercial venues in a community. The built environment may either enhance or restrict opportunity for exercise and socialization. Public health scientists have started looking to related environmental factors such as substandard housing, crime, noise, pollution, and hazardous waste as causes of the health disparities that today characterize the United States. An individual may do much to affect her own likelihood of getting sick by changes in diet and exercise. But, as community advocates often contend, only coalitions of individuals, organizations, and institutions can change the environmental forces that surround the individual.

The goals of community coalitions vary in scope. A survey of community coalitions illustrates the range of activities they undertake.[45] Community coalitions also differ in their origins and membership. Following are some examples:

■ *The Project Immunize Virginia (PIV).* A statewide partnership focused on immunization, PIV was initiated under state funding by the Eastern Virginia Medical School. PIV seeks to increase the rate at which Virginians receive vaccinations appropriate to their age and health risk profile. Participating organizations include over two hundred agencies, including local community groups, professional societies, and public health departments.

■ *The Mutual Partnerships Coalition (MPC).* A Seattle-based coalition, MPC combined the resources of the city housing authority, a community food bank, a

United Way agency, a central city minority youth organization, and a large HMO. MPC focused its efforts on reducing isolation among inner-city elders. It was expected that the elders involved would have higher-quality lives, reduce their requirements for health care, and become less dependent on social service agencies.

■ *Bethel New Life.* The Bethel New Life coalition had its start on Chicago's West Side in the wake of riots and destruction in the 1960s and 1970s. Members of the Bethel Lutheran Church passed the hat, raising $9,600 to purchase and rehabilitate a small apartment building. Over the years, the coalition leveraged its assets and expanded aid to community residents by obtaining loans and purchasing homes. Among its many functions today, Bethel New Life addresses upstream precursors of disease such as housing, employment, and community. The coalition promotes environmentally friendly housing, provides assisted living and homemaker services to elders under contract with public agencies, and makes healthy food available to community residents.

Public Policy. As detailed in Chapter Nine, public policy constitutes a powerful mechanism for determining how health care is financed and delivered in the United States. Recall that *public policy* involves the direction taken by government toward a particular public function or concern. Obviously, public policy is made through legislation and executive orders by elected officials. Less obviously, public policy is both made by and reflected in actions of the civil servants who staff agencies charged with implementing elected officials' decisions. Historically, public policy has been important in preventing disease through basic public health actions and infrastructure.

Some observers look to public policy as the key to disease prevention. Only public policy, they reason, can reduce environmental threats to health. In this connection, community residents capable of making an impact on policy may promote legislation against environmental hazards and in favor of access to health care. Policy, it is reasoned, can reduce the social and economic disparities that contribute to disparities in health.

In areas of more immediate concern, public policy has begun to address food-related issues in an effort to control overweight and associated health risks. New York City has been particularly active in using public policy in nontraditional ways for prevention purposes. Recent examples of New York's policy-based initiatives have focused on tobacco and nutrition. Tobacco-related policy has featured tax increases, a comprehensive smoke-free air law, hard-hitting anti-tobacco advertising, and cessation services. Nutrition-related interventions have included mandates banning trans fats from restaurants and requiring restaurants to post calorie information on menu boards.[46]

California has followed a similar course. Both legislative action and voter initiatives have resulted in stringent anti-tobacco laws and funding for a strong anti-tobacco publicity campaign. In 2003, the California legislature passed a law banning sales of soda in elementary schools, a move intended to address youth obesity by reducing sugar intake.

In several states, advocates have started policy think tanks to advance prevention. These organizations aim at increasing awareness among policy makers, analyzing proposed legislation, and bringing together others with a commitment to prevention. Often these organizations have received support from philanthropic foundations concerned with health. The Foundation for a Healthy Kentucky, for example, has sought to launch an "army of advocates" pressing for action by state government. In 2007, the foundation funded a unit of the University of Kentucky to provide communities across the state with "science-based strategies for advancing smoke-free policies on the local level and educating citizens and policymakers about the importance of smoke-free environments." The unit also provides technical assistance to local smoke-free advocates, including strategies for local data collection and dissemination, communication, and media.[47]

On a larger scale, the California Wellness Foundation helped launch the Center for Health Improvement in the mid-1990s. This organization conducted policy analysis and statewide polling to demonstrate the importance that Californians placed on prevention to state policy makers.[48] Within a decade of its founding, the organization expanded its scope of operation to prevention-related policy nationwide.

CHALLENGES TO PREVENTION

Both practice and science suggest that prevention is both widely applicable and of potentially great benefit. This is true of prevention-related contributions from both within and outside the formal health care system. But managers and policy makers must balance widespread enthusiasm for prevention with an understanding of its limitations. Scientific investigations have not always substantiated the efficacy of interventions believed to prevent illness. The principles that have been supported by science cannot always be applied in practical interventions. Special challenges arise when prevention depends, as it ultimately does, on human behavior. Even highly motivated people often find it difficult to change personal health practices—as those who have tried to quit smoking or lose weight can attest. Deliberately changing the behavior of millions of others is proportionately more challenging.

Scientific Concerns

As in other fields of science, progress in building a factual basis for prevention has been neither consistent nor steady. Investigations such as the Framingham Heart Study and the Alameda County Study have laid groundwork for much of the prevention-related activity taking place today. But equally or more extensive studies have failed to produce the hoped-for results. Often even positive findings are difficult to apply in a practical way because of their complexity. Presumably healthful interventions, moreover, have occasionally been found to produce serious harm.

Negative Research Findings

Instances of disappointing research results may be cited in all prevention arenas described above: medical, behavioral, and community-based. Such studies have involved numerous individual programs, followed thousands of people, and taken years to complete. Costs of the experimental interventions have in some cases involved hundreds of millions of dollars.

Chemoprevention. Ingestion of specific chemical compounds for the purpose of preventing illness is known as **chemoprevention**. Scientists in the early 1980s believed that vitamins E and A might reduce the risk of lung cancer. To determine whether individuals could lower their cancer risk through these vitamins, scientists conducted a randomized, double-blind experiment.

Subjects for this experiment were male smokers, a group at elevated risk of contracting lung cancer. A total of 29,133 men fifty to sixty-nine years of age took part in the trial. They were randomly assigned to one of four regimens: vitamin E alone, beta carotene (which is made into vitamin A in the body) alone, both vitamin E and beta carotene, or a placebo. Follow-up continued for five to eight years. No reduction in lung cancer incidence was observed among the men who received vitamin E, beta carotene, or both.[49]

Anti-Tobacco Instruction. Another major study assessed the efficacy of a sophisticated instructional approach to prevent children and youths from beginning to smoke as they grew older. The intervention was a teacher-led tobacco use prevention curriculum. Young people in the program received a total of sixty-five classroom lessons between the third and tenth grade. The curriculum emphasized development of skills for identifying prosmoking influences (such as tobacco advertising, marketing strategies, and peer influence), resisting influences to smoke (such as advertising analysis and resistance skills), and correcting erroneous normative perceptions. In addition, the curriculum sought to promote young people's self-confidence in their ability to refuse social pressure to smoke and to enlist positive family influences. The approach taken by the intervention was recommended by an expert National Cancer Institute panel and the Centers for Disease Control and Prevention.

To assess the program's efficacy, scientists randomly assigned forty school districts in Washington state to either an intervention or a control condition. Children and youths attending school in these districts were followed from third grade until two years past high school. A total of 8,388 individuals were followed until completion of the study. Children and youths in the school districts used as controls were exposed only to the health promotion and tobacco avoidance programs that were normally carried out. Smoking behavior was assessed in twelfth grade and two years after completion of high school. The experiment lasted fifteen years.

No significant difference in smoking was found between people who had attended schools in the control and experimental districts. The experimenters concluded that the trial furnished "no evidence . . . that a school-based social-influences approach [could be] effective in the long-term deterrence of smoking among youth."[50]

Community Health Promotion. Many people concerned with prevention have looked to community partnerships such as those described above to improve health on a large scale. Evaluation studies of community prevention efforts have provided some support for advocates of this approach. Researchers, for example, found encouraging results in interventions intended to reduce cardiovascular risk in the United States and elsewhere.[51,52] However, these studies were unable to demonstrate that lower risk actually resulted from the interventions.

A very large-scale community-based intervention begun in the 1980s provided an important opportunity for testing the efficacy of community health promotion programs. Funded by the Henry J. Kaiser Family Foundation, the intervention was known as the Community Health Promotion Grants Programs (CHPGP). It sought to promote health and prevent disease by modifying community norms, environmental conditions, and individual behavior. Under the intervention, communities received grants to select their own health promotion targets and devise and implement strategies of their choice. The program remained active into the 1990s and provided larger-scale funding than perhaps any previous health promotion intervention.

The Mammography Controversy

Mammography, a form of X-ray screening for breast cancer, represents one of the most widely practiced methods of prevention in the United States. For decades, the American Cancer Society has recommended that women over forty years of age receive mammography screening, although the recommended frequency of screening has varied.

The practice of mammography screening, however, has become controversial. A review of research on the effectiveness of mammography published in 2000 cast doubt on the benefits of the procedure. Two Danish scientists, Gotzsche and Olsen, carefully reviewed studies done of mammography in Europe, Canada, and the United States. They found all except two major studies to be seriously flawed.[57] Neither of these studies showed that mammography saved lives. The scientists concluded that that mammography often resulted in harm, as women without malignancies (or with malignancies unlikely to become aggressive) received unnecessary, invasive treatment.

In a 2006 update, Gotzsche and another colleague concluded that mammography "likely reduces breast cancer mortality," but that the reduction of risk of death from the disease was quite small. They wrote: "For every 2,000 women invited for screening throughout ten years, one will have her life prolonged. In addition, ten healthy women, who would not have been diagnosed if there had not been screening, will . . . be treated unnecessarily. It is thus not clear whether screening does more good than harm."[58]

As of 2003, the American Cancer Society and the U.S. Preventive Services Task Force (USPSTF) continued to recommend mammography screening, although USPSTF gave the procedure only a grade of B.

The initiative's sponsor desired a "comprehensive, independent, and rigorous" assessment of the intervention and retained a team of experts to evaluate eleven funded communities in the western United States.[53] The evaluation team used multiple research techniques, both adolescents and adults were surveyed, healthfulness of foods in local grocery stores was assessed, and communities receiving funds under the initiative were compared with control communities. Some evidence of favorable changes during the course of the intervention was detected. However, the investigators concluded that "the CHPGP, like other prominent community-based initiatives, generally failed to produce measurable changes in the targeted health outcomes."[54]

Diet. A number of dietary approaches to prevention have failed to find support when assessed by well-designed experiments and other studies. For example, fiber, fruits, and vegetables were long believed to offer protection against cancer, particularly cancers of the colon and rectum. To determine whether these food components provided actual protection, scientists pooled data from a wide range of studies of diet and health. After analyzing data on 724,628 people observed for up to twenty years, one group of scientists concluded that "high dietary fiber intake was not associated with a reduced risk of colorectal cancer."[55] Another group concluded that fruit and vegetable intake was not associated with overall colon cancer risk.[56]

Complex Conclusions

Positive findings, of course, have also been obtained from research studies on prevention. Representative findings are summarized earlier in this chapter. Even when they have obtained encouraging findings on prevention, however, researchers have often concluded that their findings are not uniformly applicable to people of different ages and lifestyles. The complexities of human biology and behavior contribute to the challenges of making prevention work.

Findings from the Women's Health Initiative (WHI) illustrate this complexity.[59] The WHI was a highly ambitious randomized controlled trial intended to identify means by which postmenopausal women could prevent adverse health developments by ingesting hormones and changing their diets. All phases of the study involved nearly 200,000 women who were followed for as long as ten years.

Relationships between dietary modification and health outcomes have proven complex. Dietary modification in the trial included a low-fat diet and increased ingestion of calcium and vitamin D. Earlier research had suggested that a low-fat diet would help prevent cancer. Generally women who were assigned to the low-fat group were no less likely, according to a widely accepted statistical criterion, to develop cancer than the controls. According to the same statistical criterion, however, women who began with a relatively high fat content in their diet and made large reductions in fat intake as part of the experiment realized a benefit. These women were less likely to contract breast cancer than those who began with a high-fat diet and did not reduce their fat intake.

The experimenters expected that increased dietary calcium and vitamin D would protect women from fractures during the postmenopausal years. But in the experiment, the women who increased their calcium and vitamin D intake generally were no less likely to experience fractures than the controls. One group of women did benefit, however. Among women over sixty years of age, those who increased dietary calcium and vitamin D did experience fewer fractures.

Harmful Outcomes

Of concern to advocates of prevention should be potential harm from interventions thought to be healthful. Findings from the WHI cited earlier illustrate this phenomenon. The scientists who designed the study had hoped that treatment with hormones (estrogen, progesterone, or both) would protect women from cancer and fractures of the hip and other bones. Women who were given the hormones experienced some expected benefits. They had fewer fractures and a lower risk of colon cancer. However, significant increases were found to occur in breast cancer, stroke, and vascular disease. Authorities terminated the hormone phase of the WHI as soon as these adverse outcomes became apparent.

Long-term follow-up of Framingham Heart Study participants also provided evidence that practices expected to prove healthful produced harmful results instead. One researcher followed 832 healthy middle-aged men for twenty years, monitoring their diet and health. He found that men who adhered to a low-fat diet were more likely to have strokes than those who did not.[60] A thirty-year follow-up of 2,421 women found that those who had been most physically active were, to a "marginally significant" degree, the most likely to develop breast cancer.[61] In an innovative experiment known as A Healthy Future, over 2,500 elders in an HMO were randomly assigned to receive special prevention services. These services included health risk assessment, counseling, and a comprehensive package of preventive interventions focused on diet, exercise, and depression. A control group received the usual array of preventive services offered by the HMO. After two years, more deaths were found to have occurred in the experimental than the control group.[62]

When Exercise Becomes Unhealthful

Middle-class Americans share a widespread belief in the benefits of exercise. But excessive exercise can be damaging to health and even fatal.

According to a *Wall Street Journal* report, doctors and psychotherapists are worried about obsessive, even addictive exercise.[63] A growing number of exercisers, some believe, are taking anti-inflammatory drugs to mask serious injuries and sacrificing their family lives and jobs in pursuit of impossible physical goals. Obsessive joggers and aerobic dancers develop tendonitis, shin splints, and stress fractures, conditions with lifelong consequences. Women who lose too much body fat may develop amenorrhea (loss of monthly menstrual periods), a condition whose ultimate impact on the body is unknown.

The report cites the following examples:

- A Miami woman in New York on business was frantic over missing her daily aerobics classes. To compensate, she paced the streets at night, even though the pain was so excruciating that she couldn't put a sheet on her legs at night. Back in Miami a stress fracture halted her exercise activity. One night she sat outside the exercise studio near her home crying as she watched others dance.

- A Dallas man, who described himself as "absolutely obsessed" with running, logged as much as one hundred miles a week. He got up at 4:30 a.m. to run, often wrapping elastic bandages around his knees to reduce the pain in his aching joints. He was sleepy by 2:00 or 3:00 in the afternoon.

- A running-obsessed homemaker started therapy and cut down. But her compulsion was still evident. She found herself frantically dancing to music while ironing, vacuuming, and mopping.

Physicians and psychologists have attributed addictive exercise to conditions such as low self-esteem, loneliness, desire to feel independent and powerful, and the need to escape from a bad marriage or a troublesome family life. Compulsive exercisers may also crave the high that comes from intense activity. When deprived of activities, these individuals experience the same depression, nervousness, and insomnia as drug users and alcoholics in withdrawal.

According to a psychologist quoted in the report, "upper and middle-class professionals wouldn't think of getting loaded in bars or copping drugs on the street," but use exercise as "the way they cope with conflicts inside themselves."

In jest, a medical writer has suggested that jogging shoes carry a warning label much the way cigarettes do.

In a more serious vein, marathon running has increased dramatically among recreational runners in recent years. Risks associated with marathon running were underscored when professional runner Ryan Shay died suddenly during a 2007 Olympic trial event in New York.[64] The athlete was only twenty-eight years old and in apparently perfect health. It is worth remembering that Pheidippides, the Greek soldier after whose feat the marathon is named, died immediately after his historic run from Marathon to Athens in 490 BC.

The science of prevention has produced findings that are sometimes favorable, sometimes unfavorable, and often mixed. However, policy makers, advocates, and health educators often race ahead of science. Zealotry of this kind results in actions that range from inconvenient to potentially harmful for the public. Examples in tobacco control and nutrition provide illustrations.

Overinterpretation of Research Findings

With the aim of reducing nonsmokers' exposure to environmental tobacco smoke (also called *sidestream* or *second-hand smoke*), municipalities throughout the United States have outlawed smoking in restaurants, bars, and workplaces. But questions have arisen about the dangers the public may actually face. In 1998, for example, a federal judge ruled that the Environmental Protection Agency (EPA) had overstated the connection between second-hand smoke and health risks to nonsmokers in an influential study. Ruling against the EPA in a suit mounted by the tobacco industry, U.S. District Judge William L. Osteen wrote that the agency had "disregarded information and made findings based on selected information" and "failed to disclose important [opposing] findings and reasoning."[65]

A group of researchers from Albert Einstein College of Medicine have commented that many public health recommendations on diet lack sufficient scientific support. Consistent with the scientific findings summarized above, they emphasize the uncertainty, complexity, and potential harm associated with dietary interventions that are popular with both health authorities and the public.[66] They comment that recommendations for a low-fat diet may have caused people to allay the resulting hunger by consuming more carbohydrates, resulting in weight gain. An individual who reduces fat intake may decrease his cholesterol levels and hence heart disease risk, but incur an increased risk of diseases such as diabetes by gaining weight. Recognizing the complexity of prevention, they comment that "public health guidelines are one-size-fits-all pronouncements that fail to account for variations in genetics, behavior, and environment." Acknowledging the ultimate limitations of prevention, they cite research demonstrating that "most heart attacks occur in . . . individuals who are at average or low risk based on any given risk factor."

Implementation Challenges

Despite inconsistencies and disappointing results, science does support selected medical, public health, and behavioral principles of prevention. Immunization and some forms of screening apparently do save lives. Avoidance of a high-fat diet, regular moderate exercise, and ingesting minimum daily rations of fiber and omega-3 fatty acids are apparently healthful. The importance of avoiding tobacco is well known. But developing effective mechanisms that enable human beings to benefit from these principles faces significant challenges.

Changing Individual Behavior. Current patterns of human behavior represent a challenge to any method aimed at disseminating prevention practices. Adverse patterns of behavior prevail in the U.S. population. As indicated in Chapter Four (see Table 4.1), over one-third of Americans are physically inactive. The vast majority are overweight. Almost 20 percent still smoke. Major trends are unfavorable for prevention. As indicated in Chapter Four, for example, 44.8 percent of Americans were overweight in the early 1960s, compared with 65.2 percent during the period 1999 through 2002. Physical activity has declined similarly, in part due to increasing average age in the United States. On average, women in their twenties interviewed for the Nurses' Health Study in 1997 spent about forty hours each week in active leisure pursuits; for women in their fifties, such activity averaged about twenty hours weekly.[67]

A number of interventions intended to promote healthful behavior have been reported as successful. However, evaluation of these interventions has not demonstrated that they can be applied beyond specially selected populations, that they are consistently effective, or that their impact is substantial. Evaluation of efforts to change behavior in some key areas via counseling interventions has reached the following conclusions:

■ Diet interventions have sometimes been effective, sometimes not. Intensive, counseling-type procedures—those that feature regular interaction of participants with counselors and use of telephone and Internet reminders—have been most effective.[68]

■ An anti-tobacco counseling intervention known as Free and Clear has shown evidence of success. This intervention includes periodic telephone calls by counselors to the participant.[69] Notably, evaluation of the program included objective measures of tobacco use via laboratory analysis of participants' saliva. Free and Clear has been widely commercialized.

Counseling interventions such as these require participants to have some degree of commitment. For most prevention purposes, these would represent a minority of individuals at risk in the population. Information dissemination and public policy interventions can reach a much wider segment of the public. Evaluation findings from such interventions include the following:

■ The state of California's multimillion-dollar effort to reduce tobacco use via mass media campaigns, enforcement of local antismoking laws, and school-based prevention programs was temporarily successful. For the first four years, tobacco use in California declined more rapidly than had been expected on the basis of a nationwide decline. However, smoking in California ceased to decline after 1994 and leveled off at a prevalence rate of 18 percent.[70]

■ The ban on soda sales in schools referenced earlier in this chapter has had only limited efficacy. A Rand Corporation study conducted a few years after the ban was instituted compared soda consumption by fifth graders in schools where the beverages were available versus those in schools where they were unavailable.[71] Only minor differences were found in soda consumption between schools where the drinks were sold versus schools where they were banned.

Even people strongly concerned with prevention may find the messages of prevention science difficult to apply in their own lives. Research articles, for example, report exercise requirements in calories and joules, which are not readily translatable into lifestyle. The research of Doll, Peto, and others suggests that exercise in adolescence and eventual childbearing protect women against some forms of cancer. But few women appear likely to plan their lives in this manner simply to lower their risk of malignant disease.

Social and Economic Disparities. Referenced several times in the preceding text, social and economic disparities in health and longevity represent a major challenge for the health care system, public health, and communities. Similar disparities in health risks are apparent and pose challenges to prevention. According to figures presented in Chapter Four (see Table 4.1), overweight was most prevalent in the early 2000s among African American women (77.1 percent) and Mexican American men (73.2 percent). A total of 37.6 percent of Americans were physically inactive at that time; however, the prevalence of inactivity among African Americans was 48.5 percent, Hispanics 51.9 percent, and Native Americans 54.7 percent. Even more striking were disparities in physical activity by years of education. Among people with education beyond high school, 28.1 percent were inactive. Among people without high school diplomas, the rate was 61.2 percent.

There is no reason to believe that poor people and minorities are less concerned with their health than the relatively advantaged. But any effective health promotion effort must address the environmental and historical reasons for unfavorable health behavior among poor people and minorities. Interviews of disadvantaged African Americans in six U.S. cities reveal a mix of social and cultural forces that create "what are in many cases dangerously poor eating habits."[72] The forces responsible for such habits include stress from crowded conditions and dangerous neighborhoods, a stigma against looking thin (connoting drug use and AIDS to some), and taste for traditional but unhealthy foods such as pork ribs and fried chicken.

Organizational and Professional Support. A key challenge in applying scientific findings on prevention in the real world concerns not consumers but institutions and professionals. Some business firms and health care organizations have allocated significant resources to prevention. But in many others commitment has been slight. Business firms, for example, may support in-house prevention programs or subsidize health club membership in boom times. These benefits help employers attract and retain employees in a tight labor market. But such programs are often abandoned when business slackens off.[73]

With the exception of delivering direct services such as immunization, clinical professionals do not appear to encourage prevention as much as they might. Some research suggests that physicians are more likely to counsel high-income patients about health behavior than low-income patients.[74] Historically, the physician's role has addressed treatment of visible illness rather than prevention. The interplay of

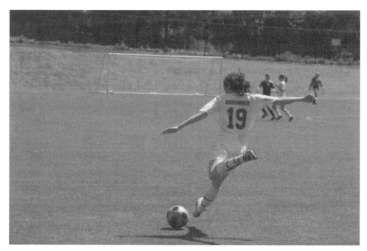

A young soccer player takes a shot. Despite concern that young Americans are increasingly adopting sedentary lifestyles and becoming obese, team sports remain popular. This is particularly true among young women, for whom athletic opportunity has increased markedly in recent years.

public expectations and medical practice seems to discourage an emphasis on prevention. These comments of Dr. Arnold Relman, a long-time editor of the *New England Journal of Medicine*, illustrate this dynamic:

> *In this sense, the traditional roles of physician and patient are changed when physicians practice preventive, rather than diagnostic and therapeutic, medicine. In the traditional relationship, a patient seeks a physician's help because he is ill, or is worried that he may be ill. The physician, in attending the patient, is providing a service that the patient feels he needs, and in a substantial percentage of cases the patient will ultimately come to believe that the service has been of some benefit to him. With preventive services, however, most patients do not seek out the physician but must be persuaded to do so by the argument that they will benefit in the long run from the preventive encounter. They rarely can be sure that they have in fact been helped. Some patients, of course, ask for checkups or other preventive services and are grateful when their physicians can reassure them that they are healthy. In most cases, however, patients are likely to receive primary preventive care with about as much enthusiasm and gratitude as they would a fire drill.[75]*

DOES PREVENTION SAVE MONEY?

As noted earlier, part of the appeal of prevention has been the presumption that it saves money. Logically, it would seem that an individual should reduce her personal health care costs by avoiding illness. Similarly, a disease detected early in its progress would be easier and less expensive to treat. In public statements, managers and policy makers at the highest level have linked prevention with cost savings. Some preventive measures do reduce health expenditures. But research suggests that while some preventive measures reduce health care costs, others may have the opposite effect.

Cost-Effectiveness of Interventions

The work of economist Louise B. Russell of the Brookings Institution illustrates the use of cost-effectiveness analysis (see Chapter Eight) for assessment of prevention.[76] She used this procedure to analyze vaccination, screening, and lifestyle interventions. In one instance, she applied cost-effectiveness analysis to a campaign to inoculate children against measles in the years following introduction of the antimeasles vaccine (1963–1968). Dollar costs directly incurred for medical care were calculated by adding expenses of administering the vaccine and treating people who contracted measles despite the campaign. These included children who were missed by the campaign or in whom vaccination did not produce immunity.

According to Russell's analysis, the campaign saved 973 lives, prevented 3,000 children from becoming mentally retarded (an occasional consequence of measles), and reduced absences from school and work by 34 million days. The campaign increased *direct* medical expenditures by $31 million. The campaign also was projected to save $200 million in institutional care for children who would have become retarded had they not received the vaccine. Taking the long view, then, the campaign had a favorable health and financial impact.

Cost-effectiveness analysis of other prevention interventions, however, resulted in less favorable findings. Vaccination for smallpox in the United States, for example, ceased in the 1970s, when efforts to eradicate the disease worldwide were well along. Russell comments that by that time the benefits of smallpox vaccination had "became equivocal at best." At the beginning of the next century, however, smallpox vaccination gained renewed attention, as bioterrorism became a public concern. U.S. authorities began administering smallpox vaccine to potential first responders. Among the 37,901 people vaccinated, there were 100 serious adverse events, resulting in 85 hospitalizations, 2 permanent disabilities, 10 life-threatening illnesses, and 3 deaths.[77] Barring a major bioterrorism attack involving smallpox, this program will rate poorly according to cost-effectiveness criteria.

Analysis of screening and related treatment is more complex. Costs include screening, actual diagnosis, medication, and repeated doctor visits. Many interventions have side effects, whose treatment requires expenditures. Additional costs result from the extended life expectancy of people who are successfully treated—death ends the individual's utilization of health services. According to Russell's analysis, hypertension control requires expenditures greater than the savings realized by prevention of heart attack and stroke.

A later cost-benefit analysis of cervical cancer screening and related treatment illustrates how increasing the intensity of prevention generally increases health expenditures. Research by a team at Georgetown University indicated that Pap tests administered every three years to women up to age seventy-five would reduce deaths by about 75 percent. If screening were done on this basis, the cost per quality-adjusted life year (QALY) gained would have been $11,839 in 2000 dollars. A more aggressive program was considered under which women of all ages would be included, screening would take place every two years, and human papillomavirus testing would be added to the procedure. Under this scenario, deaths would be reduced by over 95 percent. But cost per QALY gained would grow to $76,183.[78]

Table 10.2 summarizes the cost-effectiveness of several preventive procedures. Although cost-effectiveness varies, most interventions involve net increases in health

TABLE 10.2 Cost-effectiveness and cost impact of selected prevention measures

Intervention	Cost-Effectiveness	Cost Impact	Comment
Immunization			
Smallpox	Low	Increase	Population at low risk
Measles	High	Decrease	Widespread risk, rare side effects
Screening and treatment			
AIDS	Low	Increase	Treatment long-term, expensive
Hypertension	Moderate	Increase	Treatment long-term, potential side effects
Cervical cancer	Moderate	Increase	Low incidence, need for repeated screening
Lifestyle			
Exercise	Uncertain	Uncertain	Benefits vary by individual and type and frequency of exercise

care costs. Table entries for AIDS are based on the fact that AIDS treatment, though often effective, is expensive and requires continuation for many years. Cost-effectiveness of exercise and other lifestyle interventions is uncertain because its elements are widely diverse and impact is likely to vary among individuals.

The Case of Tobacco Control

Efforts to reduce smoking in the United States illustrate the limitations of cost control via prevention. Smoking is widely believed to create an economic burden for society as a whole. But economists have long believed that society realizes a net financial gain from tobacco use. Data from a study conducted in the 1980s appears in Table 10.3.[79]

TABLE 10.3   Costs and benefits per pack of cigarettes

	Cost per Pack ($)
Costs	
Medical care	.55
Sick leave	.01
Increased life insurance	.14
Fires	.02
Harm to others from second-hand smoke	.25
Lost taxes on earnings	.40
Total cost to society	1.37
Benefits	
Nursing home savings	.23
Pensions, Social Security payments forgone	1.19
Excise taxes on tobacco	.53
Total benefit to society	1.95

Smokers indeed require more medical care, at least while they remain alive. However, increased medical expenses are offset by the fact that smokers generally die earlier than nonsmokers, and hence incur no further medical care costs. Society recoups some of these losses from taxes on tobacco and by saving on nursing home expenses that the deceased smoker will not incur. Big savings are realized in the pension and Social Security benefits that the smoker will not live long enough to claim.

The importance of cost-benefit and other financial analyses of prevention may not be whether it does or does not save money; rather, such information should be used to decide among alternative opportunities for prevention. In this connection, Russell has written that the claims being made for prevention as a way to cut medical costs are generally untrue, but that "even when prevention does not save money, it can be a worthwhile investment in better health, and this—not cost saving—is the criterion on which it should be judged."

THE FUTURE: PREVENTION AND U.S. HEALTH CARE

Despite the limited encouragement provided by scientific research, disease prevention and health promotion continue to make sense. Over the past century, immunization against childhood diseases has done immense good. Screening for selected diseases has been indisputably beneficial. Chronic disease management systems show promise for tertiary prevention. Although the science is neither complete nor clear, improvement in diet and practices could be widely beneficial in the United States. The decline in physical activity and increase in overweight among Americans is of concern. But life expectancy continues to increase and physical function to improve throughout American society. Smoking in the United States has declined significantly.

Prevention shares characteristics with other movements in U.S. health care. Similar to health insurance and the Blue Cross movement covered in Chapter Seven, prevention is a compelling idea that has changed both individual lives and institutions. As in most movements, prevention has been most visibly embraced by a particular segment of society—in this instance, an educated elite of nonsmokers, exercisers, and consumers of low-fat diets.

To what degree will health care management and policy become involved in the prevention movement? The issue is particularly problematic for health care providers. Except for childhood immunization and other traditional interventions, little evidence exists to suggest significant economic returns from prevention services. The comments of famed economist Uwe Reinhardt underscore the challenges that providers face: "If I run a commercial [health care organization] with Wall Street breathing down my neck and there is an intervention that costs me now but will save me money in ten years, I won't do it. Or, I might do it if it wasn't too expensive and I could parlay it into a perception of quality."[80]

Ultimately, the future of prevention will depend on the decisions of individuals as both consumers and citizens, and by policy makers. If people exhibit willingness to pay for prevention by health care providers, related services will be offered. If citizens support greater expenditures for prevention, more generous coverage by public and private insurance will result. If prevention becomes part of the public discussion, policy will respond in areas such as nutrition, physical education, and built environment.

KEY TERMS

Primary prevention
Secondary prevention
Tertiary prevention
Screening
Framingham Heart Study

Alameda County Study
Disease prevention
Health promotion
Chemoprevention

SUMMARY

This chapter reviews the health care system's resources for keeping people well and assesses the likelihood that prevention of illness can help reduce health care costs.

Both the public and policy makers have looked to *prevention* as a means of safeguarding quality of life and controlling health care costs. Approaches to prevention include lifestyle and behavior of individuals (*health promotion*) and medical and public health interventions (*disease prevention*).

Researchers and clinicians have long recognized that a moderate lifestyle featuring healthy eating, exercise, and avoidance of tobacco and excessive alcohol helps maintain health and prolong life. Recent investigations have highlighted potential benefits of cholesterol-lowering pharmaceuticals and dietary supplements (such as omega-3 fatty acids). Clinical interventions such as Pap tests and colonoscopy have demonstrated efficacy in early detection of cancer.

Several challenges are notable in implementing prevention. Unfavorable practices regarding diet and exercise are widespread in the United States. Established patterns of behavior are difficult to change. Recent studies, moreover, have called into question some widely practiced interventions, such as mammography.

Prevention is valuable for promoting human health and well-being. But prevention cannot solve the U.S. health care system's financial problems. Many preventive measures increase, rather than reduce, health care costs.

DISCUSSION QUESTIONS

1. Summarize the major findings of research on prevention. Which do you consider to be the strongest from a scientific point of view? Which would be most useful to guide individual behavior?

2. To what degree can clinical medicine reduce the risk factors identified in the Framingham Heart Study? What methods currently in use are most effective, and what might be added to usual medical practice?

3. The Alameda County Study has reported that people with good social connections live longer than people who are isolated. What might account for this relationship? Can deliberate interventions be designed to make use of this finding to increase human longevity?

4. In view of the limitations discussed in this chapter, what forms of participation in prevention are health plans most likely to support in the coming years? Given the resource limitations they face, what might health plans do to better advance prevention objectives?

5. Based on the extensive research currently available on prevention, what would you advise policy makers to support for the purposes of (a) promoting the health of the U.S. population, and (b) achieving cost savings for the health care industry?

6. It has been argued that although prevention may not save money for the health care system and society as a whole, it may have significant economic benefit for individuals and their dependents. Is this true?

CHAPTER

11

GOVERNMENT, POLICY, AND POLITICS IN HEALTH CARE

LEARNING OBJECTIVES

- To understand the need for government participation in health care
- To learn how government participates in the U.S. health care system
- To become familiar with major milestones in U.S. health policy
- To see how private interests influence government actions
- To recognize effective strategies for advocacy

GOVERNMENT AND HEALTH CARE IN THE UNITED STATES

Although government plays a smaller role in health care in the United States than it does in other countries, it is still an important force in the health care industry. Funding from public sources is important, as in publicly operated systems of health insurance and subsidy. Medicare, Medicaid, and state and county programs for the indigent constitute major forces in U.S. health care. Government's role goes far beyond directly paying for health care. This role includes regulation of health care delivery and insurance, oversight and discipline of health professionals, disease surveillance and preparedness, drug and device licensure, and research into disease mechanisms and treatment.

The Case for Government Participation

A core teaching among economists asserts that goods and services are most efficiently produced and distributed by a market substantially free of dominance by powerful private parties and interference by government. Freed from such restrictions, active and sometimes boisterous interaction among buyers and sellers ensues, akin to stock and commodity exchanges in New York and Chicago or open-air markets throughout the world where bargaining is the norm. Price and quality are proclaimed and disputed. Buyers assess multiple alternatives. In theory, initiative and innovation thrive under such conditions of open competition.

But goods and services are seldom exchanged in just this fashion. Governments periodically intervene in markets. At various times in history they have encouraged or restricted production, promoted or restricted exports or imports, or inflated or stabilized the value of currency. In twentieth-century communist societies, governments attempted to replace the market entirely with state-mandated production and distribution. Private interests themselves restrict the freedom of the market. Workers decrease the availability of individuals with vital skills by forming restrictive trade unions. Professionals act similarly by restricting training opportunities and requiring licensure. Large firms make competition impossible through their ownership of patents and ability to cut prices using savings achieved through large-scale production—price cuts promptly rescinded when competition has been driven out of business.

Establishment and maintenance of a free market in health care seems especially dubious. This becomes apparent when the features of the health care market are examined in detail. It is useful to compare characteristics of health care goods and services with the conditions required for a free market. According to a classic formulation by economist Victor Fuchs, a **free market** exists in the following circumstances:

- There are many well-informed buyers and sellers, no one of whom is large enough to influence price unilaterally

- Buyers and sellers act independently (that is, there is no collusion)

- There is free entry for other buyers and sellers not currently in the market[1]

A fourth condition might be added—that buyers pay for goods and services with their own money and sellers bear the entire cost of bringing to market the goods and services they offer.

In theory, conditions that make a free market possible lead to optimal production, pricing, and distribution of goods and services. Consumers shop for the best quality at the lowest price; they are capable of detecting defects and fraud. Providers respond to informed, discriminating consumers by continuously striving to improve quality and lower prices. When prices rise, additional producers enter the market to take advantage of opportunities to profit, while consumers who find themselves priced out depart. Both the entry of new producers and departure of some consumers lead to lower prices. The producer's responsibility for covering the costs of bringing goods and services to market limits overproduction. The consumer's need to pay for goods and services through her own resources prevents excessive consumption.

Systemwide, the free market offers protection against the overproduction and shortages that plagued the communist countries. A central economic planner's error might affect the well-being of people in the hundreds of millions. But the error of a single producer or consumer has very limited impact. Overall, goods change hands, and services are delivered at their "natural price," which both buyers and sellers feel is acceptable.

Particularly in health care, actual conditions depart significantly from those required for a truly free market. Table 11.1 presents a side-by-side comparison of conditions that characterize the "ideal" free market and those that characterize health care. A great many differences are apparent.

Immediately apparent is the disparity of information between producers and consumers of health services. Few people who are not health professionals fully understand the services delivered by their providers. They have little understanding of differences in quality among services or providers.

Shockingly few health care consumers ask the price of medical goods and services prior to receiving them. This inattention arises in large part from the predominance of insurance over the years of the late twentieth century. Consumers seldom compare prices charged by hospitals and health professionals. Even an aggressive consumer may find it hard to obtain information on charges prior to treatment. Health professionals themselves often have scant information on prices. Most consumers find out what their services have cost only when they receive their insurance statements. This usually occurs weeks or months after "purchase" of the associated goods and services.

Health care consumers usually do not objectively assess the quality and efficacy of the goods and services offered to them. Few outside the health professions understand the technicalities of a specific medication or procedure. Health professionals themselves do not always make good decisions regarding the well-being of their patients. Clinicians do not always understand the pharmacology of the medications they prescribe and often order expensive imaging, hospitalization, and surgery whose benefits are open to question.

TABLE 11.1   Comparison of free-market and actual market conditions in health care

Free-Market Theory	Actual Market Conditions
Well-informed buyers and sellers predominate	Consumers seldom know much about prices and quality of the care they receive
No individual buyer or seller is large enough to influence price unilaterally	In some markets, a single hospital or HMO may strongly influence price
Buyers and sellers act independently	Buyers form cooperatives, and sellers form professional societies and networks
There is free entry into the market	Entry into the market requires extensive training and licensure
There is free exit from the market	Perceived need for health care deters exit by consumers
Buyers use their own money to make purchases	Most health care is paid for by commercial insurance or government programs
Sellers use their own resources to bring their goods and services to market	Health professionals are trained partially at public expense; publicly funded research subsidizes drug and equipment manufacturers

Consumers, moreover, usually fail to utilize indicators of quality that are readily obtainable or understandable. Mere availability of data on prices and quality through media such as the web does not ensure that comparison shopping will take place. Consumers tend to take the qualifications of their providers for granted. Few ask, for example, where their physician was trained or whether his board certification is current. Consumers may see a primary care provider for years without knowing her specialty.

Regarding another area identified in Table 11.1, entry to and exit from the health care market are far from free. This is probably true in most countries. Postcollege training for physicians normally requires eight years, plus additional time for fellowships required by subspecialties. Many nonphysician health professionals—registered nurses, physical therapists, and X-ray technicians, for example—must have at least a college degree. Reluctance of some educational institutions to expand teaching capacity promotes strong competition for available opportunities and further restricts entry into the market. The high cost of education discourages many from seeking entry into the health professions.

Exit from the health care market is likewise difficult. Consumers indeed reduce health care expenditures when they are obliged to pay costs out of pocket. But they appear willing to pay a great deal in life-or-death situations. As noted previously, health care is a commodity in "negative demand." No one *wants* health care for its intrinsic features, such as time in waiting rooms and intrusion into the body by scopes and needles. People consume health care in the conviction that they *need* it. In response to perceived need, consumers seldom delay or decline, as long as costs or an absence of providers do not bar access. Providers also find it hard to leave the market. One reason for this pattern is the need by providers (particularly physicians) to pay off debt incurred during the training years.

A third relevant detail in Table 11.1 concerns use of the provider's own resources to bring health care goods and services to market. The availability of consumers to obtain health care through mechanisms other than out-of-pocket payment has already been discussed. Likewise, providers of health care in the United States seldom, if ever, pay the full cost of production. Professional education in health care receives both direct and indirect public support. The universities that educate future health professionals receive support via state taxation, private gifts, and grants and contracts from both public and private sources. Government has provided fiscal support for residency programs in primary care specialties and in underserved locations.

Pharmaceutical companies and manufacturers of medical equipment benefit from public support of the basic sciences. Increased understanding of metabolism, microbiology, genetics, and other dimensions fundamental to human biology make development of new drugs possible. Pharmaceutical companies today contribute massively to research directly relevant to pharmacology. But research in the basic sciences remains a public enterprise, conducted by government scientists or university researchers working under government salaries or contracts.

Socially disadvantaged people make a usually unrecognized but highly important contribution to providers' capacity to deliver service. Disadvantaged people are more likely than others to receive care in public and emergency facilities. These facilities often serve as practical training grounds for health professionals. In them, trainees may be assigned tasks such as history taking, examining, and suturing. In comparison with that of an experienced practitioner, treatment by someone still in training is likely to involve more pain, less efficiency, and greater risk of error. In this fashion, disadvantaged individuals contribute to developing society's stock of medical expertise.

A strong case, then, can be made that government must act on behalf of consumers to ensure that they receive safe and effective care. U.S. public policy reflects a belief that government participation is essential. As a consequence, public-sector participation in the U.S. health care system has increased steadily since the late nineteenth century. Preceding chapters have provided numerous examples of government participation in health care. The remainder of this chapter will provide details on selected instances of this participation and issues that have arisen from them. The pages to follow will also address the origins of policy regarding health care, the mechanisms that government uses to oversee and direct health care, and the political process by which policy comes into existence.

GOVERNMENT PARTICIPATION IN HEALTH CARE

The principles through which government participates in the U.S. health care system include legislation, funding, regulation, and judicial rulings. These mechanisms are interrelated; legislation, for example, allocates funding resources, and regulatory actions may be challenged in the courts. Government in the United States has always had an interest in health. Early examples include establishment of quarantine facilities for seamen, which dates from 1790. Government funds were used to build water and sewer systems throughout the nineteenth century. In the latter half of that century, government took a major step in influencing health care through licensing of physicians, which was not a requirement of practice in all states until 1901 (see Chapter Two). For generations, localities have funded hospitals and health departments. All hospitals except facilities of the federal government must have licenses, typically obtained from state agencies. Today direct funding of care for elders and indigent people absorbs more government resources than any purpose except for the federal Social Security program.

Legislation

Legislation is the most visible form of policy making. Table 11.2 recapitulates some of the most important health legislation of the past few generations. These measures illustrate the range of mechanisms by which government has sought to make health care more accessible and to control its cost, as well as to protect the safety and privacy of patients. It is important to note that some major pieces of legislation have produced not only the intended impact but unanticipated, adverse consequences. In this manner, a generation of lawmakers may create tangles that later generations must live with or remedy.

Several federal measures illustrate the impact that legislation has had on health care in the United States. Regulation of pharmaceuticals was initiated in the early twentieth century and successively expanded over the ensuing decades. The first of the National Institutes of Health was established just prior to World War II. As in the case of pharmaceuticals, successive pieces of legislation expanded the federal role. Medicaid and Medicare date from the mid-1960s. Both programs originated as additions to the periodic process of renewing the Social Security program, and both have seen increases in their mandates and costs over time.

Other policy created through legislation, though, has proven changeable and transient. The Health Professionals Educational and Assistance Act (1963) is an example. This measure provided grants for increasing enrollment in medical schools and financial support to medical students. Subsequent versions of this measure provided funds for training in nursing and other health fields. By the mid-1970s, the version passed by Congress and signed by President Gerald Ford asserted that the United States had

TABLE 11.2   Major U.S. health policies, intended impact, and unanticipated outcomes

Policy	Era	Intended Impact	Unanticipated Outcome
Hospital building and reconstruction	1940s–1960s	Modernize hospitals, increase public access	Excess hospital supply, increased cost
Health care subsidies for elderly and poor	1960s	Promote access to health care by disadvantaged groups	Extreme inflation as new demand exceeds resources
Health manpower training	1960s–1970s	Increase supply of primary care physicians	Excess supply of family practitioners and general internists
Central health planning	1970s–1980s	Coordination of resources, cost savings	Ineffective implementation agencies, increasing health care capacity beyond apparent need
HMOs	1970s–1990s	Reduced health care costs	Public dissatisfaction and abandonment
State-level insurance mandates	1980s–2000s	Universal access, cost control	Conflicts of laws, excess demand

overcome its shortage of doctors and nurses. Renewal of this act shifted emphasis to increasing the supply of health professionals in underserved areas and physicians in the specialties of family practice, general internal medicine, and pediatrics.

Policy that originated as legislation and that proved transient included federally mandated health planning. Beginning in the 1960s, Congress passed a series of bills intended to encourage development of statewide and local plans to promote efficient use of health resources. These plans were intended in part to reduce duplication of expensive health care facilities within health care market areas. Passed in 1975, the National Health Planning and Resource Development Act was the strongest measure of the health planning era. Under this law, localities were mandated to establish health systems agencies (HSAs) that would draw up regional health plans and estimate the levels of resources such as hospital beds and CT scanners required by residents. A hospital or physician group wishing to add significant capacity was required to apply for and obtain a certificate of need (CON) from the HSA for this purpose.

Unlike the kind of centralized government that predominates in Europe, the system in the United States is *federal*. The U.S. federal system allocates considerable independence to states and local units of government. This has led to measures that reflect local concerns and social outlook. California has mandated structural retrofitting of hospital facilities to withstand future seismic events. The National Health Planning and Resource Development Act had expired by the early 1980s. Over twenty years later, however, half the states had kept CON review on their books. New York state retained a law that prohibits for-profit hospitals as corporatization grew elsewhere. In an era when federal law severely restricted use of Medicaid funds for abortion, a number of states provided funds that enabled poor women to terminate their pregnancies.[2]

Aside from substantive bills, legislation also often focuses purely on appropriation of funds. Appropriations legislation specifically concerns financial allocations to government agencies or for particular purposes. Normally, appropriations and substantive matters are addressed in separate bills. Most legislation cannot be carried out unless the legislature allocates sufficient funds for its purposes. Congress typically votes on a series of appropriations bills that, when taken together, comprise the entire federal budget. Careful study of the huge federal budget is needed to determine how much money is being allocated to a particular mandated action of government.

Appropriations legislation is perhaps even more contentious than substantive legislation. An appropriations bill provides a second chance for opponents who have failed to block a relevant substantive measure. People who want to see a government function dropped can do so by ensuring that its funding is reduced or eliminated. In Congress, the allocations arena has at times become so heated that no money has been allocated for any agency's functioning. Developments of this kind have resulted in suspension of government operations pending passage of a budget. On other occasions, legislators have ensured funding of government functions through temporary measures known as *continuing resolutions*.

Ballot Propositions

In some states, measures that are essentially legislative are decided by the voters. *Ballot propositions* of this kind can be of great importance. Interest groups supporting a proposition spend heavily to have it placed on the ballot, a process usually requiring the collection of thousands of voter signatures in its support. Increasingly, these signatures are collected by paid contractors rather than public-spirited volunteers. Interests supporting the ballot measure then spend additional millions to attain voter approval. Some state laws require supermajorities of voters for passage of certain measures, particularly those with major fiscal implications.

California likely leads the nation in the number of propositions appearing on its ballots. Health-related propositions have included measures to increase the tax on cigarettes, the proceeds earmarked for antitobacco publicity and education, research on tobacco-related diseases, and health care for the indigent. An unusual measure passed in the early years of the twenty-first century imposed a 1 percent tax on all incomes over $1 million, with proceeds dedicated to mental health services. The most far-reaching measures, had they passed, would have mandated health care for all in California.

In a similar fashion, legislatures place items in appropriations bills that amount to substantive mandates. A government agency may receive extra millions for purposes not explicitly mandated in substantive bills. Influence over the budget process can enable a legislator to introduce and obtain financial allocations for items she favors. Powerful legislators force provisions into appropriations bills for projects benefiting their jurisdictions or individuals who have given them political or financial support. Known as *earmarking*, this process is widely criticized, but still frequently used.

Funding

Preceding chapters have demonstrated the importance of direct government payments for health care. For decades, federal spending on health care has exceeded outlays for defense. As long ago as 1993, for example, federal funding of health programs approximated $402 billion, compared with $359 billion for defense.[3]

The influence exercised by government through health care funding is even greater than that suggested by the percentage of the health care dollars that government generates. Hospitals must be accredited by The Joint Commission or a state agency in order to receive Medicare and Medicaid payments. Medicare patients tend to be high-volume consumers and thus valued by hospitals. Virtually all hospitals in the United States, then, seek accreditation. This is true even of facilities in which only a low percentage of patients are covered by Medicare. Universities that receive training funds from the federal government are required to meet a variety of associated public mandates. Medical schools that received funding under the federal Health Professionals Educational and Assistance Act were required to establish specific numbers of residency training slots in primary care. Changes in payment rules under Medicare require that doctors accept the Medicare fee schedule, often lower than prevailing fees. In effect, doctors participating in Medicare are forced to give discounts to all their Medicare patients, even if some of these might be willing and able to pay higher fees.[4]

Regulation

Regulation is the exercise of governmental power over an individual's or organization's conduct of an otherwise legal activity. Technically, for example, it is possible for anyone to open a hospital and offer health services. But hospitals may operate only according to rules asserted and enforced by government agencies or private organizations empowered by government. Regulation may involve assessment of competence, performance oversight, and imposition of restrictions on range of acceptable activities. For many health care organizations and providers, regulation constitutes the most direct and frequently experienced form of contact with government.

State licensing boards have historically operated as regulatory agencies in the United States. These boards have possessed the power not only to license health professionals but also to prohibit or encourage certain forms of professional behavior. As recently as the 1970s, for example, boards of optometry in some states prohibited licensed optometrists form operating branch offices, working for corporations, and advertising prices. Other regulations imposed by boards of optometry addressed the minimum equipment needed for office practice, the requirements for continuing education to maintain licensure, and the qualifications for admission to practice by optometrists licensed in other states.[5] The Medical Board of California still prohibits the so-called *corporate practice of medicine,* that is, employment of physicians by firms other than professional corporations controlled by physicians.

Regulation also takes place under less restrictive legal constructs such as *accreditation* and *certification*. **Accreditation** is a concept usually applied to a facility such as a hospital or a free-standing surgical center. Various agencies award accreditation status to health care facilities as diverse as hospitals, nursing homes, free-standing surgical centers, and laboratories. The term **certification** is usually applied to individuals and is awarded on the basis of training, peer review, and completion of continuing education. As described in an earlier chapter, most U.S. physicians are certified by their specialty boards. As in the case of non-board-certified physicians, facilities and individuals without accreditation or certification often provide health services, though under restricted scope.

Judicial Rulings

Rulings from the judge's bench on points of law have profound effects on health care. Typically, the decisions that have the most far-reaching effects are made in *appellate* courts. These courts review decisions that are made in courts of original jurisdiction or trial courts, where verdicts are often formulated by juries. Appellate courts deal with challenges based not on facts but on rules implicit in statutes or legal precedent. Legal decisions of this kind themselves have the force of law. Whole areas of law are relevant to health care, including decisions related to incorporation, governance, liability, and nonprofit status.

Thousands of cases are relevant in this connection, and systematic review is beyond the scope of this textbook. A few historical examples illustrate the importance of court decisions in determining how health care is organized and delivered in the United States. In *Dent v. West Virginia* (1888), the U.S. Supreme Court upheld a state law reestablishing licensure of physicians, a concept that had gone into eclipse as a consequence of the Thompsonian movement earlier in the century. The court ruled that the state of West Virginia had the right to require the practitioner worthy of licensure "to hold a degree from a reputable medical college, pass an examination, or prove that he had been in practice in the state for the previous ten years."

Several generations later, in 1943, another landmark decision helped clear the way for the managed care revolution that was to come. When the first fledgling HMOs began operation in that era, organized medicine responded with extreme hostility. Doctors associated with these plans were excluded or expelled from local medical societies, denied privileges at local hospitals, and even slandered. In response, the U.S. Department of Justice launched an antitrust suit against the American Medical Association, known as *American Medical Association v. United States.* As a consequence of this lawsuit and subsequent negotiations, the American Medical Society agreed to cease its opposition.

Rather than resolve issues, court decisions can initiate continuing controversy. The famous case of *Tarasoff v. Regents of the University of California,* which pitted concerns for personal privacy against public safety, provides an example. This 1974 case concerned the murder of University of California student Tatiana Tarasoff by another student, Prosenjit Poddar. The emotionally disturbed Poddar had told a university psychologist that he intended to kill Tarasoff. Against the advice of the psychologist, the university did not restrain Poddar, who proceeded to commit the murder. In response to legal action by the Tarasoff family, the California Supreme Court ruled that health professionals have a *duty to warn* potential victims of deranged individuals, even though this principle contradicts that of patient-provider confidentiality.

The issue, however, remained controversial. Rehearing the case some years later, the California Supreme Court formulated a broader doctrine, the *duty to protect.* Under this doctrine, health care providers could take steps to safeguard potential victims without disclosing medically confidential information. Such action might, for example, take the form of placing the potential perpetrator in custody or alerting law enforcement officials to the danger. Still, courts throughout the United States still uphold the stricter duty to warn concept in applying the *Tarasoff* precedent.[6]

Administrative Actions

Although government participation in health care may begin with legislation, it often ends with decisions by administrative agencies. Agencies of the executive branch of government, unkindly known as the *bureaucracy,* are mandated to take the actions required to make legislative intent a reality. Officials in these agencies are legally required to act in a manner consistent with legislation. As a practical matter, day-to-day actions of officials are governed by regulations addressing matters too specific to be expressed in the language of legislation. Directives, memos, and circulars continuously enter the in-boxes of officials updating them on decisions by higher-ups, outcomes of hearings concerning the agency's mandate, or legal opinions and decisions.

Administrative agencies, however, do not merely respond to externally imposed direction. Most agencies and the individuals within them enjoy a degree of *discretion*— decision-making latitude in areas not explicitly addressed by statute, regulations, or established agency policy. In administering the highly complex Medicare and Medicaid programs, the Centers for Medicare and Medicaid Services (CMS) inevitably have significant opportunities for discretion. At the initiation of the Health and Human Services Secretary in 2004, for example, CMS officials developed new rules requiring that skilled nursing facilities report detailed data on staffing and quality of care.[7] At operational levels of CMS, civil service personnel make decisions regarding specifics such as how licensed staff and FTEs will be defined and how inspection data are reported. Although these decisions may be small in scale, they may determine the day-to-day concerns of health care providers and ultimately the efficacy of the enabling legislation.

Privatization of Government Functions

Government significantly participates in the U.S. health care system through several mechanisms. But ironically, much of this participation occurs through private intermediaries or agents. Privatization is an important feature of public life in the United States. Consistent with U.S. political culture (see Chapter Two), government funnels a high percentage of the dollars it pays for health care through private firms. In addition, government delegates important parts of its regulatory responsibilities to the private sector. The direct participation of private interests in government decision making further illustrates the integration of public and private actions in U.S. health care.

The Joint Commission (See Chapter 2) is the poster child of delegation of public responsibility to a private entity. This organization was formed in the early 1950s for the purpose of accrediting hospitals. It has always operated as a private nonprofit organization. The Joint Commission name reflects its origin as a consortium of organizations vitally interested in the quality of hospital care. These included the American College of Physicians, the American College of Surgeons, the American Hospital Association, the American Medical Association (AMA), and the Canadian Medical Association. The Joint Commission no longer accredits only hospitals, having added accreditation of organizations such as nursing homes and certain free-standing medical facilities as such entities have become more important in the health care industry.

The Joint Commission's founders commented that they needed support of all these interests to attain sufficient resources and achieve a unified voice.[8] Others expressed the opinion that they knew a high-quality and well-recognized system of hospital inspection and surveillance would have to evolve as the industry became more and more important. These individuals said that The Joint Commission's founders were intent on seeing these functions remain in private hands rather than be taken over by a government agency. Political considerations important in The Joint Commission's founding remain important today. The hospital industry and medicine originally held a majority of the seats on The Joint Commission's governing board. In recent years, representatives from fields such as nursing and labor have been added, but hospital administrators and medical professionals still predominate.

The Joint Commission determines the accreditation of hospitals by extensive reviews of a hospital's staffing, equipment, cleanliness, and management practices. The Joint Commission requires hospitals to complete a detailed self-study report and then sends a site-visit team to examine facilities and question personnel. Accreditation status is determined in discussion among the commissioners, informed by the hospital's self-study and the site-visit team's report. Hospitals may receive accreditation for up to three years.

Initially, The Joint Commission offered accreditation on a voluntary basis. With the inception of Medicare and Medicaid in the 1960, though, The Joint Commission accreditation has become essentially mandatory for the majority of U.S. hospitals. The federal agencies that administer these programs—CMS and its precursors—accept Joint Commission accreditation as signifying full compliance with Medicare and Medicaid requirements. Highly dependent on Medicare and Medicaid funds, most hospitals in the United States feel compelled to maintain Joint Commission accreditation. Although a private organization, The Joint Commission can be seen as carrying out key inspection and screening functions on behalf of government and the public.

The Joint Commission represents only one instance of privatization in the implementation of U.S. health policy. Many U.S. health care concerns subscribe to the accounting rules of the Financial Accounting Standards Board (FASB), which, like The Joint Commission, is a private nonprofit. Hospital laboratories are accredited by the College of American Pathologists, yet another private organization. The programs and requirements for board certification of physicians are also in the hands of private organizations. Since 1933, specialty boards have been approved jointly by action of American Board of Medical Specialties, a private nonprofit organization, and AMA's Council on Medical Education, another private nonprofit.

Though largely absent from the public view, these and many other private organizations function, formally or informally, with the authority of government in health care. In a complementary fashion, government agencies often operate under the direction of private interests. It may be argued that dominance by hospital industry representatives on local planning boards reduced their ability to represent the public interest. The same may be alleged of state-level agencies responsible for licensing and disciplining health professionals. These boards are composed largely of the same health professionals over whom oversight is exercised. It may be suspected that these boards represent the interests of the professions from which they are drawn, rather than those of the public.

The degree to which private organizations or individuals should be entrusted to carry out public mandates is controversial. It is possible to argue that career government officials could do the job better. But it is also true that firms and individuals commercially involved in health care know more about the field than any government agency or bureaucrat. Without depending on organizations such as The Joint Commission, moreover, the government would have to establish additional regulatory units, accelerating an already rapid growth in the size of government.

THE PUBLIC ENVIRONMENT

Rightly or wrongly, health professionals and organizations operate in an environment crowded with laws and regulations. Figure 11.1, focusing on the hospital, illustrates only a few features of this environment. The Joint Commission, CMS, and FASB represent only a few of the agencies that hospital managers must deal with. Hospital management personnel must be conversant with these features of the public environment, maintain contact with responsible officials, write reports, respond to interrogatives, and pay fees.

As indicated in Figure 11.1, laws and regulation originating at every level of government affect hospital operations. Areas of federal concern include Medicare and Medicaid regulations, Food and Drug Administration (FDA) rulings, and Drug Enforcement Agency (DEA) practices. State law controls the licensure of hospitals and health professionals, and state agencies have the power to investigate, inspect, and discipline organizations and personnel found in violation. State government administers worker compensation laws. Either state or local government, or agencies of both, may have the power to approve or disapprove hospital construction and retrofit plans. Local government (county and city jurisdictions) passes ordinances that affect

FIGURE 11.1   *The regulatory environment of the U.S. hospital*

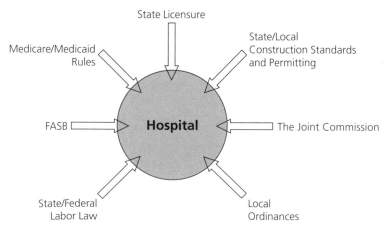

hospital operations in areas such as traffic, noise, and waste disposal. Hospitals operate in an environment crowded with local agencies, from zoning boards to fire marshals' offices.

THE MEANING OF PUBLIC POLICY

This chapter has described several important ways in which government participates in or affects the health care industry. Government participates in the industry by directly providing care and indirectly by funding health services. Government influences the delivery of services through laws and regulatory activities that encourage or limit the activities of direct service providers or payers. The actions of government may be said to reflect *public policy,* the intent of governmental decision makers in passing laws and formulating regulations.

Public policy is by no means always explicit or clear. Recall that the framers of the U.S. Constitution stated—in words familiar to every child who has had to memorize the Preamble—that the document's purpose was "to form a more perfect union." Policy associated with the Second Amendment to that document, however, is much less clear. The language of this amendment would seem to guarantee only the right of individuals "to keep and bear arms" as part of a "well-regulated militia." But people today argue that the amendment guarantees the right of all Americans—excepting the juvenile, the criminal, and the clearly insane—to own and carry guns. Policy explicit enough to guide government action often requires new legislation, judicial interpretation, or decisions of limited scope by managers in public bureaucracies.

Health-related legislation provides important examples of explicit and implicit policy intent within the same measure. Legislation known as the Employee Retirement Income Security Act (ERISA), passed in 1974, provides an illustration. As the title implies, most of the language in ERISA addresses the rights of employees in the pension plans to which they have contributed and the responsibilities of employers to guarantee these rights. But of greater importance to health policy is a clause proclaiming that federal law preempts state law regarding employee benefits. This clause was originally included to make it easier for firms to administer employee benefit programs. Preemption of state laws would simplify plan administration, since firms operating in multiple states would need to deal with only a single federal law, as opposed to multiple (and possibly conflicting) state laws. In practice, however, preemption of state laws regarding employee benefits made it difficult, if not impossible, for states to require that private-sector firms provide health insurance for their workers. ERISA proved a continuing challenge for states wishing to enact *employer mandates* of this kind.[9]

Public policy comes about through a number of processes. Researchers and experts may contribute to policy by identifying and highlighting risks to public well-being. Thus, Surgeon General Everett C. Koop successfully challenged the administration of President Ronald Reagan to adopt more activist policies toward the AIDS epidemic in the 1980s. Judges help establish public policy by "discovering" implications in statutes and earlier court decisions. In this fashion, a "duty to warn," discovered in the *Tarasoff* case described earlier in this chapter, became an element of public policy.

But the process by which policy is established is predominantly political. It is a rare instance where even the findings of scientists or jurists are free from this process. As Chapter Twelve demonstrates, politics plays an important part in the funding and career progress of most or all scientists. The same is true of jurists or, more specifically, appellate judges who interpret legislation or law of other origin. Judges of all kinds obtain their positions through the ballot or via political appointment.

POLITICS: THE DRIVER OF POLICY

Politics may be thought of as a process by which an individual or group attempts to determine the actions of a jurisdiction whose decision makers are free to agree or disagree. A jurisdiction is usually understood as a nation, state, city, or geopolitical entity. But politics also takes place within organizations, as members jockey for leadership positions or other personal advantages. Politics takes place within families, as the occurrence of palace revolutions continually attests. In a middle-class family, a young person's attempt to gain a privilege by first convincing the less resistant parent may not be newsworthy. But it is politics all the same.

The Nature and Function of Politics

Although politics is most apparent in contests over money and power, people also engage in politics for less egotistical reasons. Advocates of social change use politics to pursue their objectives. Techniques ranging from conventional electioneering to civil disobedience helped bring about the antidiscrimination laws that transformed the United States in the late twentieth century. Politics also serves as a resource for people desiring to change a nation's commitments, objectives, and strategies, as is seen in lobbying for or against educational reform, public borrowing, or war. The same process occurs at the local level, as members of a neighborhood association argue over resolutions regarding the actions of police officers or zoning board officials.

Politics is present in the organizations described in Chapter Five. The organizational complexity of hospitals provides fertile ground for politics. The governance structure of a hospital is often the venue for political intrigue. In many instances, medical personnel have become dissatisfied due to economy measures instituted by the administration. On a hospital board of trustees, the medical staff president might form an alliance with other interests to oust the CEO and other top administrative personnel. Within university-based medical centers, specialty-based advocates seek to dominate the allocation of funds and the hiring of personnel.

Wherever it is practiced, politics has certain essential elements. Competition is one of these. In politics, people promote the thinking or action they desire over the preferences of others. Another feature of politics is informality. The most effective forms of politics seem to involve personal persuasion and exchanges of favors. This is true even in settings like the U.S. Congress, where highly specific rules govern proceedings.

As senate majority leader, Lyndon B. Johnson was famed for giving colleagues the "Johnson treatment," draping one arm around a colleague's shoulder and firmly grasping his lapel with the opposite hand. Thus immobilized, many a senator was forced to hear Johnson's proposal or argument. Along these same lines, House Speaker Tip O'Neill's comment that "all politics is local" continues to be widely quoted. O'Neill meant that no matter how much power one attains, face-to-face relationships never lose their importance.

Politics may seem at best inefficient and at worst sneaky and dishonest. But politics performs an important function for society. No jurisdiction can be run entirely on the basis of rules. People resort to politics when standard operating procedures do not produce the results they desire. Politics is an alternative to truly destructive forms of competition, such as sabotage, assassination, or civil war. Thus, politics promotes social stability. Finally, politics is often the only mechanism through which change can occur. Government bureaucrats may not agree with the standard operating procedures they are handed, but still act consistently with them. Only politics can alter the focus and mission of government—the carrying out of public policy.

Like buying and selling in markets, politics seldom, if ever, takes place as a free-for-all. Rather, it is bound by the traditions and rules of the organizations or institutions in which it takes place. On the national level, politics takes place within the broader social environment. Elements of the environment include several already mentioned: political culture, political climate, public opinion, and rules governing legislatures. It should be noted that legislatures have the power to suspend and revise the very rules under which they operate—except in instances where such changes result in provisions inconsistent with the U.S. Constitution or relevant state constitutions.

Essentials of Political Action

Consensus and Coalitions. Successful politics in the United States comprises achievement of an effective consensus regarding a particular issue. The importance of consensus is often clearest in legislative sessions. No legislation passes unless a majority of voting members approves the measure or lacks sufficient motivation to impede its progress. Politics is successful when people and groups believe that items in a bill affect their interests in a net positive fashion and form a coalition to press for its passage.

Consensus is also crucial for the passage of ballot measures placed before the public. Consensus must be achieved among organized interest groups regarding the measure. In health matters, for example, agreement among parties such as the state medical association, the state hospital association, and the state chamber of commerce may form the basis of a powerful consensus. Parties to the consensus must include a sufficient number of organized interest groups to raise the funds necessary for an effective campaign. An effective consensus among interest groups can induce legislators to form a consensus of their own. Finally, consensus must be achieved among "publics" in the jurisdiction. Organized interest groups can promote such a consensus by influencing their members. But the grand consensus must include voters who are not part of organized interest groups. Such individuals, however, may be addressed as groups defined by income, race, gender, and other social background factors.

In the case of routine legislation, building consensus among key groups often occurs simultaneously with the drafting of actual legislation. Most legislation is in fact routine. Most health-related bills aim only at bringing a minor business advantage to one or more players in the industry. A state hospital association, for example, may seek changes in the way nurses' overtime hours are calculated. The association's legislative representative vets the idea to the representatives of other players, such as insurance, medicine, and large hospital systems. In round-robin fashion, these representatives negotiate acceptable language for the forthcoming bill. Some of the parties may have provisions of interest to their constituencies added. A friendly legislator is then contacted; his staff then drafts an actual bill to be introduced by the legislator. Often the industry representatives will themselves draft the bill, simply submitting it to the legislator for her consideration.

Consensuses and coalitions are seldom permanent. Each individual player may need to join or construct a new coalition associated with each successive issue. Politics of this kind, which predominates in the United States, does not often seek annihilation of adversaries. Rather, relationships must remain cordial and doors kept open for future consensus building.

Advocacy and Lobbying. Although consensus and coalitions drive politics in the United States, decision makers such as legislators and executive branch officials—including chief executives such as presidents and governors, agency heads, and bureaucrats—ultimately determine policy. Interest group representatives must motivate legislators to introduce and support their bills. Once laws have been enacted, these same representatives often pressure executive branch officials to ensure that the measures are carried out in a manner consistent with their interests.

Interest group representatives attain the required access through advocacy. **Advocacy** is a sustained effort to convince decision makers and alter public perceptions regarding a political position. Advocacy employs a wide variety of methods. Advocates visit legislators. Sometimes visitation occurs *en masse*; special interest groups, for example, organize "state capitol days," during which members meet with legislators from their districts to push their positions. Advocates sponsor policy analyses and scientific studies whose results they believe will support their objectives. Well-heeled interest groups retain public relations firms to popularize their ideas. Advocates organize letter-writing campaigns and demonstrations, complete with speakers and placards, to underscore their arguments.

Lobbying is one form of advocacy. People may use the terms *advocacy* and *lobbying* interchangeably. But unlike other forms of advocacy, lobbying involves giving money and other resources to legislators. Lobbyist money is typically given to elected officials in the form of campaign contributions. Lobbyists write checks on behalf of their employers and encourage others who share their interests to contribute. Just as advocates require the services of elected officials, these officials require contributions from advocates. Campaigns are expensive. In 2004, for example, the average winner of a seat in the U.S. House of Representatives incurred over $1 million in campaign expenses.[10] In large jurisdictions such as California or New York, an effective campaign for the state house may easily cost this much. Senate campaigns cost many millions, and the 2008 presidential race cost over $1 billion.

The requirement of extensive financial resources for election campaigns has opened the door of many a legislator's office to visits by lobbyists for various health care interests. Money may not directly buy a legislator's vote or an executive official's decision. But it causes the official to listen to the interest group's voice. These officials may be expected to seriously consider the desires of key contributors. In the 2004 election cycle, health care professionals contributed $74.1 million to presidential and congressional candidates; pharmaceutical and health care product companies, $18.0 million; hospitals and nursing homes, $16.6 million; and health services and health maintenance organizations, $7.9 million. In the 2006 cycle, health care professionals contributed $53.9 million to congressional candidates; pharmaceutical and health care product companies, $19.3 million; hospitals and nursing homes, $13.7 million; and health services and health maintenance organizations, $7.6 million.

Funds spent lobbying at the federal level in an off-election year provide additional clues to the locus of lobbying power in the United States. Organizations concerned with health care comprised the second most generous players in the early twenty-first century. Among these interests, manufacturers of drugs and medical equipment provided the most money, dominating the financial side of the health lobbying field. Top-spending organizations in all areas demonstrate the diversity of powerful health care interests. The U.S. Chamber of Commerce, with strong interests in gaining relief from the health insurance obligations of its members, led the pack. The American Association of Retired People, AMA, Pharma (a pharmaceutical lobbyist), and the American Hospital Association were among the top ten givers.

In addition to money contributions, lobbyists and the organizations they work for may help sponsor the elected official's travel. Lobbyists hire the spouses of elected officials or funnel business to the firms where they are employed. Gifts such as sports tickets and vacation trips may be given. Today, campaign finance laws restrict gifting to members of Congress; still, such practices continue to take place, as evidenced by their periodic discovery and ensuing scandals.

Despite its sleazy reputation, lobbying plays a key role in policy making. Lobbyists are legally barred from purchasing favors or exchanging cash for favorable legislative actions. But in most instances, resources contributed by lobbyists simply buy access to elected officials. Dependent on the lobbyists' money, the official is compelled to return lobbyists' phone calls, schedule meetings, and hear concerns and requests for action.

Lobbying, then, is a fundamental part of U.S. politics. Some political observers consider the lobbying community as equivalent in importance to the Senate and the House themselves, or their equivalents in state government. Thus, lobbyists are sometimes thought of as a "third house," forging consensus and writing legislation to be carried by elected officials with whom they have ties.

Nonprofit Advocacy. Lobbying in Congress and state legislatures may constitute the most visible form of advocacy. But other forms of advocacy may be equally effective. An episode in first years of the twenty-first century illustrates how effective advocacy can be without the cash transfers that characterize lobbying. This episode also illustrates techniques that may be used to influence executive branch officials. The example given here involved career civil servants at the Office of Rural Health Policy (ORHP), a unit of the federal Health Resources and Services Administration (HRSA).[11]

The availability of adequate health care personnel and resources to people living in rural areas has long been an issue in the United States. For decades, the federal government has directly and indirectly supported rural hospitals and clinics. Controversy arose in the 1970s about which areas in the United States should be designated as rural for purposes of federal funding. Originally, federal policy makers designated places as urban or rural on the basis of county. Areas within a county that contained a city were considered urban; those without a city were designated as rural.

This designation system became less meaningful as more cities developed in the western United States. Within a single county there might be both a large city and vast tracts of sparse, rural settlement. In the 1980s, the federal government modified its classification system so that rural areas in counties containing cities would become eligible for rural health funding. Eventually, a system evolved under which individual census tracts (small areas with about five thousand residents) relatively close to cities could be classified as rural. Known as rural-urban commuting areas (RUCAs), these geographical unit designations reflected the fact that many rural residents commuted long distances to jobs in the city. Still, these people were residents of rural areas, rightly entitled to health care supported by federal monies.

Controversy arose over whether a sufficient number of areas had been designated as rural under the RUCA system. Rural health interests throughout the United States advocated for expansion of RUCA-designated eligibility. This effort was spearheaded by the California State Rural Health Association (CSRHA). California's rural residents living in counties containing urban centers outnumbered their counterparts in any other state.

Barred from conventional lobbying by laws governing nonprofits, CSRHA raised the issue's visibility and pressured ORHP to expand eligibility through methods that included the following:

- Publicizing a state agency study demonstrating that large numbers of Californians lived in essentially rural places that were not officially designated as rural

- Hosting federal officials at a conference in California, one feature of which was a tour of actual, though not officially, rural areas

- Obtaining a letter to officials at ORPH signed by forty-one California Assembly and Senate members

- Obtaining a similar letter from members of Congress representing rural areas throughout the United States

- Visiting ORPH officials in Washington, D.C., and ranking officials of HRSA with authority over ORPH

Ultimately, RUCA designations were liberalized, making areas that were home to hundreds of thousands of people newly eligible for rural health assistance. The degree to which pressure from CSRHA caused the change to occur is uncertain. Government officials do not readily acknowledge that they have been pressured into decisions. But advice from agency executives, fear of angry members of Congress inclined to trim funding, concern over the possibility of a congressional hearing, and desire simply to avoid bad publicity appear likely to have contributed to the eventual decision.

Specialized and technical concerns such as RUCA designation usually remain unrecognized by the broader public. Advocates seldom expend major resources on mobilizing the public in such cases. Other issues, however, lend themselves strongly to public involvement. Public involvement, in turn, helps generate political and financial resources for direct advocacy of government officials. A process described by Susan Brown of the Susan B. Komen Foundation, a key breast cancer advocacy group, includes steps involving the public much more closely than did RUCA. These steps include the following:[12]

- *Priming the market:* creating awareness of a problem that needs to be addressed

- *Energizing consumers:* mobilizing people and dollars to support the cause; these resources may be used to sponsor events that attract media attention, enabling more people and funds to be mobilized

- *Taking political action:* using the clout achieved by the previously described means to work for legislative changes, such as mandating coverage of screening in health insurance and increasing budgets for breast cancer research

- *Going mainstream:* keeping the message strong and fresh by expanding ties with business, government, and science; creating leadership training programs; and obtaining appointments to commissions and boards

Consumer Advocacy. It would be a mistake to identify lobbying as solely the province of large commercial interests. Consumers or their relatives have played the advocacy game with considerable expertise. Consumer groups organized around specific health concerns have fought with the same intensity as often-vilified branches of the health care industry. Political agitation is behind the favored status of end-stage renal disease patients with regard to Medicare benefits. The emphasis on AIDS research at NIH appears to have arisen from the political organization of gays and other groups at elevated risk for the disease.

Writing in the journal *Health Affairs,* political scientist Daniel P. Carpenter describes how consumers concerned with a specific illness pressure FDA officials to accelerate approval of relevant medications.[13] According to Carpenter, the power of consumer lobbies with the FDA today exceeds even that of the pharmaceutical companies typically blamed for muscling through legislation or regulatory action. But consumer action may be only the most visible force addressing this agency. Carpenter also documents action taken by pharmaceutical companies in helping patient advocacy groups get started and in financially supporting their operation.

WINNING AND LOSING IN HEALTH CARE POLITICS: THREE CASE STUDIES

The following three case studies on health legislation illustrate the principles of policy and politics discussed earlier. These case studies involve legislation introduced in successive decades of the late twentieth century. Two of the measures were successful, eventually being signed into law and profoundly affecting the financing and delivery of health services throughout the United States. The third measure infamously failed. Both the winning and losing cases provide lessons for attaining political success in the struggles bound to emerge in the decades to come.

These cases underscore several key features of U.S. politics. First, politics in the United States operates by seeking consensus among individuals and organized interest groups. Second, advocacy and lobbying from multiple quarters play a crucial role in achieving consensus—or, in some cases, making consensus impossible. Third, the political culture of the United States favors limited, step-by-step actions rather than immediate, revolutionary change. *Political climate,* an atmosphere favoring some policy directions over others, exercises influence alongside the more stable political culture. At times and to varying degrees, public opinion and expert input have emerged as factors of importance.

The Health Maintenance Organization Act (1973)

The Health Maintenance Organization Act of 1973 initiated an era of rapid expansion of HMOs in the United States. Lawrence D. Brown, then of the Brookings Institution, conducted a detailed study of this major development in U.S. health policy.[14] Controversy associated with policy development introduced the term *health maintenance organization* (HMO) into the nation's vocabulary. Prior to the Nixon-era legislation, such plans had been known simply as prepaid group health plans or practices. Framers of the legislation believed a sexier label was needed to capture public attention and approval. Paul Ellwood, a physician and technical advisor to the Nixon White House, had coined the term HMO in the 1960s. Along with many others, Ellwood believed that the fee-for-service system rewarded providers for each unit of service they delivered. On the contrary, prepayment would motivate providers to keep their patients healthy, since no additional income could be earned by treating the diseases they might develop. The term HMO achieved public currency when used as the title for the ensuing legislation.

Ultimately, the legislation provided grants and loans to start, expand, or promote the interests of health maintenance organizations that qualified as such under the HMO Act. The act preempted state laws that made it more difficult to start or operate a federally qualified HMO. It exempted federally qualified HMOs from actions by the health systems agencies soon to be established. Initially, the act required that federally qualified HMOs establish premiums via community rating, although waiver provisions enabled HMOs to use experience rating. Organizations seeking to become federally qualified HMOs had to offer a comprehensive range of services. In a departure from traditional prepaid plans, the legislation permitted for-profit organizations and independent practice associations (IPAs) to become federally qualified HMOs and enjoy the related benefits. The legislation required firms with twenty-five or more employees that provided health insurance as a benefit to offer a federally qualified HMO along with traditional indemnity insurance if (a) one or more federally qualified HMO existed nearby and (b) such a plan requested that it be offered.

The Political Process. The legislation that would ultimately become the HMO Act was initiated by the Nixon White House. Like other Republicans of the time, President Richard M. Nixon generally opposed government participation in health care, branding it "socialized medicine." But as the reelection campaign approached in 1971, the Nixon administration felt it needed to address health care. It appeared likely that Senator Edward Kennedy would become a leading contender for the presidency, and Senator Kennedy was widely identified in the voters' minds with health care reform. A health policy initiative based on support for the HMO concept seemed like a good Republican alternative.

The concept appealed to Republicans because it did not mandate fundamental change in the organization and delivery of health services. The legislation promoted new options for a public concerned with the availability and cost of care. Old options were preserved. In addition, the measure enabled physicians to take advantage of new options (such as the IPA) while continuing to concentrate on the traditional fee-for-service approach. Overall, the proposed legislation had a voluntaristic character.

Opposing the measure from its early days was the Group Health Association of America (GHAA). Having for decades served as advocate for independently formed prepaid plans, GHAA argued that public support should not be given to new and untested types of plans. Both the GHAA and organized labor opposed provisions in the measure to give federal monies to profit-seeking organizations, as some of the new HMOs were expected to be. The AMA, traditionally suspicious of change, expressed considerable skepticism. Administration officials such as Ellwood, however, were excited about the experiment, and transmitted this excitement to President Nixon.

Why the Measure Succeeded. From the start, the limited nature of the HMO Act defused much potential opposition. The measure instituted only a small change in the U.S. health care scene, compelled no one to practice in or join a plan, and involved no significant growth in governmental presence. But the emergence of a sufficiently comprehensive coalition in its support best explains the bill's eventual passage.

Opponents to the administration concept proved willing to compromise. Senator Edward Kennedy introduced a rival bill (SB 14) that after much modification eventually became law. The initial Kennedy bill crystallized liberal objections to the Nixon plan. The original Kennedy measure demanded that federally supported HMOs offer a very specific range of benefits, whereas the administration had proposed open and market-based offerings. Kennedy's bill required community rating of enrollees and enrollment of certain high-risk (and thus potentially expensive) patients. The bill also entailed vastly greater financial outlays than the White House had envisioned.

Significant compromise ultimately secured passage of HMO legislation in the form of a highly modified version of Senator Kennedy's SB 14. Kennedy and his allies agreed to significantly lower financial allocations than those they had originally proposed; the Nixon administration agreed to higher allocations than they had originally proposed. The Nixon administration agreed to provisions they had initially fought against that obliged federally supported HMOs to offer specific types of services. The administration, historically pro states' rights, agreed to provisions overriding state laws viewed as anti-HMO.

According to Brown, a successful coalition and compromise-building process took place, giving rise to a measure acceptable to the president and federal legislators of widely different political persuasions. As he describes the process, "On a very long list of very wide disagreements [legislators] had reached middle ground time and again." And perhaps most important, "On each of the many controversial provisions, accommodations had been reached by careful, patient, repeated applications of the politician's art" (p. 275).

California Medicaid Reform (1982)

Legislation emerged from California in 1982 that had profound national impact. Since the 1970s, California had faced an increasing financial burden due to its Medicaid program, known in that state as Medi-Cal. Medicaid receives joint funding from federal and state coffers. The program placed a particularly difficult burden on California's state budget. Federal law calibrates a state's share of Medicaid costs according to the state's per capita income, and Californians on average earn more than people in most other states. To address this financial burden, California tightened Medi-Cal eligibility requirements, reduced benefits, and tried a number of HMO-type experiments. But ultimately the state resorted to a solution that was to have profound national significance and impact well beyond the public sector—*competitive contracting.*

Addressing a Medicaid Crisis. Several factors coalesced to produce a major fiscal crisis for the Medi-Cal program in the early 1980s. A taxpayer revolt had prompted measures greatly reducing resources at several levels of government. Economic recession further reduced tax revenues and increased enrollment in welfare programs such as Medi-Cal. At the same time, the cost of providing medical care was increasing at an alarming rate, with inflation in medical care running twice that in the general economy.

At the conclusion of the 1982 legislative session, two bills, AB 799 and AB 3489, passed the California legislature and were signed into law. AB 799 made it legal for state agencies to solicit competitive bids from individual hospitals for their services and to sign exclusive contracts with the winning bidders. AB 3489 accorded the same liberty to private insurance companies and HMOs. These two measures represented a departure from prior law, which required both state agencies and private insurers to pay "any willing provider" for health services rendered and billed to the state or private firm. The opportunity to seek competitive bids promoted price competition among providers, reportedly saving many millions of dollars in the years that followed.

The Political Process. Powerful forces opposed the market reform eventually brought about by AB 799 and AB 3489. These forces included two interests of historically great power in California—the hospital industry and organized medicine. Although some hospitals welcomed the idea of competition, the California Hospital Association did not want to see large numbers of its members excluded from potentially lucrative business. According to Linda Bergthold, who chronicled these events, the California Medical Association in the past had characterized similar initiatives as "communistic" and "un-American."[15]

Advocates of the reform measures included California's HMOs, for-profit chains, business in general, and the health insurance industry. Proponents of competitive contracting had the most to lose by continuing the foregoing system. California state government, of course, had a strong interest in any reform that would reduce its fiscal obligations. The insurance industry, and the industrial concerns that paid insurance premiums, placed predominant emphasis on the tie-in of AB 3489 with AB 799. These interests believed, with good reason, that competitively contracted Medi-Cal vendors would shift the costs of their Medi-Cal clients into the bills of privately insured patients. In this fashion, the Medi-Cal vendor would profit from the state business without truly having to cut costs. AB 3489 made such cost shifting unlikely, since private entities could also invite competitive bids, which would seldom be successful if they reflected costs shifted from Medi-Cal clients.

To some, the rapid passage of AB 799 and AB 3489 in the closing hours of a legislative session have seemed a miraculous exception to the tedium and delay that often characterizes lawmaking. But viewing the politics involved from behind the scenes reveals much deliberate political organization. Legislative staff and elected officials had worked for months on options, particularly ones acceptable to the insurance and business communities. Once the procompetitive strategy embodied in the two bills was decided upon, action began to make it a reality. According to Bergthold:

The strategy which the Medi-Cal reform legislation was introduced and passed is noteworthy for its intricacy. Every trick in the legislative manual was used; every possible parliamentary maneuver was brought in to help steer passage. Much of the credit for the strategy goes to [the extraordinarily powerful] Speaker of the Assembly Willie Brown and his staff. . . . Business interests were used by legislators to counteract the power of the physician and hospital lobbies. Speaker Willie Brown used the power of his office to obtain assent from Democrats in the legislature. . . . Policy Committees, in which most reform bills are ground up and spit out by special interests, were bypassed [p. 207].

In a parliamentary *coup de grace*, AB 799 and AB 3480 were scheduled for vote in such a way that "legislators had to vote for both bills in order to pass the budget." Passage of the budget represents the crux of all sessions of the California state legislature. Once the legislative and executive branches have worked out substantive differences, moves to delay final disposition of the budget seldom take place. Beyond the normal end of the legislative session loom the torrid months of the central California summer.

The Health Security Act (1993)

An initiative in the early 1990s by the administration of President William J. Clinton deserves special attention. The so-called Clinton Health Plan was introduced into Congress as the Health Security Act. The Health Security Act represented the most comprehensive attempt ever made to overhaul the U.S. health care system. It aimed at covering many, if not all, uninsured people in the United States and containing health care costs for all Americans. The failure of the Health Security Act to become law illustrates the snags and pitfalls that important and controversial legislation can encounter. The fate of the Health Security Act illustrates the power of skilled and well-financed lobbying and public relations assets to derail legislation. The measure's failure also illustrates the challenges that U.S. political culture (see Chapter Two) poses to far-reaching change. Most important, the failure of the measure illustrates the importance of building effective coalition support for achieving policy objectives in the U.S. political system.

Plan Development and Provisions. The administration appointed a task force to develop a reform proposal and legislation to make the proposal into law. First Lady Hillary Rodham Clinton headed the task force, assisted by Ira Magaziner, a brilliant management consultant and crony of the president from their days as Rhodes Scholars. The task force included hundreds of individuals, including White House staff and invited experts and consultants. Time-consuming and contentious, the task force worked in secret, although leaks to the media occurred from time to time. Ultimately, the Health Security Act emerged, a mammoth 1,342 pages in length.

A few provisions illustrate the scope of the proposed act. A *National Health Board* would be appointed by the president to oversee the health care system. Its powers would have included the pricing of health insurance premiums, the approval of new benefits in a standard national health plan, and enforcement of public and private spending limitations at the national and state level. *Regional Health Alliances* would be established that would offer plans to consumers. All employers would be required to provide at least a standard package of health benefits and to pay at least 80 percent of its cost. Finally, the plan contained several provisions for spending caps and price controls to be exercised by government agencies.

Rejection of the Plan. Large and complex, the Health Security Act represented a major achievement in technical policy formation. Within the hundreds of pages comprising the measure, it was said, an answer to every question regarding the proposed system could be found. The answer to each such question, moreover, would be consistent with the answers to all others.

But the venture was fatally flawed from a political standpoint. President Clinton, a Democrat, had the advantage of control by his party of both the House of Representatives and the Senate. Still, insurmountable challenges arose in the attempt to gain favorable action from Congress. The process by which the plan was developed contributed to its ultimate failure. After the dust had settled, Haynes Johnson and David S. Broder, two experienced Washington reporters, published a detailed retrospective.[16] Following are some of the factors they cited in the Health Security Act's failure.

■ *Loss of momentum.* Clinton had promised action within the first hundred days of his administration. Newly elected presidents generally enjoy a "honeymoon period," during which their policies are more likely to gain approval than later on. The Health Security Act was not introduced until well into the new administration's first year. This delay allowed opposing interests to organize and public suspicion to develop.

■ *The task force process.* The process by which the Health Security Act was developed took place in a manner hidden from both the public and Congress's view. Congress, accustomed to leading the development of legislation, felt slighted and hostile. A number of Democrat and a few Republican Congress members and Senators introduced their own health care reform bills in direct opposition to the Health Security Act.

Key interest groups such as the Health Insurance Association of America may have lent support if their concerns regarding price controls had been heard. But, excluded from the process, they moved toward active opposition. At its most visible, opposition took the form of a series of television ads featuring a middle-class couple ("Harry and Louise") expressing concerns about the pending legislation.

Flaws in organization and leadership became evident within the task force itself. Rivalry occurred among consultants and staff for influence with Magaziner and Hillary Clinton. The diary of a staffer singled out Ms. Clinton's leadership style as a barrier to progress: "She [can be faulted] because of her drive and capriciousness. It sounds sexist but it's also very true. Every decision is changed at least twice and she bounces up and down before setting her answer in concrete. [She has] an unerring conviction that she is right" (p. 19).

■ *Strong public opposition.* In the absence of clear understanding, the U.S. public tends to oppose policy change. This has been demonstrated repeatedly in initiative elections. Newspapers such as the *Wall Street Journal* carried out tortuous analyses of who would be financially helped and who would be hurt by the Health Security Act. Outside experts and even government agencies questioned the accuracy of the measure's financial impact as presented by the administration.

Commercial and small-business interests spearheaded organized opposition. These were joined by evangelical groups opposed to abortion coverage by the plan. Organizations representing these interests intensely lobbied Congress. The Health Insurance Association of America and individuals in its network made 450,000 contacts with Congress, including telephone calls, visits, and letters, "amounting to almost a thousand to every member of the House and Senate" (p. 213).

Uncertainty bred public suspicion and, ultimately, opposition. Although initially favorable, public opinion polls showed declining support for the plan as time went by. As summarized by Johnson and Broder, "The majority of those polled said the plan would do more harm than good to retirees, the middle class, people with insurance, and people like themselves . . . [and that] they felt 'big concern' over the possibility that it would add to bureaucracy, damage the quality of medical care, boost costs, limit the choice of doctors and hospitals, raise taxes, and cost jobs" (p. 193).

■ *Excessive complexity.* As a piece of legislation, the Health Security Act was big and complex. The measure's hundreds of pages challenged the understanding of even those close to the legislation. People eager for health care reform themselves questioned whether it could be effectively implemented. In the months that followed the measure's introduction, a White House communications official commented:

> The plan itself was disastrously complex. We did a count of the number of new councils or commissions or bodies that this thing sets up. It's in the nineties. I mean, that's a joke.
>
>   . . . We came up with such a big, fat, ugly bill that it was an easy target. We created a target the size of Philadelphia. I mean, Harry and Louise were good ads, but come on, they weren't that difficult to create. Somewhere, somebody . . . should have come in and said, "We cannot send this fucker up to the Hill" (p. 229).

LESSONS LEARNED

The two successes and one failure described above underscore the factors necessary for successful efforts to change health care–related policy in the United States. These include effective coalition-building, collaboration with key policy decision-makers, support (or at least lack of strong opposition) by the public, and consistency with the political culture.

Effective Coalitions. Effective coalitions are bound together by a common interest in a proposed government action. Issues around which coalitions gather take many forms. These may include bills in Congress or state legislatures, policy within government agencies, or confirmation of cabinet officials and judges. The success of a political coalition depends on giving each member enough of what it desires to maintain its commitment, yet not so much as to alienate others in the coalition. Seldom, if ever, does a single group or interest get everything it wants. Coalition building requires compromise.

The Clinton team missed important opportunities to create a winning coalition. Representatives of business and commercial insurance interests who might have helped bring about compromise legislation were rebuffed. Some coalition partners were recruited, such as the American Federation of State, County, and Municipal Employees. But firm commitments were seldom, if ever, achieved. Natural allies such as the American Association of Retired People were never brought on board.

The coalition formed to *oppose* the Clinton plan was much more powerful. The amount of money (cash and in-kind) spent on molding public opinion and lobbying Congress against the Health Security Act has been estimated at $100 million. Members of this coalition had a clear, common interest: defeating health care reform as it was presented in the Clinton plan.

Compare the experience of the Clinton years with the Nixon years. The Nixon White House and its congressional allies worked directly with forces led by Senator Kennedy, perhaps Nixon's chief ideological foe and political rival. A similar phenomenon was observed in California's successful Medicaid reform. The successful effort to pass versions of the Obama-inspired Patient Protection and Affordable Care Act in the House and the Senate was similarly coalition-based. Alliances were forged with powerful interests including organized medicine and the pharmaceutical industry. Developing and maintaining a coalition within the U.S. Senate required extensive deal-making with key senators. To help secure Louisiana's Senator Landrieu's support, for example, a special subsidy of $300,000 for her state was included in the legislation. Critics of the agreement dubbed it the "Louisiana Purchase."

Support by Decision Makers. Whatever the merits of a proposed policy, it must be supported by legislators to be enacted. Legislators jealously guard their right to formulate bills, assess their merits, and form coalitions in support or opposition. The Clinton team seemed insufficiently aware of these facts in its work with Congress. Key members of the House and Senate felt excluded from the planning process, which caused significant resentment. Again, the Nixon era success is notable. The HMO Act should be viewed as a Republican success; however, the measure that finally passed had been originally introduced by Democrat Ted Kennedy. The Obama Administration's strategy acknowledged the importance of Congress from the very beginning, initiating action on health care but leaving specifics to several key congressional committees and leaders.

Public Support. Many policy objectives do not require mass public support. But a concern as widely shared as health care certainly does. As the months of planning went by, public suspicion of the Clinton health plan increased. This was fueled in part by "Harry and Louise" ads and other public relations work by the plan's opponents. But the secrecy and complexity of the plan and its formulation also played a part.

Again, a relatively simple message by the plan's opponents made their job easier. These opponents raised the specter of government bureaucracy encroaching onto the historically intimate realm personal health services. Such an emphasis may have been inaccurate. But it was more easily grasped by the public than the complex array of boards, alliances, and insurance options in the Clinton plan. The Clinton team could not turn public opinion in its favor. Similarly, public opinion polls conducted as the House and Senate deliberated their respective versions of the Patient Protection and Affordable Care Act indicated that only a minority of Americans felt that the measure would benefit them personally. Lack of public support presented a huge barrier to reconciliation of the House and Senate versions of the measure and its eventual enactment into law.

Political Culture and Climate. As noted earlier, long-standing political culture in the United States discourages rapid, comprehensive change. Moves to place larger parts of civic and economic life under the control of government are particularly suspect in the United States. The Clinton plan was manifestly abrupt, comprehensive, and bureaucracy-laden. Note that neither the federal HMO Act nor California's AB 799–AB 3489 combination was intended as comprehensive change. They were conceived as tactical adjustments rather than basic revisions. Likewise, the Patient Protection and Affordable Care Act left most of the U.S. health care system intact—the financing and delivery of most Americans' health care were neither directly nor immediately affected.

Political climate, the backdrop to policy making, also needs to be considered by people seeking policy change. Political climate concerns the prevailing orientation of policy makers and concerns of the public. In the opinion of some, an atmosphere of confrontation rather than collaboration arose between Democrats and Republicans as the Clinton plan developed. In the Nixon era, by contrast, political rivals appeared willing to work together for limited purposes. A favorable political climate was even more apparent in the California Medicaid reform episode. Potential opponents became allies in a effort to address a fiscal crisis heightened by the cost of providing California's poor with health services. Supporters of health care reform in 2009 faced a political climate no less partisan than in the Clinton years.

THE CASE AGAINST GOVERNMENT IN HEALTH CARE

The most fundamental issues in U.S. health policy concern the degree and manner in which government involvement should take place. Early on, this chapter presented a strong case for government involvement. In closing, the opposite case should be represented as well.

Most economists recognize that the market for health care goods and services is quite imperfect, therefore requiring government participation. Not all observers, however, come to this conclusion. Libertarians believe that government (insofar as it exists at all) should interfere as little as possible in people's private affairs, including the health care they provide and receive. At the extreme, such thinking would support abolition of laws requiring medical licenses and perhaps government approval of drugs and devices. More moderate individuals suspicious of government have argued against compulsory health insurance programs and government-mandated insurance paid for by employers.

Those opposed to government participation in health care have argued that government does not represent a neutral force. Rather, government falls prey to society's powerful individuals, corporations, and interest groups. Licensure laws protect the privileges of doctors, chiropractors, and other health professionals. Regulatory agencies become captives of those whose activity they are intended to regulate.

Some convincing research supports this assessment. As late as the 1970s, it was unusual for health care providers of any kind to engage in advertising. Health care providers and their organizations claimed that advertising was "unprofessional." According to this position, advertising and other practices normal in general commerce led to diminished quality of care. Health professional organizations also applied this argument to employment of their members by corporations, alleging that such employment would weaken professional independence and hence the quality of services provided. These organizations lobbied hard for passage of state laws prohibiting advertising and the "corporate practice" of medical care.[17] Skeptics, however, argued that the real reason for such prohibitions was to protect practitioners from price reductions that often result from such practices. Findings from the study of optometry by Begun and colleagues discussed earlier support this contention, reporting lower consumer prices in states that permitted advertising and corporate practice.

Skeptics on both the right and left side of the political spectrum have contended that regulation of any kind largely benefits the industry regulated, resulting in higher costs and reduced choice for consumers. In this perspective, regulatory agencies and similar bodies typically become *captives of their constituencies.*

In a classic study, historian Gabriel Kolko examined the development of regulation in interstate commerce in the early twentieth century.[18] Most have viewed this era as a time when "progressives" used governmental mechanisms to control the excesses of monopolists and robber barons. However, argued Kolko, the regulatory agencies established during that era were dominated by industry representatives. These representatives divided up territories and fixed prices in a manner advantageous to their industries. What railroading and banking had done on their own during the gilded age (late nineteenth century) was merely repeated in the progressive era under the aegis of government.

In time, developments currently taking place in the United States may produce conditions closer to a free market in health care than they have been in the past. Cost sharing has made consumers more conscious of price. An increasing level of educational attainment has reduced the knowledge and prestige gap between health care providers and consumers. Reduced social distance encourages consumers to ask difficult questions and critically evaluate the answers they receive. The twenty-first century information revolution definitely promotes a free market. Hundreds of web and print-based media now offer information on doctors and hospitals, enabling consumers to make better-informed choices than ever before.

KEY TERMS

Free market

Regulation

Accreditation

Certification

The Joint Commission

Politics

Advocacy

Lobbying

SUMMARY

The role of government in U.S. health care is small by world standards but still critical. A free market in health care does not exist in the United States, nor would most Americans desire to see one established. Government programs help correct imperfections in the health care market. But government intervention has also had adverse effects on some dimensions of health care.

Government actions in health care have included licensure of health care organizations and personnel, training of health professionals, support for research and development, financing of construction and expansion of health care facilities, and oversight of health care delivery. In some instances, arguments can be made that government actions have created more problems than they have solved. Although some U.S. health policy initiatives have achieved permanence, others have seen initial enthusiasm followed by abandonment.

Political decision making in the United States takes place through consensus formation. Most health legislation emerges from coalitions seeking to advance the interests of coalition members. This principle is applicable to political action carried out by both narrow industry groups and organizations representing the broad public interest.

DISCUSSION QUESTIONS

1. To what degree can incrementalism in U.S. health policy be seen as positive versus negative for the public's well-being?

2. Should privatization in application of U.S. health policy be reduced?

3. Should the role now played by government in the U.S. health care system be increased, reduced, or allowed to remain the same?

4. What lessons for the future can be learned from past reform efforts, both successful and unsuccessful?

5. Does the policy-making process in the United States, emphasizing the action of self-interested coalitions, bypass a broader "public interest"?

CHAPTER

12

CHOICES FOR THE FUTURE

LEARNING OBJECTIVES

- To assess the implications of American values and expectations for health care as a continuing public issue
- To understand the challenges faced by non-U.S. health care systems
- To appreciate the lessons of state-level experiments in health care delivery and finance
- To review recent comprehensive reform efforts
- To anticipate future controversies and explore options

OPPORTUNITIES AND BARRIERS TO CHANGE

While describing the characteristics and operations of the U.S. health care system, the foregoing chapters have identified a wide variety of problems. Despite these problems, the system has delivered high-quality care to the vast majority of Americans for generations at a cost society has been willing to pay. Few, however, would challenge the need for policy initiatives capable of controlling costs, ensuring quality, and covering the uninsured.

Any initiative for change must take place within limits placed by American values and political culture. To review, values that have contributed to the system's stability include meritocracy and belief in private property and the free market. The American belief in meritocracy dictates that society should most generously reward people who have personally achieved the most in business, professions, science, or art. Meritocracy supports such phenomena as high pay for executives, superior elementary education for children in affluent suburbs, and more convenient (if not higher quality) health care for the privately insured. Widespread belief in private property and the free market has been instrumental in keeping the system from becoming government-run. Americans, moreover, believe in personal choice and maximization, values that have limited the success of innovations that, like HMOs, are often experienced as constraining.

Yet Americans also believe in equality. Traditionally, this belief has been confined to matters such as equal treatment under the law and freedom of speech. In modern times, belief in equality has come to include material resources. Few Americans feel comfortable seeing their fellow citizens deprived of basic necessities, which in today's thinking include health care. Americans may not support complete equality on this or any other dimension. But the belief is widespread that all humans have enough in common to merit access to certain fundamentals.

It is important to remember that even the strongest social values periodically undergo realignment. Such revision has generally occurred in response to national crisis. In a major departure from tradition, U.S. policy makers in the 1930s enacted large-scale programs to combat the Great Depression. To remedy a banking and credit crisis in the twenty-first century's first decade, the U.S. government became a partial owner of major corporations. These actions signified reduced confidence in the free market. The principle of individual choice has been periodically suspended in wartime, when men have been conscripted and individual economic activity preempted and constrained. Incrementalism, itself a value that has helped prevent rapid change in health care, comes under pressure in national crises such as these. People are more open to significant change when they feel their own well-being to be at risk.

Economic instability in the early twenty-first century made possible loss of health insurance a cause for anxiety among many previously secure Americans. Ensuing public discussion brought widespread attention to dilemmas that had concerned health care specialists for generations. Controversies regarding care for the disadvantaged, the appropriate role for government, and who should pay appear to defy permanent resolution. History suggests this to be the case. Solutions to major issues in U.S. health care have been proposed and at times enacted, only to remain controversial. Major public policy innovations have given rise to adverse, unanticipated consequences and have undergone revision or repeal. In a democratic society valuing maximization and personal choice there is no reason to expect that this pattern will change.

In seeking answers to challenges facing the U.S. health care system, analysts and policy makers have often looked abroad or to a number of U.S. states that have developed innovative programs. A few examples from these venues have provided leads that Americans have been tempted to follow in search of national reforms. But these examples illustrate the evasiveness of straightforward and enduring solutions to U.S. health care dilemmas.

Policy Is Not Permanent

It is important to note that legislation and other public decisions are often transitory. By the 1960s, the post–World War II Hill-Burton Act, which had provided funding to hospitals in exchange for an obligation to serve the indigent, was no longer operative. Government-run central health planning legislation was enacted in the 1970s but permitted to expire in the 1980s under conservative President Ronald Reagan. The popular State Children's Health Insurance Program (SCHIP) program, once seen as a potential means for covering not only poor children but their families, underwent significant retrenchment when state funding declined in the early 2000s.

The potential volatility of public policy is perhaps best illustrated by short-lived legislation enacted in 1988 that required relatively well-off elders to pay a Medicare surtax. Revenue from the surtax was intended to cover catastrophic hospital expenses from which Medicare beneficiaries were not protected. The 40 percent of Medicare beneficiaries with the highest incomes would have been subject to the surtax, a maximum of $800 in the year it was enacted.[1]

A strident backlash ensued. "Jeering senior citizens" surrounding the Chicago office of powerful House Ways and Means Committee Chairman Dan Rostenkowski.[2] The surtax was rapidly repealed.

NON-U.S. HEALTH CARE SYSTEMS: CHALLENGES AND LESSONS LEARNED

From afar, it is tempting to think of non-U.S. systems as better organized, more convenient, less expensive, and at least as effective as the United States. Some evidence suggests that health policy involves less controversy elsewhere. Although selected features of non-U.S. health care systems indeed have appeal, the general assumption of their superiority is questionable.

It is important to restrict the range of countries to which the United States is compared to those with advanced industrial economies and democratic political institutions. Critics of the U.S. health care system have not always done so. Some, for example, have looked back in history and settled on the *feldsher* of Tsarist and early Communist Russia as a model for the United States. The feldsher was an individual whose limited medical education was thought sufficient to care for ordinary medical needs in a friendly and inexpensive manner.[3] Dr. J. S. Horn, an English surgeon, once captured the imagination of Americans with his description of China's *barefoot doctors,* medical itinerants with limited capabilities deployed by the government to provide rural health care.[4] However romantic, neither the feldsher nor the barefoot doctor is relevant to U.S. health policy. The use of such personnel reflects health care systems much more primitive than any remotely acceptable to Americans.

A Variety of Systems

Table 12.1 summarizes the variety of health care systems operating in countries comparable economically and politically to the United States. All the countries represented in this table have national insurance systems of some kind that provide universal coverage. The systems in Germany and France are relatively private sector-oriented. Germany's system comprises a network of private sickness funds associated with employers, unions, and other private organizations. Government subsidizes these funds and operates a system to cover people for whom an individual fund is not available. A somewhat similar system operates in France. Hospitals in Germany are owned by the sickness funds, while those in France are owned by local governments.

Government plays a more central role in English and Canadian health care. Funding for the health care systems in these countries is predominantly governmental. In England, the Ministry of Health owns the hospitals and allocates an annual fixed sum for the operation of each. In Canada, hospitals are owned by private, nonprofit organizations but funded by the government. Although a single agency (the Ministry of Health) directly allocates budgets to English hospitals, provincial governments perform this function in Canada.

In none of the countries represented in Table 12.1 are physicians employees of the government. In all these countries, however, most receive a good part, if not all, of their income (directly or indirectly) from government programs. Mechanisms of payment differ from country to country. In England, for example, general practitioners receive payment via capitation, while specialists ("consultants"), who are associated with individual hospitals, receive salaries. Canadian doctors are paid on a fee-for-service basis.

Not addressed in Table 12.1 is the availability of private health insurance. In several European countries, private health insurance systems operate alongside the public system. The presence of private systems enables residents with sufficient personal means to receive health care at facilities that are independent of government and to receive services unavailable to them under government programs. Germany, Italy, and Austria, for example, have government-financed health care systems but

TABLE 12.1   Types of non-U.S. health care systems

System Type	Hospital Ownership	Funding
Private sector		
Germany	Private and government	Private insurance payments and government subsidies to sickness funds and hospitals
Government participant		
France	Government	Nongovernment agencies subsidized by government
Government-financed		
United Kingdom	Government	Central government agency
Canada	Nonprofit organizations	Joint federal and provincial government

permit private systems to operate alongside. Public policy in England and Canada discourages private systems. Laws in some Canadian provinces prohibit private health insurance.

Global Cost Control

Most if not all economically advanced democracies (other than the United States) apply *global measures* to contain health care costs. The term here means a single or integrated set of procedures applied to an entire health care system to restrain costs. In the words of one commentator, a global cost control mechanism can be characterized as "a coherent decision-making apparatus for controlling costs—or attempting to."[5]

Expenditure caps and *expenditure targets* are the most widely applied global cost control methods. Under **expenditure caps,** government agencies allocate a fixed amount of money per year to hospitals or physicians in a jurisdiction, or for all health services in the country as a whole. If indications appear that the expenditure cap is likely to be exceeded, the agency pays the hospitals and physicians at a lower rate in an attempt to remain in budget for the year.

Expenditure targets are less stringent than expenditure caps. Like expenditure caps, expenditure targets specify a ceiling on health care expenditures. Under **expenditure targets,** however, officials do not reduce payments to health care personnel and facilities in a given year to ensure that expenditures remain below the ceiling. Rather, officials deduct the excess from the next year's allocations for health care.

Setting of expenditure caps and targets takes place through negotiation. Depending on the country, for example, physician organizations negotiate with local sickness funds, provincial governments, or national ministries of health. Negotiations of this kind have strong potential to be controversial, as government agencies seek to restrain expenditures and physicians and hospitals desire to see their income levels maintained and their resources sufficient to provide for the public's needs.

System Performance

Better performance by European-style health care systems in preventing illness and healing patients would argue strongly for their emulation in the United States. Critics of the U.S. health care system, in fact, cite apparently superior performance by non-U.S. systems in areas such as infant mortality. Studies comparing performance of non-U.S. systems with the United States have been conducted on a number of other health concerns.

Several researchers have argued that care for people with established illnesses is the most relevant focus for cross-national comparison. The work of one research group addressed the question of possible social disparities in health care utilization in countries whose health care systems ensured universal access. According to these researchers, economically advantaged people utilize more specialty care than the relatively disadvantaged. In countries that provide universal access, consumers usually must obtain specialty care via referral from primary care doctors. The researchers speculate that physicians have a prorich bias in referring patients to specialists.[6]

Provision of specific elements of care in countries that have universal coverage also helps shed light on differences between U.S. and non-U.S. health care systems. A study conducted in the late 1980s and early 1990s compared treatment and survival experiences of heart attack patients treated in Quebec and the United States. Trends observed in both locales suggested a more rapid increase among U.S. patients in treatments such as angiography and coronary artery bypass graft. Survival rates increased among patients treated in both locales during the period observed. But the trend toward increased survival was stronger in the United States.[7]

According to an important study by an international team, individuals with some of the most common forms of cancer have a greater likelihood of survival when treated in the United States than in European health care systems. Data were obtained from the cancer registries of fourteen European countries and the U.S. Surveillance, Epidemiology, and End Results system. Analysis of these data showed that U.S. patients with cancers of the colon, rectum, breast (female), lung, or prostate had a greater likelihood of surviving five or more years than patients treated in any European country. Survival differences in some forms of cancer were quite large. In comparison with Americans treated for prostate cancer, for example, European patients were nearly three times as likely to die fewer than five years after diagnosis. The study's authors suggest that, at least for some cancers, more aggressive treatment helps explain the U.S. survival advantage. In Europe, for example, elderly patients are less likely to receive anticancer surgery than in the United States.[8]

Avoidable ill health and preventable mortality unquestionably result from faulty aspects of the U.S. health care system. But at least for some disease, it would appear that the U.S. system performs better than many non-U.S. systems. European and Canadian systems assure universal access to health care. However, this access does not ensure equal utilization of care. This observation is consistent with a classic in epidemiology known as the *Black Report.* A document produced by an expert panel chaired by Sir Douglas Black, a prominent English physician, the *Black Report* demonstrated significant socioeconomic disparities in health and life expectancy even in countries where universal access to health care was legally mandated.[9]

A SYSTEM TO BE EMULATED? CONCERNS ABOUT CANADA

Among non-U.S. health care systems, Canada deserves special attention. More closely than any other country, Canada resembles the United States in political economy and culture. The physical proximity of Canada has provided opportunity for close observation by U.S. health care researchers.

A single program provides financial support for most health services utilized by Canadians. The program is known as *Medicare,* but bears no resemblance to the U.S. program for the elderly beyond the name. For decades, Medicare has enjoyed wide popularity in Canada and served as a source of national pride for Canadians.

U.S. commentators have expressed admiration for the Canadian system because it provides universal coverage. Under Medicare, moreover, Canada's health care costs have increased less rapidly that those of the United States. Contributing to the relatively slow growth of Canada's health care costs have been various methods of upstream resource allocation. Budgetary control over health care organizations has restrained purchases of expensive equipment. Canada's federal government has limited the country's supply of physicians by restricting licensure of doctors from abroad. At least one province, British Columbia, for a time refused to issue billing codes (necessary for payment under Medicare) to new physicians even if they were legally qualified to practice.

Canada is often held up as a paradigm for U.S. health care reform. However, U.S. reform advocates should be aware of increasingly apparent shortcomings in Canada. Some of the most widely recognized of these are described next.

Excessive Wait Times

According to official sources, Canadians waited twenty-five weeks for cataract surgery in 2007 from the time their primary care doctor referred them for treatment to the time they received treatment, and forty-two weeks from referral to treatment for joint replacement. Wait times for these and other procedures are far longer than official targets. An expert in health system performance studies at the Fraser Institute commented as follows in 2008:

> *According to the Pan-Canadian Benchmark Wait Times announced jointly by the federal, provincial and territorial governments in December, 2005, being treated within*

twenty-six weeks from the time a Canadian sees a specialist to the time they receive treatment for hip or knee replacement surgery is considered reasonable. So is being treated within twenty-six weeks for level 3 cardiac bypass surgery, or sixteen weeks for cataract surgery for patients at "high risk," or four weeks for radiation therapy. Yet many of the provincial wait times guarantees announced earlier this year are much longer than even these generous targets.[10]

Wait times are a consequence of resource allocation restraint. An insufficient number of doctors in the community results in more consumers seeking care at hospital emergency departments. Fewer CT scanners mean longer waits for diagnosis. Intentional or not, policies that result in increased waiting for services amount to **rationing** of care. Some consumers lose interest in an intervention during an extensive queuing period. Others may die before their turn for service comes. In a notable development, the Province of Quebec now pays for care received outside the province or outside Canada itself for residents who would have waited excessive lengths of time to obtain the services in Quebec.

Mixed Performance

A comprehensive comparison of Canadian and U.S. health statistics suggests that overall, Canadians enjoy better health.[11] Table 12.2 presents data on two basic indicators of health, life expectancy and infant mortality, for 2004. Life expectancy is higher and infant mortality lower in Canada.

According to other measures, however, the U.S. system appears to perform better. Data in Table 12.3 indicate the percentages of Canadians and Americans with specific chronic diseases who report receiving treatment for these conditions. The data are based on the 2002–2003 Joint Canada/U.S. Survey of Health, a collaborative effort by Canadian and U.S. government agencies. As shown in Table 12.3, Americans in the eighteen to sixty-four age group were more likely than Canadians to receive treatment for conditions such as high blood pressure and coronary heart disease. Differences in the likelihood of receiving care were even greater among individuals aged sixty-five and over. Among individuals sixty-five and over, Americans were more likely to receive treatment for all chronic conditions with the exception of heart disease.

The 2002–2003 Joint Canada/U.S. Survey of Health found that people in the United States not were not only more likely to receive treatment for chronic diseases but were more likely to receive interventions intended to prevent such conditions. Among U.S. men ages forty through forty-nine, 49.5 percent had had a prostate-specific antigen (PSA) test for early prostate cancer within the past three years. Almost 30 percent had ever had a colonoscopy or sigmoidoscopy for detection of colon cancer. Among Canadian men in the same age group, 15.2 percent had had a PSA within the past three years and 4.6 percent had ever had a colonoscopy or sigmoidoscopy. Among U.S. women twenty through sixty-nine years old, 86.3 percent had had a Pap test within the past three years, compared with 75.1 percent of Canadian women. Among

TABLE 12.2 Life expectancy and infant mortality in Canada and the United States

	Infant Mortality (per 1000 live births)	Life Expectancy			
		At Birth		At Age 65	
		Male	Female	Male	Female
Canada	5.3	77.7	82.5	17.7	20.9
U.S.	6.8	75.2	80.4	17.1	20.0
White	5.7	75.7	80.8	17.2	20.0
Black	13.5	69.5	76.3	15.2	18.6

Sources: Statistics Canada, Catalogue no. 85F0211X; CDC-NCHS, National Vital Statistics Reports.

U.S. women aged forty through sixty-nine, 88.6 percent had ever had a mammogram, compared with 72.3 percent of Canadian women.[12]

The data in Tables 12.2 and 12.3 leave open an important question: Do people in the United States overconsume health care or are Canadians relatively deprived of beneficial services? Resolution of this issue is beyond the scope of the present text. Whatever may be the answer, service delivery in Canada does not match expectations of U.S. consumers or the treatment preferences of U.S. physicians. Disparities between the United States and Canada are particularly apparent among individuals sixty-five and over. This observation is consistent with treatment for cancer in Europe which, as referenced above, appears to be less aggressively applied to elders.

Public Controversies

Despite the universal coverage it offers, Canada's Medicare system is a frequent object of contention and dissatisfaction. Examples of regularly recurring complaints and controversies include the following:

■ *Limited scope of coverage.* Among long-standing concerns of Canadians has been the limited scope of coverage offered by Medicare. People in the United States take insurance coverage for pharmaceuticals for granted. Canada's Medicare program does not cover this increasingly important area of health care. Certain supplies in addition to medications are likewise not covered.[13]

■ *Unavailability of a private health care alternative.* As indicated earlier, a number of European countries with national health care systems allow private health insurance plans to operate and permit physicians to treat patients under private coverage.

TABLE 12.3 Percentage who receive treatment for selected chronic conditions in Canada and the United States

	Percentage Who Receive Treatment			
	Ages 18–64		Ages 65 and over	
	U.S.	Canada	U.S.	Canada
Asthma	78.8	80.3	91.6	82.5
High blood pressure	88.3	84.1	97.7	95.1
Emphysema or related diseases	73.1	53.0	73.6	64.3
Diabetes[a]	83.9	80.3	91.3	80.4
Coronary heart disease	94.8	88.9	96.3	90.5
Heart disease, not otherwise specified	69.6	67.2	90.8	91.4
Angina	61.0	74.6	77.7	73.0

[a]Treatment includes either insulin or "diabetic pills."

Canada has slowly begun to permit such a system to develop. It still represents a very small part of Canada's health care sector. Proponents of privatization argue that such an innovation would bring more money into Canada's health care system. Others, however, contend that even limited privatization would foster development of a two-tiered health care system. Some Canadians have expressed the concern that a two-tiered system would allow development of the inequalities that are perceived to characterize the United States.

■ *Conflict over funding.* Controversy regularly erupts over the level of finding made available for health care. Editorial writers in Canada's newspapers have contended that too little money is made available by the federal government and that the money allocated has not improved services. Regular controversy takes place between the federal and provincial governments regarding funding allocations. Legally, the provinces have are obliged to provide health care to their residents. But the provinces depend heavily on the federal government for funds. Finally, Canadian policy makers share the concern of their U.S. counterparts over rising health care costs.

Like other non-U.S. health care systems, that of Canada cannot be categorically accepted as a model for the United States. It is unlikely that U.S. consumers would accept the queuing for services that is commonplace in Canada. U.S. clinicians appear unlikely to feel comfortable with the health services their Canadian counterparts are accustomed to providing. Controversy over the levels of funding made available to the provincial governments occurs regularly. Such controversy would likely be even more acute in the United States.

STATE-LEVEL INITIATIVES IN THE UNITED STATES

As comprehensive health care reform eluded federal policy makers in the late twentieth century, policy makers at the state level took independent action. They formulated innovative solutions and conducted experiments of national significance. Accomplishments and issues of these initiatives later influenced health care policy debates at the national level. Challenges in implementing and maintaining these programs provide clues to those likely to effect recent federal health care reform legislation.

One of the most valuable experiments took place in Hawaii. That state instituted a "play-or-pay" mandate for employers. Employers were required to provide health insurance coverage for their employees or pay into a state insurance fund. From the early 1970s on, this and other mechanisms enabled Hawaiians to enjoy near-universal health care coverage.

The **Oregon Health Plan** attracted significant national attention in the early 1990s. Like Hawaii, Oregon passed legislation instituting a play-or-pay system. Coupled with this provision was a significant expansion of the state's Medicaid program for people not covered by employers. To control the cost of its expanded Medicaid program, Oregon developed a rationing system. It was planned that the program would pay only for care that was sufficiently high on a priority list. Priorities were established through a highly democratic process, involving series of town meetings throughout the state.

In 2006, the state of Massachusetts instituted a program to cover all state residents. Elements of this plan included an employer play-or-pay system and several other measures to enable people without insurance to obtain coverage. In a unique feature among state-level programs, Massachusetts required nearly all residents to obtain health insurance.

An innovative component of the Massachusetts plan was the **insurance connector**. The insurance connector was designed as a publicly accessible electronic resource enabling consumers to shop for insurance plans. Plans accessible through the insurance connector were to include an array of private-sector products developed under state auspices. For individual consumers or small-business owners, such plans are especially advantageous. In effect, consumers shopping through the insurance connector comprise risk pools of thousands of individuals. Costs of insuring large risk pools are far lower than those of insuring individuals. Thus, consumers may obtain insurance far more cheaply.

Other state-level programs featured insurance-related legislation. Over the years, several states established insurance programs for high-risk individuals and small employers. New York, New Jersey, Maine, and Vermont, for example, passed measures requiring health insurers to use community rating, resulting in lower insurance costs for high-risk individuals.[14]

Several factors limited the success of state programs or their adoption outside the state of origin. Many state innovations were preempted by federal law. Provisions of the federal Americans with Disabilities Act prevented Oregon from implementing its priority list of covered items. Classification of some services as low priority differentially affected severely ill, and hence, disabled individuals. Most important was the Employee Retirement Income Security Act (ERISA). From 1974 into the twenty-first century, ERISA prohibited employer mandates, thus making play-or-play plans unlawful. Only Hawaii was able to sustain such a mandate, because appropriate state laws were on the books before ERISA's enactment.

Most if not all of these state-level programs encountered difficulties due to unexpectedly high costs, both to the state and the consumer. This problem results at least in part from national trends. The first two years of the Massachusetts program evidenced greater access and utilization. But costs to individuals were observed to have risen, jeopardizing their newfound access. In addition, a shortage of health care providers was found to have developed as an influx of newly insured people sought services.[15]

RECENT HEALTH CARE REFORM EFFORTS

Following upon a high level of public concern and campaign promises by several presidents, the U.S. House of Representatives and Senate passed separate reform bills in 2009. Alluded to at several points in the preceding text, this legislation was known as the Patient Protection and Affordable Care Act. More than 2,000 pages in length, the measure sought to reduce the number of Americans who lacked health insurance by more than 30 million. Key provisions of the measure included a significant expansion of Medicaid, employer and individual insurance mandates, subsidies for the purchase of private health insurance, an insurance exchange similar to the Massachusetts insurance connector, and reform of certain private insurance industry practices.

Following action in Congress, however, the reform effort encountered an atmosphere of extreme political volatility. Both houses of Congress needed to pass identical versions of the bill, an eventuality which had not occurred at this writing. However, future enactment of elements of the legislation appeared likely, and thus merit examination.

Provisions of the Reform

Expansion of Medicaid. The core of the legislation involved expansion of Medicaid eligibility to include people of limited income but above the federal poverty level. Medicaid, of course, was originally enacted to cover the health care needs of poor people. But often, Medicaid eligibility has been limited to families qualifying for welfare programs such as TANF, SSI, or SCHIP. Because Medicaid programs are enacted and operated by individual states, eligibility and benefits differ from state to state. For the first time, reform would have allowed adults to enroll who did not necessary qualify for other public programs and who did not have children.

Employer and Individual Mandate. In a marked reversal of earlier policy, the Patient Protection and Affordable Care Act required all but the smallest employers to offer health insurance to their employees and most individual Americans to obtain insurance. Employers affected by the legislation who did not offer insurance plans were to be subject to fines, as were individuals who did not obtain insurance.

Subsidies for Insurance. To assist individuals and small businesses in complying with the new insurance mandates, the Patient Protection and Affordable Care Act included subsidies to defray the cost of the required policies. Persons qualifying for the subsidies were not merely the poor. Qualifying individuals could earn several times the federal poverty level. The size of subsidies made available under the law would have run into the thousands of dollars for some potential beneficiaries.

Insurance Exchanges. Also to assist individuals and small businesses in complying with the insurance mandate, the Patient Protection and Affordable Care Act sought to establish insurance exchanges similar to the Massachusetts insurance connector within each state. The exchanges were intended to allow individuals to comparison shop among an array of insurance plans offered by private companies. To appear on an exchange, insurance plans had to offer a comprehensive range of benefits larger in scope than many plans traditionally offered in the commercial market.

Private Insurance Reform. New regulations on the health insurance industry included the requirement that all applicants be offered policies. Individuals with pre-existing conditions could not be denied coverage, nor could beneficiaries be dropped from a plan because they had incurred high costs. Insurance companies were barred from specifying lifetime limits on benefits in their policies. Insurance companies remained free to set rates corresponding to age-related risk. However, the difference between premium levels offered to younger versus older people were to be restricted to a range narrower than they historically had been.

The Reform's Limitations

As Congress deliberated, journalists characterized the forthcoming legislation as a "revamp" and "overhaul" of health care in the United States. The characterization was an inaccurate one. Only restricted features of the U.S. system of health care finance were addressed by the Patient Protection and Affordable Care Act. None of the basic characteristics of organization and delivery of services was changed. Placing emphasis on enrolling the uninsured in plans, the legislation did not decisively address controlling expenditures, making coverage less expensive for those already insured, or limiting future increases in the price of health insurance policies.

The measure clearly focused on covering groups that have historically lacked health insurance (see Chapter 7). Expanded Medicaid was to provide a key resource for the working poor. Subsidies for purchase of private insurance were to enable self-employed individuals and people employed by firms that did not offer plans to obtain coverage. Prohibition of denial due to pre-existing conditions was intended to enable the sick and disabled to buy policies or, if their income was sufficiently low, to obtain coverage through Medicaid. The individual mandate was designed to bring low users, gamblers, and free riders into the insurance pool. Generous subsidies were proposed to help individuals overcome the barrier to coverage represented by the continuing high cost of policies.

Both in its enactment and provisions, the Patient Protection and Affordable Care Act reflected values and dimensions of the political culture that have long prevailed in the United States. Leaving most of the pre-existing finance and the entire delivery system intact, the measure is consistent with the degree of incrementalism with which Americans feel comfortable. To pass the bills, coalitions were assembled in Congress based not on ideology but on trade-offs of components favored by different members. Financial inducements, some quite large, were offered to officials who were most reluctant to join the coalition (see Chapter 11).

Concretely, the Patient Protection and Affordable Care Act sought to continue rather than depart from solutions that had been considered earlier in Congress or enacted within individual states. In the incrementalist tradition, expansion of Medicare to the "near elderly" was proposed during the Congressional deliberation. Under this proposal, persons fifty-five and over would have been permitted to buy into the program. Much research evidence has been presented to demonstrate the desirability of Medicare expansion.[16,17] Medicaid expansion had also been considered earlier by Congress, several bills in earlier sessions having called for a large expansion of eligibility for Medicaid as a means of moving toward universal coverage.[18]

Other proposals made in Congress included establishment of a new government-run insurance entity intended to compete with the private insurance industry, a feature of the Massachusetts plan.[19] Congressional support was evident from early 2009 for a measure that would have required all but the smallest firms to provide health insurance to their employees or pay a special tax.[20] At that time, support was also present for the individual mandate, requiring every American to have health insurance or incur a penalty.[21] Ultimately, the required votes could not be obtained for Medicare expansion or a government-operated insurance plan.

FUTURE CONTROVERSIES AND OPTIONS

The political roadblocks encountered by the Patient Protection and Affordable Care Act re-enact past controversies and foreshadow those likely to accompany future reform efforts. A system-wide perspective helps to comprehend future controversies and formulate solutions.

Likely Issues

Paying for expanded coverage of Americans under any comprehensive reform legislation will be foremost among emergent issues. Costs for the first ten years of the

Patient Protection and Affordable Care Act were estimated at around $1 trillion. Experience with past health care programs suggests that costs could have risen much higher. Decision-makers in the 1960s never publicly contemplated the eventual costs of Medicare and Medicaid, today well on their way to the trillion dollar mark. It is important to emphasize that the Patient Protection and Affordable Care Act contained no provisions for comprehensive application of proven cost control methods.

Controversies over payment are likely to pit state-level agencies and officials against their federal counterparts. Expansion of Medicaid—a program jointly funded by federal and state monies—places significant financial responsibilities on state governments. For years, states have struggled to pay for their Medicaid programs. State-level officials are likely to resist future financial obligations.

Intergenerational conflict among Americans over payment is a strong possibility. Younger, working individuals already pay substantial Medicare taxes to support health care for the elderly. Any requirement that younger individuals also buy insurance for themselves would increase the burden on younger Americans. Young people are less likely to become ill and incur high charges for health care than older ones. Movements may arise to redress the resulting imbalance of payment and risk.

Moving beyond costs, the readiness of the system of health care delivery for comprehensive reform is uncertain. Expansion of the health care labor force and construction of new facilities are not necessarily attractive policy options. At best, these measures would be time-consuming and expensive. Questions about quality of care, moreover, are likely to arise. Chapter 7 has suggested the possibility that Medicaid, particularly when delivered under managed care, may be developing into a second-tier delivery system. Protests by the Medicaid-insured could ensue if suspicion of second-rate care in Medicaid managed care operations becomes widespread.

Options for the Future

Paying for existing commitments and restraining future cost increases will require Americans to consider options they have been historically reluctant to entertain. New sources of revenue are quite likely necessary. To restrain future cost growth, restriction of service may be unavoidable.

Fundamentally, augmentation of the existing tax base may be necessary. Many analysts have long advocated full taxation of health care benefits, including those less generous than the so-called "gold plated" or "Cadillac" plans. A value-added tax (VAT) mechanism has been suggested, amounting to a national tax on producers of goods and services.[22] A tax on sugar-containing soda pop has been proposed, supported by the assertion that ingestion of sugar increases the consumer's health risks and thus his likely health care expenses.

Controversial as it may be, expansion of the U.S. tax base may be easier than controlling the entire system's costs. In this connection, it is useful to recall Henry Aaron's thinking (see Chapter Two) about the high cost of marginally useful medical interventions. Ultimately, control of costs may require administrative restriction of such interventions. The concept of **comparative effectiveness** may become increasingly relevant to such choices. An application of evidence-based medicine, comparative effectiveness research makes side-by-side comparisons of alternative methods of treating a given condition. One might envisage a future in which comparative effectiveness research significantly reduces marginally or less-effective interventions, thus making a major contribution to cost control.

This approach, however, has rapidly drawn criticism from health professionals.[23] Not all patients, it has been argued, benefit from the treatment choice that evidence-based medicine suggests is generally the better. Some large-scale studies have shown that patients treated under evidence-based guidelines did no better or even worse than those treated otherwise.[24,25] Whatever studies may find, patients will still demand treatments that they believe beneficial, even if marginally so. To the degree that comparative effectiveness and other evidence-based medicine is applied in efforts to control costs, news reports will be filled with stories of patients who believe they have been denied care they should receive.

Whatever technical expertise and statesmanship is applied to the issues raised in this chapter, controversy will remain active. The emotion, uncertainty, and mystery essential to health care will ensure continuation of today's controversies and development of new ones. The history of health care has been one of increasing human well-being. Balancing the use of resources and sustaining an underlying social consensus may be even more important than progress in medical science for continued improvement of human health.

KEY TERMS

Expenditure caps

Expenditure targets

Rationing

Insurance connector

Oregon Health Plan

Comparative effectiveness

SUMMARY

Widespread satisfaction with health care in the United States has contributed to the system's stability, as have several key American values. However, few can ignore the need for steps to safeguard access, quality, and affordability of health care now and in the future. U.S. policy makers have looked for guidance to health care systems abroad and experiments within individual American states. None of these can serve as a model for innovation in America. Canada, once seen as a paragon, has experienced outcomes unlikely to prove attractive to most Americans. State plans have encountered many challenges and a number have failed or been rescinded.

For the foreseeable future, the United States will maintain basic features such pluralism and private sector dominance. But government will play an increasing role in the system's financing. Significant, new inflation in the health care sector is possible.

Actual policy choices and related controversies are likely to be concentrated in two areas. First, the U.S. tax base will likely need to expand to ensure adequate funding and equity of responsibility for the new health care coverage. Second, effective mechanisms must be adopted to restrain increases in the cost of health care in the United States.

The basic nature of health care makes it likely that related controversies will occur periodically, if not continuously, in U.S. public life.

DISCUSSION QUESTIONS

1. Does China's experience with "barefoot doctors" have any applicability in the twenty-first century United States?

2. Of the non-U.S. health care systems discussed in this chapter, which might serve as the best mode for the United States?

3. Would Americans benefit from adopting expenditure caps or expenditure targets such as those used in some non-U.S. systems?

4. To what extent can persons newly insured under Medicaid expect the same quality of care as those who are privately insured?

5. In addition to those discussed in this chapter, what health care-related controversies might be expected to develop in the near future?

GLOSSARY

A

Accreditation   Assertion by a professional or industry association that an organization offering services to the public meets the accrediting association's standards of capacity and performance.

American Association of Medical Colleges (AAMC)   An organization representing the interests of schools of medicine in the United States.

Ad Council   A nonprofit organization of advertising industry firms dedicated to developing and sponsoring public interest announcements and campaigns.

Advanced practice nurse   An individual who, in addition to a basic nursing degree, has an advanced degree or other certification to perform more specialized and independent work. Examples include nurse practitioners, nurse midwives, and nurse anesthetists.

Alameda Study   A large-scale longitudinal investigation begun in 1965 that focused on behavioral and social correlates of mortality.

Allopathic   Medicine as practiced by mainstream physicians in the United States and Europe based on factual observation, scientific experimentation, and disciplines such as anatomy, physiology, immunology, and pharmacology.

Ambulatory care   Office-based or outpatient care, as distinguished from care delivered to patients in hospitals or other residential facilities (derived from the Latin root *ambulare,* to walk).

Ambulatory care–sensitive condition   A condition that, if treated in an ambulatory setting, is less likely to require eventual emergency care or hospitalization (for example, asthma, diabetes, or congestive heart failure).

American Medical Women's Association (AMWA)   An organization founded by female physicians in 1915 with the mission of advancing women in medicine and improving women's health.

Attending staff   Fully trained physicians who, in addition to hospital admitting privileges, usually have an outside office–based practice.

B

Backward-bending labor supply curve   A concept in labor economics suggesting that people will reduce their contributions to the market (such as hours worked or patients seen) once they have achieved a particular income target.

Balance billing   The practice by which a health care provider charges patients the difference between the compensation paid by an insurance company or government program and a higher rate that the provider considers justified.

Bioterrorism   A technique applied for the purpose of creating terror or social disorganization utilizing pathogenic microorganisms or the toxins they produce (akin to the term *germ warfare*).

Blood work   Laboratory techniques applied to blood drawn from a patient for diagnostic purposes.

Board certification   A credential granted to a physician usually requiring successful completion of an examination by a specialty board certifying that the physician is qualified to practice a particular specialty.

Built environment   Objects of human construction such as buildings, streets, and other infrastructure that potentially affect an individual's health or well-being.

C

Caduceus A widely recognized symbol of medicine in the form of a winged staff around whose shaft are wound one or two serpents.

Capitation Payment by an insurer or other sponsor to an individual health care provider or organization on the basis of a flat fee for each individual enrolled.

Carve-out The practice by a health plan or integrated delivery system of contracting with an outside organization to provide a particular type of service such as laboratory services or mental health.

Case control A research design based on comparing individuals exposed to an experimental intervention with individuals selected from the population who are not exposed to the intervention but have characteristics (such as demographic features) that are the same as those exposed.

Catastrophic A degree of financial liability or loss of very high magnitude.

Centers for Medicare and Medicaid Services (CMS) The federal agency that administers the Medicare and Medicaid programs.

Certificate of need (CON) A document issued by a public sector planning or regulatory agency allowing a health care facility to be constructed, a new service to be offered, or new high-cost equipment to be deployed.

Certification Assertion by a professional or industry association that an individual practitioner or organization is qualified to perform specific services.

Charge nurse The supervisor of a nursing shift on a hospital service, whose duties include assigning individual nurses to specific patients.

Chiropractic A health profession first organized in 1895 that uses musculoskeletal manipulation to treat a wide variety of complaints, the best known of which is back pain.

Clinical trial A research design intended to test the safety and efficacy of a medical or surgical intervention, typically conducted by randomly assigning patients to an "experimental" and "control" group and statistically comparing health status indicators between these two groups following the intervention.

Cobweb feedback cycle A concept in labor economics that captures fluctuations in prices of goods and services based on delayed impact of periodic oversupply and undersupply.

Cohort A set of individuals with a time-related characteristic in common, such as year of birth or onset of a disease.

Community rating Establishment of insurance premiums based on the risks estimated for the entire population within a specific geographic area without regard to individual factors of gender, age, employment, or current health status.

Community or voluntary hospital A nonprofit hospital whose primary mission is to serve residents of nearby neighborhoods.

Copayment A form of cost sharing in which an insured patient pays a percentage of the cost of a specific unit of service or health-related product (such as a visit with a physician or a prescription filled by a pharmacist).

Corporate practice of medicine According to some state laws, the practice of medicine as an employee of an organization owned or controlled by individuals who are not physicians.

Cost-benefit A positive or negative number obtained by subtracting the cost of providing an intervention from the value of its outcome expressed in monetary terms (such as posttreatment income of an individual able to retain employment due to the intervention).

Cost-effectiveness The financial cost of a desired health or health-related outcome; formally, a ratio of dollars to number of successful outcomes achieved (such as cases of measles avoided or quality-adjusted years of life obtained).

Cost-plus Payment from a sponsor of health care comprising the provider's cost of delivering the good or service plus a negotiated additional percentage of that cost.

Cost sharing Any of several arrangements under which an insured individual is required to pay a portion of the costs associated with a unit of health care (such as a doctor visit); familiar examples of cost sharing are deductibles and copayments.

Cost shifting The practice of covering the costs of uninsured or poorly insured patients by increasing the charges to patients who have better insurance coverage or are personally wealthy.

D

Deductible   A form of cost sharing under which an insured person receives no benefits in a given year until his medical expenses have exceeded a specified amount.

Disease prevention   Medical or public health activity carried out to reduce individuals' likelihood of developing illness, such as immunization or screening.

Double blind   A feature of clinical trials design in which both researchers and subjects are "blinded"—unaware of the arm of the study into which any individual subject has been placed.

E

Elective procedure   A procedure undertaken according to a plan and on a scheduled date as opposed to an emergency procedure.

Emergent condition   A condition that immediately threatens the life or may cause significant deficit in the health or function of an individual if not immediately treated.

Employer mandate   A legal requirement that employers provide a benefit such as health insurance to their employees.

Endemic   The occurrence of a disease in numbers that are normally expected in a given population.

Entitlement   A public program to whose benefits an individual is entitled on the basis of specific standards such as employment history, age, and disability status.

Epidemic   Extraordinarily large incidence of a disease or occurrence of a disease in segments of the population where it does not normally occur.

Evidence-based medicine   Restriction of medical interventions to those whose efficacy is supported by research studies.

Experience rating   Establishment of insurance premiums based on the risks estimated for a restricted population or group, typically individuals employed by a firm.

F

Fecal occult blood testing   A procedure to detect the presence of blood in stool as a potential indication of gastric or bowel disease or cancer.

Fee for service   Payment to a health care provider by an individual or insurer on the basis of a separate fee for each service performed.

Fiscal intermediary   A private-sector organization that contracts with the Centers for Medicare and Medicaid Services to manage accounts and pay reimbursements to Medicare and Medicaid providers.

Foreign medical graduate   A physician who has received her degree from a medical school outside the United States.

Framingham Study   A longitudinal study in Framingham, Massachusetts, begun in 1948, that has provided significant information about the individual characteristics that lead to cardiovascular disease (including heart attacks, heart failure, and stroke).

Free clinic   A type of community health center providing services (directly or by referral) on a low- or no-fee basis.

Full-time equivalent (FTE)   An administrative term denoting the availability, presence, or need for a full-time employee with specific responsibilities or for a specific project (typically two thousand hours per year); the full-time equivalent function may obtained from a single individual, by two or more individuals working part-time, or two or more individuals occupied in part of their work time in other functions or projects.

G

Global cost control   A mechanism for controlling costs applied to all health care providers in a country, typically applied by a central government agency.

H

Health maintenance organization (HMO)   A type of managed care organization providing comprehensive services funded primarily by capitated contracts, employing or contracting with a specific group health professionals to deliver services, and traditionally not making insurance benefits available for services obtained outside the plan.

Health promotion   Individual behavior or lifestyle features intended to reduce the likelihood of future illness, such as exercise, healthy eating, weight control, and avoidance of tobacco, excessive alcohol use, and high-risk sex.

Health savings accounts (HSAs)   Tax-free programs for paying health care charges not covered by insurance.

Health systems agency (HSA)   A local agency empowered to conduct health planning activities and regulate building of facilities and deployment of expensive equipment under the National Health Planning and Resource Development Act (1975–1980).

Healthcare Effectiveness Data and Information Set (HEDIS)   Maintained by the National Committee for Quality Assurance, a database on the quality of care in employee health plans widely used by employers to guide selection of plans.

Hill-Burton Act   A 1946 law, the Hospital Survey and Construction Act, that provided federal grants and guaranteed loans to build and improve the physical plant of hospitals in the United States.

Homeopathic   A form of medicine that is practiced under the principle that interventions that produce the symptoms of a disease in fact cure that disease; modern homeopathic remedies include highly diluted solutions of agents believed to be curative and water from which such agents have been filtered.

House staff   Interns and residents in a hospital (also known as *house officers*).

I

Imaging   Any electronically or radiation-assisted device or procedure providing clinicians with views of internal structures or processes within the body, including X-ray, CT scan, and MRI technology.

Indemnity   An insurance setup under which beneficiaries are reimbursed for actual payments for health care.

Independent practice association (IPA)   An organization that packages service capacity from independent physician practices and markets these packages to health plans or managed care organizations.

Institutional review board (IRB)   A federally accredited unit in an organization performing biomedical research responsible for assuring the safety of human subjects.

International Classification of Disease (ICD)   A system widely used in insurance billing and epidemiology that assigns unique codes to diagnosed diseases and a wide variety of signs, symptoms, abnormal findings, complaints, social circumstances, and external causes of injury or disease.

Intravenous   Inserted or injected into a vein.

J

Joint Commission on Accreditation of Healthcare Organizations (JCAHO)   A private nonprofit organization whose partners include the American Hospital Association, the American College of Surgeons, and the American Medical Association that accredits and certifies organizations involved in the delivery of health care (more recently known as the Joint Commission).

M

Managed care   An arrangement for financing or delivery of care under which an administrative entity intervenes between the consumer and the provider through utilization review, scheduling, case management, or other means.

Managed care organization (MCO)   An organization that carries out the functions required for providing managed care.

Managed services organization (MSO)   A firm that performs managed care administrative functions for organizations that choose to outsource these functions.

Margin   The excess of revenue over expenses.

Mass market   A good or service which a very high percentage of individuals in society may at least on occasion find useful or desirable.

Means test   A standard of eligibility for a public program based on income or wealth below a specified minimum.

Medicaid   A program jointly funded by the federal and individual state governments for indigent individuals.

Medical director   A member of the management team in a hospital or other health care organization appointed by the governing board and responsible for activities of and relationships with the medical staff.

Medical savings accounts (MSAs)   Accounts that allow individuals with high-deductible health plans to establish tax-free funds to pay for the deductibles and other medical expenses.

Medical staff president   A physician elected by the medical staff of a hospital or other health care organization to represent the interests of her colleagues to the organization's governing board.

Meta-analysis   An analysis of preexisting studies intended to produce highly generalizable and valid answers to questions of scientific or therapeutic importance.

Multispecialty practice   A medical practice organization in which members of several different specialties practice.

Myocardial infarction   A heart attack.

N

National Committee for Quality Assurance (NCQA)   A private, nonprofit organization that reviews, accredits, and certifies managed care organizations, utilization review organizations, and several other types of health care organizations.

Naturopathic medicine   A form of medicine that uses naturally occurring agents such as botanicals and techniques such as therapeutic nutrition and lifestyle counseling to prevent and treat illness.

Niche market   Highly restricted segments of the population who use a given product or service.

Nurse staffing ratio   The ratio of nursing personnel to patients in a facility or one of its specialized units (for example, intensive care).

Nursing director   A member of the management team in a hospital or other health care organization appointed by the governing board and responsible for activities of and relationships with the nursing staff.

Nursing registry   A private agency that provides nursing personnel to hospitals and other health care organizations on a per diem basis.

Nursing supervisor   A nurse performing second-level supervision, directly supervising charge nurses.

O

Outbreak   A small, localized epidemic.

P

Pandemic   Worldwide occurrence of a disease in larger numbers than normally expected; a worldwide epidemic.

Payroll tax   A tax that employers are required to withhold from employees' pay or that an employer is required to pay computed on the basis of the employee's salary, such as Social Security and Medicare taxes.

Peer review   Review of a scientific report, research proposal, or individual's professional performance by fellow professionals.

Per member per month (PMPM)   The amount paid by a health plan to a provider (individual or organization) for care of each enrolled individual under a capitated contract.

Physician extender   A health professional who, working under a physician's supervision, extends his capacity to care for patients, such as physician assistants and nurse practitioners.

Placebo effect   The impact of an inert substance or procedure known to have no physiological effects on a patient's perception of a disease or its signs and symptoms.

Pluralism   The presence in a society of many distinct repositories of power and centers of decision making or the belief that society should be organized in this fashion.

Practice act   State-level legislation that covers qualifications, legal scope of practice, surveillance, and disciplinary procedures for health and other professionals.

Preferred provider organization (PPO)   An organization or unit established by a parent organization that makes contracts with individual physicians or physician groups to provide discounted care on a fee-for-service basis.

Premium   A payment for insurance coverage.

Primary care   Routine diagnostic, therapeutic, and referral services usually obtained from a generalist practitioner in the consumer's community.

Procedure-oriented specialty   A medical or surgical specialty that emphasizes technologically assisted interventions such as surgery, imaging, and anesthesia.

Prostate-specific antigen (PSA) test   A test for early prostate cancer based on the presence of excessive prostate gland secretions.

Q

Quality-adjusted life year (QALY)   A measure used in cost-effectiveness analysis based on the expenditures required for enabling an individual to live for an additional year and experience high quality of life during that period.

Quasi-experimental   A research design intended to mimic classic experimentation by using nonequivalent control groups, time series, and other techniques.

Quaternary care   Services that are both highly specialized and rarely used.

Quitline   A telephone service intended to help smokers quit.

R

Randomization   A component of experimental procedure that randomly assigns subjects to specific arms of the study.

Randomized controlled trial (RCT)   An experimental procedure characterized by randomization of subjects to specific interventions (sometimes including a control) and statistical comparison of outcomes assessed according to standard measures.

Rationing   Withholding of goods or services of potential value to a patient for the purpose of conserving supply or controlling costs.

Regulation   The exercise of governmental power over an individual's or organization's conduct of an otherwise legal activity.

Reliability   In research methodology, the likelihood that the same information obtained by one method or individual will be obtained by another individual or method.

Request for proposals (RFP)   In business or research, a call for bids on a body of work, including proposed methods, cost, and time required for performance.

Resource-based relative value scale (RBRVS)   A method of determining payment for a physician service according to the total work of the physician in providing the service and associated practice and training-related costs.

Risk pool   The individuals whose insurance premiums are added together for the benefit of any individual member who incurs a loss (such as charges for medical care).

S

Safety net provider   An organization or individual who provides care for uninsured, underinsured, or otherwise disadvantaged people.

Screening A test, procedure, or examination that can be readily applied to large numbers of individuals for early detection of diseases such as diabetes and cancer.

Secondary care Health services obtained from community-based specialists or hospitals, such as routine surgery.

Selective contracting An arrangement by an insurance company or government agency for the services they fund to be delivered solely by an entity that has won a bidding competition to provide the services.

Sequelae Pathological conditions resulting from a prior disease or injury.

Service benefit An insurance benefit received in the form of service, rather than payment to a health care provider or reimbursement for such payment.

State Children's Health Insurance Program (SCHIP) A joint federal-state program begun in the 1997 to provide insurance coverage for children whose families are economically disadvantaged but have incomes too high to allow them to qualify for Medicaid.

Study arm The treatment protocol to which an experimental subject is assigned, possibly including a placebo group.

T

Target income The income level that an individual seeks and at which he may reduce working hours.

Tertiary care Highly specialized or scientifically advanced interventions usually unavailable outside large, regional medical centers or university-operated facilities.

Third-party payer An entity other than the patient herself that pays for health care, including insurance companies, government agencies, and self-insured employers.

Triage A process by which patients are sorted according to the seriousness or urgency of their condition.

U

Underserved area A geographical area, typically rural or urban poor, that has too few health care facilities or personnel to serve the comprehensive needs of its residents in a timely manner.

Underwriting Based on estimates of health risks, the process by which an insurer determines whether to accept a client, the premium the client is to be charged, and exclusions and caps on claims in an ensuing policy.

Upstream control A method of controlling health care costs that relies on restricting the supply of health professionals, health care facilities, and advanced technology.

Utilization review A process by which a third-party payer or health care delivery organization assesses the appropriateness of procedures, medications, specialty care, or other services requiring expenditure of resources.

V

Validity The ability of a research design to definitively test a hypothesis or an indicator used in research to truly measure a phenomenon of interest (such as pain or emotional well-being).

LIST OF ABBREVIATIONS

AAMC American Association of Medical Colleges
AMWA American Medical Women's Association

CAM Complementary and alternative medicine
CON Certificate of need
CMS Centers for Medicare and Medicaid Services

FMG Foreign medical graduate
FOBT Fecal occult blood testing
FQHC Federally qualified health center
FTE Full-time equivalent

HEDIS Healthcare Effectiveness Data and Information Set
HMO Health maintenance organization
HSA Health systems agency or health savings account

ICD International Classification of Disease
IPA Independent practice association
IRB Institutional review board

JCAHO Joint Commission on Accreditation of Healthcare Organizations (also known as The Joint Commission)

MCO Managed care organization
MI Myocardial infarction
MRI Magnetic resonance imaging
MRSA Methicillin-resistant *Staphylococcus aureus*
MSA Medical savings account

NCQA National Committee on Quality Assurance
NIH National Institutes of Health

PMPM Per member per month
PPO Preferred provider organization
PSA Prostate-specific antigen

QALY Quality-adjusted life year

RBRVS Resource-based relative value scale
RCT Randomized controlled trial

NOTES

CHAPTER ONE

1. Kung HC, Hovert DL, Xu J, Murphy SL. Deaths: Preliminary data for 2005. NCHS Health E-Stats. 2005. www.cdc.gov/nchs/products/pubs/pubd/hestats/prelimdeaths05/prelimdeaths05.htm. Accessed December 15, 2007.

2. Himmelstein DU, Warren E, Thorne D, et al. Illness and injury as contributors to bankruptcy. *Health Affairs* 2005;24:w63–w73.

3. Lueck S. Critical condition: surging costs for Medicaid ravage state, federal budgets. *Wall Street Journal* (Eastern edition). Feb. 7, 2005:A1.

4. Roan S. The nation: in an ailing economy, the doctor can wait: more people, even the chronically ill, forgo preventive care. *Los Angeles Times,* April 8, 2009:A1.

5. National Center for Health Statistics. *Health, United States, 2007 with Chartbook on Trends in the Health of Americans.* Hyattsville, MD: National Center for Health Statistics; 2007: Table 25.

6. National Center for Health Statistics. *Health, United States, 2007 with Chartbook on Trends in the Health of Americans.* Hyattsville, MD: National Center for Health Statistics; 2007: Table 26.

7. Kohn LT, Corrigan JM, Donaldson M, eds. *To Err Is Human: Building a Safer Health System.* Washington, DC: Institute of Medicine; 1999.

8. Institute of Medicine. *Crossing the Quality Chasm: A New Health System for the 21st Century.* Washington, DC: National Academy Press; 2001.

9. McGlynn EA, Asch SM, Adams J, et al. The quality of health care to adults in the United States. *New England Journal of Medicine.* 2003;348:2635–2645.

10. Eisenberg JM. Quality research for quality healthcare: the data connection. *Health Services Research.* 2000;35:12–17.

11. Caldicott H. Obama and the opportunity to eliminate nuclear weapons. *Canadian Medical Association Journal.* 2009;180(2):151.

12. Üstün B, Jakob R. Calling a spade a spade: meaningful definitions of health conditions. *Bull World Health Organ.* 2005;83:802.

13. Wilmoth JR, Horiuchi S. Rectangularization revisited: variability of age at death within human populations. *Demography.* 1999;36(4):475–495.

14. Vaupel JW, Carey JR, Christensen K. It's never too late. *Science.* 2003;301(5640):1679–1681.

15. Sanders L. Gut problem. *New York Times Magazine,* December 16, 2007:42.

16. Posen S. *The Doctor in Literature.* San Diego, CA: Radcliffe; 2005.

17. Street RL, Gordon H, Haidet P. Physicians' communication and perceptions of patients: is it how they look, how they talk, or is it just the doctor? *Social Science and Medicine.* 2007;65:586–598.

18. Berry PA. The absence of sadness: darker reflections on the doctor-patient relationship. *Journal of Medical Ethics.* 2007;33:266–268.

19. Pear R. Doctors shun patients with Medicare. *New York Times.* March 17, 2002.

20. Wysocki B. The rules: at one hospital, a stark solution for allocating care. *Wall Street Journal* (Eastern edition). September 23, 2003:A1.

21. Ansberry C. Despite federal law, hospitals still reject sick who can't pay. *Wall Street Journal.* (Eastern edition). Nov 29, 1988:A1.

22. Grady D. Lung patients see a new era of transplants. *New York Times.* September 24, 2006:1.

23. Hall MA, Dugan E, Zheng B, et al. Trust in physicians and medical institutions: what is it, can it be measured, and does it matter. *Milbank Quarterly.* 2001;79(4):613–639.

24. Beauchamp TL, Walters L, Kahn JP, et al., eds. *Contemporary Issues in Bioethics.* Belmont, CA: Wadsworth; 2008.

CHAPTER TWO

1. Pear R. Spending rise for health care and prescription drugs slows. *New York Times.* Jan. 6, 2009:A17.

2. Economy Watch. Top ten world economies. 2008. www.economywatch.com/economies-in-top. Accessed May 22, 2009.

3. National Center for Health Statistics. *Health United States, 2008, with Chartbook on Trends in the Health of Americans.* Table 112. Hyattsville, MD: National Center for Health Statistics; 2008.

4. National Center for Health Statistics. *Health, United States, 2007 with Chartbook on Trends in the Health of Americans.* Table 26. Hyattsville, MD: National Center for Health Statistics; 2007.

5. National Center for Health Statistics. *Health, United States, 2008 with Chartbook on Trends in the Health of Americans.* Table 116. Hyattsville, MD: National Center for Health Statistics; 2008.

6. National Center for Health Statistics. *Health, United States, 2008 with Chartbook on Trends in the Health of Americans.* Figure 19. Hyattsville, MD: National Center for Health Statistics; 2008.

7. National Institutes of Health. NIH Awards to Medical Schools by Rank Fiscal Year 2005. 2005. http://report.nih.gov/award/Rank/medttl05.htm. Accessed May 22, 2009.

8. Carlson M, Blustein J, Fiorentino N, Prestianni F. Socioeconomic status and dissatisfaction among HMO enrollees. *Medical Care.* 2000;38(5):508–516.

9. Mooney SE, Weeks WB. Where do women veterans get their inpatient care? *Women's Health Issues.* 2007;17(6):367–373.

10. Kelborn PT. Largest HMOs cutting the poor and the elderly. *New York Times,* July 6, 1998:1.

11. Garrett B, Davidoff AJ, Yemane A. Effects of Medicaid managed care programs on health services access and use. *Health Services Research.* 2003;38(2):575–594.

12. Isaacs SL, Jellinek P. Is there a (volunteer) doctor in the house? Free clinics and volunteer physician referral networks in the United States. *Health Affairs.* 2007;26(3):871–876.

13. Nichols J. Indian health care: separate, unequal. *The Arizona Republic.* April 14, 2002.

14. Romer y Huesca A, Moreno-Rojas JC, Soto-Miranda MA, et al. Teaching of medicine of the University of Bologna in the Renaissance. *Rev Invest Clin.* 2006;58(2):170–176.

15. Royal College of Physicians. History of medicine links. http://www.rcplondon.ac.uk/heritage/HistoryLinks.htm. Accessed December 25, 2007.

16. Holborn H. *A History of Modern Germany: 1840–1945.* Princeton, NJ: Princeton University Press; 1969:291–293.

17. Starr P. *The Social Transformation of American Medicine.* New York: Basic Books; 1982:298.

18. United States General Accounting Office. Health professions education: clarifying the role of title VII and VIII programs could improve accountability (GAO testimony before the Subcommittee on Public Health and Safety, Committee on Labor and Human Resources, U.S. Senate, April 25, 1997). www.gao.gov/archive/1997/he97117t.pdf. Accessed December 26, 2007.

19. Department of Health and Human Services. Advancing the health, safety, and well-being of our people. 2007. www.hhs.gov/budget/docbudget.htm. Accessed December 26, 2007.

20. Sorkin AR. Big private hospital chain may be close to record sale. *New York Times.* July 24, 2006:A15.

21. Hurley RE, Strunk BC, White JS. The puzzling popularity of the PPO. *Health Affairs.* 2004;23(2):56–68.

22. Schoen C, Osborn R, Trang P, et al. Taking the pulse of healthcare systems: experiences of patients with health problems in six countries. *Health Affairs.* 2005:W5-509–W5-525.

23. Helman R, Fronstin P. 2006 Health confidence survey: dissatisfaction with health care system doubles since 1998. *EBRI Notes.* 2006;27:11.

24. Blandon RJ, Benson J. Americans' views on health policy: a fifty-year historical perspective. *Health Affairs.* 2001;20:33–46.

25. Kaiser Family Foundation/Harvard School of Public Health. Pre-election poll: voters, health care and the 2008 election. 2008. www.kff.org/kaiserpolls/upload/7829.pdf. Accessed May 24, 2008.

26. The Pew Research Center for the People and the Press. Survey report: beyond red and blue, part 6. Issues and shifting coalitions. 2005. http://people-press.org/report/?pageid=948. Accessed January 21, 2009.

27. Aaron H. *Serious and Unstable Condition: Financing America's Health Care.* Washington, DC: Brookings; 1991.

CHAPTER THREE

1. World Health Organization. International Classification of Diseases (ICD). http://www.who.int/classifications/icd/en. Accessed February 11, 2008.

2. Balon R, Segraves RT, Clayton A. Issues for DSM-V: Sexual dysfunction, disorder, or variation along normal distribution   toward rethinking DSM criteria of sexual dysfunctions. *Am J Psychiatry.* 2007;164:198–200.

3. Goolsby MJ. National Kidney Foundation guidelines for chronic kidney disease: evaluation, classification, stratification. *J Am Acad Nurse Pract.* 2002;14(6):238–242.

4. Karnofsky DA, Burchenal JH. The clinical evaluation of chemotherapeutics in cancer. In: MacLoed CM, ed. *Evaluation of Chemotherapeutic Agents.* New York: Columbia University Press; 1949:191–205.

5. Melzack R. The McGill pain questionnaire: from description to measurement. *Anesthesiology.* 2005;1–3(1):199–202.

6. McNair DM, Lorr M, Droppleman L. *Manual for the Profile of Mood States.* San Diego, CA: Educational and Industrial Testing Service; 1971.

7. Ware JE Jr, Kosinski MA, Keller SD. *SF-36 Physical and Mental Health Summary Scales: A user's manual.* Boston: The Health Institute, New England Medical Center; 1994.

8. Snow LF. Traditional health beliefs and practices among lower class black Americans. *West J Med.* 1983;139(6):820–828.

9. Weller S, Pachter LM, Trotter RT, Baer RD. Empacho in four Latino groups: a study of intra- and intercultural variation in beliefs. *Medical Anthropology.* 1993;15:109–136.

10. Zbrowski M. Cultural components in response to pain. *Journal of Social Issues.* 1952;8(4):16–30.

11. Kramer PD. *Listening to Prozac.* New York: Viking; 1993.

12. Landers P. Waiting for Prozac: drug firms push Japan to change view of depression. *Wall Street Journal* (Eastern edition). October 9, 2002:A1.

13. Whiting P, Bagnall A, Sowden AJ, et al. Interventions for the treatment and management of chronic fatigue syndrome: a systematic review. *Journal of the American Medical Association.* 2001;286:1360–1368.

14. Bovard J. MCS: a name still in search of a disease. *Sacramento Bee.* Jan. 14, 1996.

15. Conrad P. *Deviance and Medicalization: From Badness to Sickness.* Philadelphia: Temple University; 1992.

16. Scott CL, Holmberg T. Castration of sex offenders: prisoners' rights versus public safety. *Journal of the American Academy of Psychiatry and the Law.* 2003;31:502–509.

17. International Agency for Research on Cancer (IARC). *IARC Monographs on the Evaluation of Carcinogenic Risk to Humans: Human Papillomavirus.* Vol. 64. Lyons, France: IARC Press; 1995.

18. International Agency for Research on Cancer (IARC). *IARC Monographs on the Evaluation of Carcinogenic Risk to Humans: Hepatitis Viruses.* Vol. 59. Lyons, France: IARC Press; 1994.

19. Griffin BE. Epstein-Barr virus and human disease: facts, opinion, and problems. *Mutation Research.* 2000;462:395–405.

20. Chandra RK. Nutrition and the immune system: an introduction. *American Journal of Clinical Nutrition.* 1997;66:460S–463S.

21. Cohen J. Is AIDS in Africa a distinct disease? *Science.* 2000;288:2153–2155.

22. McCreanor J, Cullinan P, Nieuwenhuijsen MJ, et al. Respiratory effects of exposure to diesel traffic in persons with asthma. *New England Journal of Medicine.* 2007;357(23):2348–2358.

23. Pope CA, Barnette RT, Thun MJ, et al. Lung cancer, cardiopulmonary mortality, and long-term exposure to fine particulate air pollution. *Journal of the American Medical Association.* 2002;287:1132–1141.

24. Belpomme D, Irigaray P, Hardell L, et al. The multitude and diversity of environmental carcinogens. *Environmental Research.* 2007;105:414–429.

25. Marra G, Boland CR. Hereditary nonpolyposis colorectal cancer: the syndrome, the genes, and historical perspectives. *Journal of the National Cancer Institute.* 1995;87:1114–1125.

26. Lichtenstein P, Volm NV, Verkasalo PK, et al. Environmental and heritable factors in the causation of cancer. *New England Journal of Medicine.* 2000;343:78–85.

27. Kendler KS, Myers JM, Neale MC. A multidimensional twin study of mental health in women. *American Journal of Psychiatry.* 2000;157:506–513.

28. Couzin J. To what extent are genetic variation and personal health linked? *Science.* 2005;309(5731):81.

29. Melchior M, Moffitt ME, Milne BJ, et al. 2007. Why do children from socially disadvantaged families suffer from poor health when they reach adulthood? A life course study. *American Journal of Epidemiology.* 2007;166(8):966–974.

30. Cousins N. *Anatomy of an Illness as Perceived by the Patient: Reflections on Healing and Regeneration.* New York: Norton; 1979.

31. Siegel BS. *Love, Medicine, and Miracles.* New York: Harper & Row; 1990.

32. Cohen S, Janicki-Deverts S, Miller GE. Psychological stress and disease. *Journal of the American Medical Association.* 2007;298(14):1685–1687.

33. Fuchs VR. *Who Shall Live?* New York: Basic Books; 1974.

34. Berkman LF, Syme SL. Social networks, host resistance, and mortality: a nine-year follow-up study of Alameda County residents. *American Journal of Epidemology.* 1979;109:186–204.

35. Wolf S, Bruhn JG. *The Power of Clan: The Influence of Human Relationships on Heart Disease.* New Brunswick, NJ: Transaction; 1992.

36. Lynch JW, Kaplan GA, Pamuk ER, at al. Income inequality and mortality in metropolitan areas of the United States. *American Journal of Public Health.* 1998;88:1074–1080.

37. Horwitz T. Beer-belly blues: in New Orleans, fat is where it's at, and it shows in grim reports. *Wall Street Journal* (Eastern edition). February 23, 1998:A1.

38. Jaffe HW, Bregman DJ, Selik RM. Acquired immune deficiency syndrome in the United States: the first 1,000 cases. *Journal of Infectious Diseases.* 1983;148(2):339–345.

39. Shaw PK, Brodsky RE, Lyman DO, et al. A communitywide outbreak of giardiasis with evidence of transmission by a municipal water supply. *Annals of Internal Medicine.* 1977;87:426–432.

40. Centers for Disease Control and Prevention. Possible transmission of human immunodeficiency virus to a patient during an invasive dental procedure. *Morbidity and Mortality Weekly Report.* 1990; 39:489–493.

41. Klausner JD, Wolf W, Fischer-Ponce L, Zolt I, Katz MH. Tracing a syphilis outbreak through cyberspace. *Journal of the American Medical Association.* 2001;284:477–479.

42. Mohle-Boetani, JC, Reporter R, Werner SB, et al. An outbreak of salmonella serogroup saphra due to cantaloupes from Mexico. *Journal of Infectious Diseases.* 1999;180:1361–1364.

43. Bregman DJ, Langmuir AD. Farr's law applied to AIDS projections. *Journal of the American Medical Association.* 1990;16:1522–1525.

44. Yelin EH, Nevitt M. Epstein W. Toward an epidemiology of work disability. *Milbank Quarterly.* 1980; 58:386–415.

45. Bindman AB, Chottopadhyay A, Osmond DH, et al. Preventable hospitalizations and access to health care. *Journal of the American Medical Association.* 1995;274(4):305–311.

46. Greenwald HP. *Who Survives Cancer?* Berkeley: University of California Press; 1992.

47. Huston HR, Anglin D, Pratts MJ. Adolescents and children injured or killed in drive-by shootings in Los Angeles. *New England Journal of Medicine.* 1994;330:324–327.

48. Reynolds G. The flu hunters. *New York Times Magazine.* November 7, 2004.

49. Horton R. Infection: the global threat. *New York Review of Books.* 1995;42(6).

CHAPTER FOUR

1. Parsons T. The sick role and the role of the physician reconsidered. *Milbank Quarterly.* 1975;53(3): 257–278.

2. Gijsbers van Wijk CMT, Kolk AM, van Den Bosch WJM, Van Den Hoogen HJM. Male and female morbidity in general practice: the nature of sex differences. *Social Science and Medicine.* 1992;35(5):665–678.

3. Mechanic D, Volkart ED. Stress, illness behavior, and the sick role. *American Sociological Review.* 1961;26(1):51–58.

4. Cole S, Lejeune R. Illness and the legitimation of failure. *American Sociological Review.* 1972;37(3): 347–356.

5. Galea S, Ahern J, Tardiff K, et al. Race/ethnic disparities in overdose mortality trends in New York City, 1900–1998. *Journal of Urban Health.* 2003;80(2):201–211.

6. Singh S, Smith GA, Fields SK, McKenzie SB. Gymnastics-related injuries to children treated in emergency departments in the United States, 1990 2005. *Pediatrics.* 2008;121(4):954–960.

7. Koehle MS, Lloyd-Smith R, Taunton JE. Alpine ski injuries and their prevention. *Sports Medicine.* 2002;32(12):785–793.

8. Schmitt H, Gerner HJ. Paralysis from sport and diving accidents. *Clinical Journal of Sports Medicine.* 2001;11(1):17–22.

9. Zalavras C, Nikolopoulou G, Essin D, et al. Pediatric fractures during skateboarding, roller skating, and scooter riding. *American Journal of Sports Medicine.* 2005;33(4): 568–573.

10. Klein A. Safety gear: some pros and cons. *Skateboarder.* 2002:73.

11. Prodromos CC, Han Y, Rogowski J, et al. Arthroscopy: a meta-analysis of the incidence of anterior cruciate ligament tears as a function of gender, sport, and a knee injury-reduction regimen. *Arthroscopy.* 2007;23(12):1320–1325.

12. Al-Mayouf SM. Familial arthropathy in Saudi Arabian children: demographic, clinical, and biomedical features. *Seminars in Arthritis and Rheumatism.* 2007;36(4):256–261.

13. Bahakim HM, El-Idrissy IM. Epidemiological observations of consanguinity and retinoblastoma in Arabia: a retrospective study. *Tropical and Geographic Medicine.* 1989;41(4):361–364.

14. Jorde LB. Consanguinity and prereproductive mortality in the Utah Mormon population. *Human Heredity.* 2001;52(2):61–65.

15. Khoury MJ, Cohen BH, Diamond EL, et al. Inbreeding and prereproductive mortality in the Old Order Amish. I. Genealogic epidemiology of inbreeding. *American Journal of Epidemiology.* 1987;125(3):453–461.

16. Maynard RJ. Controlling death, compromising life: chronic disease, prognostication, and the new biotechnologies. *Medical Anthropology.* 2006;20(2):212–234.

17. Chowdhury PP, Balluz L, Murphy W. Surveillance of certain health behaviors among states and selected local areas—United States, 2005. *Mortality and Morbidity Weekly Review.* 2007;56(4):1–160.

18. Pearson WS. Ten-year comparison of estimates of overweight and obesity, diagnosed diabetes and use of office-based physician services for treatment of diabetes in the United States. *Preventive Medicine.* 2007;45(5):353–357.

18. Gazmararian JA, Foxman B, Yen LT, et al. Comparing the predictive accuracy of health risk appraisal: the Centers for Disease Control versus Carter Center program. *American Journal of Public Health.* 1991;81(10):1296–301.

20. Hnizdo ED, Sullivan PA, Bang KM, Wagner G. Association between chronic obstructive pulmonary disease and employment by industry and occupation in the US population: a study of data from the Third National Health and Nutrition Examination Survey. *American Journal of Epidemiology.* 2002;156(8):738–746.

21. Violanti JM. Dying from the job: the mortality risk for police officers. www.cophealth.com/articles/articles_dying_a.html. Accessed June 7, 2008.

22. Kroenke CH, Spiegelman D, Manson J, et al. Work characteristics and incidence of type 2 diabetes in women. *American Journal of Epidemiology.* 2007;165(2):175–183.

23. Sharkey J. Business travel: the World Bank gauges the toll travel takes on employees and looks for ways to soften the effect. *New York Times.* May 10, 2000:C8.

24. Epstein H. Enough to make you sick? *New York Times Magazine.* Oct. 12, 2003:75.

25. Wingo PA, Calle EE, McTiernan A. How does breast cancer mortality compare with that of other cancers and selected cardiovascular diseases at different ages in US women? *Journal of Women's Health.* 2000;9(9):999–1006.

26. Stein K, Zhao L, Cranner C, Gensler T. Prevalence and sociodemographic correlates of beliefs regarding cancer risks. *Cancer.* 2007;110(1):1139–1147.

27. Steinhauer J. It's infectious: fear that's out of proportion. *New York Times.* Oct. 10, 1999:16.

28. Slovic P. Perception of risk. *Science.* 1987;236(4799):280–285.

29. Starr C. Social benefit versus technological risk. *Science.* 1969;165(889):1232–1238.

30. Ames BN, Magaw R, Gold LS. Ranking possible carcinogenic hazards. *Science.* 1987;236(4799):271–280.

31. Adelman RC, Verbrugge LM. Death makes news: the social impact of disease on newspaper coverage. *Journal of Health and Social Behavior.* 2000;41(3):347–367.

32. Merrill RA. Food safety regulation: reforming the Delaney clause. *Annual Review of Public Health.* 1997;18:313–340.

33. Wang J, Zuckerman IH, Miller NA, et al. Utilizing new prescription drugs: disparities among non-Hispanic whites, non-Hispanic blacks, and Hispanic whites. *Health Services Research.* 2007;42(4):1499–1519.

34. Dunlop DD, Manheim LM, Song J, et al. Age and racial/ethnic disparities in arthritis-related hip and knee surgeries. *Medical Care.* 2008;46(2):200–2008.

35. Echeverria SE, Carrasquillo O. The roles of citizenship status, acculturation, and health insurance in breast and cervical cancer screening among immigrant women. *Medical Care.* 2006;44(8):788–792.

36. Kim SE, Perez-Stable EJ, Wong S, et al. Association between cancer risk perception and screening behavior among diverse women. *Archives of Internal Medicine.* 2008;168:728–734.

37. Hughes SC, Deborah DL. Parental beliefs and children's receipt of preventive care: another piece of the puzzle? *Health Services Research.* 2008;43(1):287–299.

38. Chen AY, Escarce JJ. Family structure and the treatment of childhood asthma. *Medical Care.* 2008;46(2):174–184.

39. Aday LA, Andersen RM. A framework for the study of access to medical care. *Health Services Research.* 1974;9(3):208–220.

40. Bandura A. Self-efficacy: toward a unifying theory of behavioral change. *Psychological Review.* 1977;84(2):191–215.

41. Andersen R. Revisiting the behavioral model and access to medical care: does it matter? *Journal of Health and Social Behavior.* 1995;36(1):1–10.

42. Goff SL, Mazor KM, Meterko V, et al. Patients' beliefs and preferences regarding doctors' medication recommendations. *Journal of General Internal Med.* 2008;23(3):236–241.

43. Gordon HS, Paterniti DA, Wray NP. Race and patient refusal of invasive cardiac procedures. *Journal of General Internal Medicine.* 2004;19:962–966.

44. Basson MD, Butler TW, Verma H. Predicting patient nonappearance for surgery as a scheduling strategy to optimize operating room utilization in a Veterans' Administration hospital. *Anesthesiology.* 2005;104:826–834.

45. Ibrahim SA, Kwoh KC, Krishnan E. Factors associated with patients who leave acute-care hospitals against medical advice. *American Journal of Public Health.* 2007;97(12):2204–2208.

46. Madden JM, Graves AJ, Feng Z. Cost-related medication nonadherence and spending on basic needs following implementation of Medicare Part D. *Journal of the American Medical Association.* 2008;299(16):1922–1928.

47. Greenwald HP, Becker SW, Nevitt MC. Delay and noncompliance in cancer detection: a behavioral perspective for health planners. *Milbank Quarterly.* 1978;56(2):212–230.

48. Linnard-Palmer L, Kools S. Parents' refusal of medical treatment for cultural or religious beliefs: an ethnographic study of health care professionals' experiences. *Journal of Pediatric Oncology Nursing.* 2005;22(1):48–57.

49. Fried T, Badley EH, Towle VR, et al. Understanding the treatment preferences of seriously ill patients. *New England Journal of Medicine.* 2002;346(14):1061–1066.

50. Institute of Medicine. *Health Literacy: A Prescription to End Confusion.* Washington, DC: Institute of Medicine, Board on Neuroscience and Behavioral Health, Committee on Health Literacy; 2004.

51. Parker RM. Health literacy: a policy challenge for advancing high-quality health care. *Health Affairs.* 2003;22(4):147–153.

52. Sharif IS, Reiber S, Ozuah PO. Exposure to Reach Out and Read and vocabulary outcomes in inner city preschoolers. *Journal of the National Medical Association.* 2002;94:171–177.

53. Betancourt JR, Green AR, Carrillo JE, et al. Defining cultural competence: a practical framework for addressing racial/ethnic disparities. *Public Health Reports.* 2003;118: 293–302.

54. Van Ryn M, Burke J. The effect of patient race and socio-economic status on physician's perceptions of patients. *Social Science and Medicine.* 2000;50:813–828.

55. Schulman KA, Berlin JA, Harless W, et al. The effect of race and sex on physicians' recommendations for cardiac catheterization. *New England Journal of Medicine.* 1999;340:628–626.

56. Pignone MP, DeWalt DA. Literacy and health outcomes: is adherence the missing link? *Journal of General Internal Medicine.* 2006;21(8):896–897.

57. Caballero AE. Building cultural bridges: understanding ethnicity to improve acceptance of insulin therapy in patients with type 2 diabetes. *Ethnicity and Disease.* 2006;16(2):559–568.

58. Tindle HA, Davis RB, Phillips RS, et al. Trends in use of complementary and alternative medicine by US adults: 1997–2002. *Alternative Therapies.* 2005;11(1):42–49.

59. Eisenberg DM, Davis RB, Ettner SL, et al. Trends in alternative medicine use in the United States, 1990–1997. *Journal of the American Medical Association.* 1998;280:1569–1575.

60. George M, Birck K, Hufford DJ, et al. Beliefs about asthma and complementary and alternative medicine in low-income inner-city African-American adults. *Journal of General Internal Medicine.* 2006;21:1317–1324.

61. Greenwald HP, O'Keefe S, DiCamillo MD. The importance of public sector health care in an underserved population. *Journal of Health and Human Services Administration.* 2004;27(1):142–157.

62. Cassileth BR. Contemporary unorthodox treatment in cancer medicine. *Annals of Internal Medicine.* 1984;101:105–112.

63. Grzywacz JG, Suerken CK, Nieberg RH, et al. Age, ethnicity, and use of complementary and alternative medicine in health self-management. *Journal of Health and Social Behavior.* 2007;48:84–98.

64. Greenwald HP, Chen RJ, Johnston-Zamora M. Putting a new face on managed care. *Marketing Health Services.* 2002;22:15–19.

CHAPTER FIVE

1. Greenwald HP. *Organizations: Management Without Control.* Thousand Oaks, CA: Sage; 2008.

2. Checkley AM, Pepin J, Gibson WC, et al. Human African trypanosomiasis: diagnosis, relapse and survival after severe melarsoprol-induced encephalopathy. *Transactions of the Royal Society of Tropical Medicine and Hygiene.* 2007;101(5):523–526.

3. Terz JJ, Schaffner MJ, Goodkin TR, et al. Translumbar amputation. *Cancer.* 1990;65:2668–2675.

4. Mellow J, Greifinger RB. Successful reentry: the perspective of private correctional health care providers. *Journal of Urban Health.* 2007;84(1):85–98.

5. Van Noort DE, Nicolai JA. Comparison of two methods of vagina construction in transsexuals. *Plastic and Reconstructive Surgery.* 1993;91:1308–1315.

6. Tarlov AR, Schwartz B, Greenwald HP. University center and community hospital: problems in integration. *Journal of Medical Education.* 1979;54: 70–378.

7. Hughes R, Hunt S, Luft H. Effects of surgeon volume and hospital volume on quality of care in hospitals. *Medical Care.* 1987;25(6):489–503.

8. Faturcechi R. Swedish Medical Center to do liver transplants. *Seattle Times.* July 11, 2008.

9. Freidson E. *Profession of Medicine.* New York: Dodd, Mead; 1975.

10. Pomrinse SD, Goldstein MS. Group practice in the US. *Group Practice.* 1960;9:854–859.

11. Hing E, Burt CW. Characteristics of office-based physicians and their medical practices: United States, 2005–2006. National Center for Health Statistics. *Vital and Health Statistics.* 2008;13(166).

12. Hing E, Burt CW. Characteristics of office-based physicians and their medical practices: United States, 2005–2006. National Center for Health Statistics. *Vital and Health Statistics.* 2008;13(166).

13. Rubin HR, Gandek WH, Rogers WH, et al. Patients' rating of outpatient visits in different practice settings: Results from the medical outcomes study. *Journal of the American Medical Association.* 1993; 270(7): 835–840.

14. Casalino LP, Pham H, Bazzoli G. Growth of single-specialty medical groups. *Health Affairs.* 2004;12(2):82–90.

15. Isaacs SL, Jellinek P. Is there a (volunteer) doctor in the house? Free clinics and volunteer physician referral networks in the United States. *Health Affairs.* 2007;26(3):871–876.

16. Cook NL, Hicks LS, O'Malleu AJ. Access to specialty care and medical services in community health centers. *Health Affairs.* 2007;26(5):1459–1468.

17. Gusmano MK, Fairbrother G, Park H. Exploring the limits of the safety net: community health centers and care for the uninsured. *Health Affairs.* 2002;21(6):188–194.

18. Rosenblatt RA, Andrilla CH, Curtin T, et al. Shortages of medical personnel at community health centers: implications for planned expansion. *Journal of the American Medical Association.* 2006;295(9):1042–1049.

19. Weinick RM, Betancourt RM. *No Appointment Needed: The Resurgence of Urgent Care Centers in the United States.* Oakland: California HealthCare Foundation; 2007.

20. Vesely R. Wal-Mart not discounting health: retail giant partnering with hospitals to boost clinics. *Modern Healthcare.* November 19, 2007:8.

21. Herzlinger RE, Krasker WS. Who profits from nonprofits? *Harvard Business Review.* 1987;65(1):93–106.

22. National Center for Health Statistics. *Health, United States, 2008.* Table 116. Hyattsville, MD: National Center for Health Statistics; 2009.

23. Lawsuits challenge charity hospitals on care for the uninsured. *Wall Street Journal* (Eastern Edition). June 17, 2004:B1.

24. Langley M. Really operating: nonprofit hospitals sometimes are that in little but name. *Wall Street Journal* (Eastern Edition). July 14, 1997:A1.

25. Langley M. Money order: nuns' zeal for profits shapes hospital chain, wins Wall Street fans. *Wall Street Journal* (Eastern Edition). January 7, 1998:A1.

26. Engel M. Hospitals' charity work hard to assess; State auditor concludes uniform guidelines are needed in reporting the dollar valuations of community care. *Los Angeles Times.* December 14, 2007:B5.

27. Mackenzie EJ, Hoyt DB, Sacra JC, et al. National inventory of hospital trauma centers. *Journal of the American Medical Association.* 2003;289(12):1515–1522.

28. Greenwald HP, O'Keefe S, DiCamillo M. The importance of public sector health care in an underserved population. *Journal of Health and Human Services Administration.* 2004;27(1):142–157.

29. Hoot NR, Aronsky D. Systematic review of emergency department crowding: causes, effects, and solutions. *Annals of Emergency Medicine.* 2008;52(2):126–136.

30. O'Driscall J. Changing the face of emergency medicine. *The Physician Executive.* January–February 2004:12–15.

31. Patel KK, Butler B, Wells KB. What is necessary to transform the quality of mental health care? *Health Affairs.* 2006;25(3):681–693.

32. National Center for Health Statistics. National Nursing Home Survey. 2006. http://www.cdc.gov/nchs/data/nnhsd/nursinghomefacilities2006. Accessed May 22, 2009.

33. National Center for Health Statistics. *Health, United States, 2007, with Chartbook on Trends in the Health of Americans.* Tables 104 and 117. Hyattsville, MD: National Center for Health Statistics; 2007.

34. Robinson JC. Consolidation of medical groups into physician practice management organizations. *Journal of the American Medical Association.* 1998;279(2):144–149.

35. Robinson JC, Casalino LP. Reevaluation of capitation contracting in New York and California. *Health Affairs* (Suppl web exclusives). 2001:W11–9.

36. Bazzoli GJ, Shortell SM, Dubbs N, et al. A taxonomy of health networks and systems: bringing order out of chaos. *Health Services Research.* 1999;33(6):1683–1717.

37. Johnson C. US targets health-care fraud, abuse: new Medicare task force wins 3rd conviction of 2007. *Washington Post.* July 19, 2007:D1.

38. Robinson JC, Casalino LP. Reevaluation of capitation contracting in New York and California. *Health Affairs* (Suppl web exclusives). 2001:W11-9.

CHAPTER SIX

1. Bindman AB, Grumbach K, Osmond D, et al. Preventable hospitalizations and access to health care. *Journal of the American Medical Association.* 1995;274(4):305–311.

2. Wilensky HL. The professionalization of everyone? *American Journal of Sociology.* 1964;70(2):137–158.

3. Freidson E. *Profession of Medicine.* New York: Dodd, Mead; 1975.

4. Edelstein L. *The Hippocratic Oath: Text, Translation, and Interpretation.* Baltimore: Johns Hopkins Press; 1943.

5. Smith RJ. Scope of practice: where things stand. *Podiatry Today.* 2007;20(5):36–44.

6. Michal MH, Pekarske MSL, McManus MK. Corporate practice of medicine doctrine: 50 state survey summary. Madison, WI: Reinhart Boerner Van Deuren; 2006. www.nhpco.org/files/public/palliativecare/corporate-practice-of-medicine-50-state-summary.pdf. Accessed May 22, 2009.

7. Shaw B. *The Doctor's Dilemma, with Preface on Doctors.* New York: Dodd, Mead; 1941.

8. Freidson E. *Profession of Medicine.* New York: Dodd, Mead; 1975.

9. Fuchs VR. *Who Shall Live?* New York: Basic Books; 1983.

10. Gorman J. Take a little deadly nightshade and you'll feel better. *New York Times Magazine.* Aug. 30, 1992:23–28, 73.

11. Parkman CA. A look at naturopathic medicine. *Case Manager.* 2001;12(5):29–31.

12. Meeker WC, Haldeman S. Chiropractic: a profession at the crossroads of mainstream and alternative medicine. *Annals of Internal Medicine.* 2002;136:216–227.

13. Davis RM. Medicare payment reform and balance billing. *AMA eVoice.* May 1, 2008. www.ama-assn.org/ama/pub/category/18533.html. Accessed May 22, 2009.

14. Landon BE, Reschovsky J, Blumenthal D. Changes in career satisfaction among primary care and specialist physicians, 1997–2001. *Journal of the American Medical Association.* 2003;289(4):442–449.

15. Ashley JA. *Hospitals, Paternalism, and the Role of the Nurse.* New York: Teachers College Press; 1976.

16. Freidson E. *Profession of Medicine.* New York: Dodd, Mead; 1975.

17. Gill CJ, Gill G. Nightingale in Scutari: her legacy reexamined. *Clinical Infectious Disease.* 2005;40:1799–1805.

18. Strachey L. *Eminent Victorians.* New York: Penguin; 1986.

19. Malpas P. Florence Nightingale: appreciating our legacy, envisioning our future. *Gerontology Nursing.* 2006;29(6):447–452.

20. Aiken LH, Clarke SP, Sloane DM, et al. Hospital nurse staffing and patient mortality, nurse burnout, and job dissatisfaction. *Journal of the American Medical Association.* 2002;288:1987–1993.

21. US Department of Labor, Bureau of Labor Statistics. Health diagnosing and treating practitioners. 2008. http://www.bls.gov/oco/reprints/ocor008.pdf. Accessed May 22, 2009.

22. O'Brien JM. How nurse practitioners obtained provider status: lessons for pharmacists. *American Journal of Health System Pharmacy.* 2003;60:2301–2307.

23. Goodman GR. The occupation of healthcare management: relating core competencies to growth as a distinct profession. *Journal of Health Administration Education.* 2003;20(3):147–165.

24. Bugbee GA. *Recollections of a Good Life.* Chicago: Hospital Research and Education Trust; 1987.

25. Wilensky HL. The dynamics of professionalism. *Hospital Administration.* 1962;7:6–24.

26. Filerman GA. Andrew Pattullo and "a strategy for building a profession." *Journal of Health Administration Education.* 1997;15(4):99–104.

27. Adelson A. Maxicare Health hires a movie accountant. *New York Times,* Aug. 9, 1988.

28. Evans M. Turning over in their suites: at 15%, hospital CEO turnover has barely wavered in the past five years, and it's expected to stay that way for a while. *Modern Healthcare.* 2007;37(15):6–7, 15.

29. Schneller ES, Greenwald HP, Richardson ML, Ott JA. The physician executive: role in the adaptation of American medicine. *Health Care Management Review.* 1997;22(2): 90–96.

30. Romano M. The doctor is in: to quell physician unrest, some hospitals are dumping lay executives and replacing them with doctors. *Modern Healthcare.* 2002;32 (39):6–7, 12, 1.

31. Hsiao WC, Braun P, Dunn DL, et al. An overview of the development and refinement of the resource-based relative value scale. *Medical Care.* 1992;30:NS1–NS12.

32. Weeks WB, Wallace AE, Wallace MM, Welch HG. A comparison of the educational costs and incomes of physicians and other professionals. *New England Journal of Medicine.* 1994;323:1280–1286.

33. Pearse WH, Haffner WHJ, Primack A. Effects of gender on the obstetric-gynecologic workforce. *Obstetrics and Gynecology.* 2001;97:794–797.

34. Schwartz WB, Mendelson DN. No evidence of an emerging physician surplus. *Journal of the American Medical Association.* 1990;263(4):571–572.

35. Fry WB. Cardiology workforce: a shortage, not a surplus. *Health Affairs.* 2004;W4:64–66.

36. Rubin R. Boomers may see doctor shortage. *USA Today.* Sept. 10, 2008:1A.

37. Auerbach DI, Buerhaus PI, Staiger DO. Better late than never: workforce supply implications of later entry into nursing. *Health Affairs.* 2007;26(1): 178–185.

38. Bach PB, Pham HH, Schrag D, et al. Primary care physicians who treat Blacks and Whites. *New England Journal of Medicine.* 2004;35:575–584.

39. White G. The code of ethics for nurses: responding to new challenges in a new century. *American Journal of Nursing.* 2001;101(10):73–75.

40. American Medical Association. Principles of medical ethics. 2001. http://www.ama-assn.org/ama/pub/category/2512.html. Accessed October 3, 2007.

41. American College of Healthcare Executives. Code of ethics. 2007. http://www.ache.org/ABT_ACHE/code.cfm. Accessed October 3, 2008.

42. Medical Board of California. 2006–2007 Annual Report. Sacramento: California Department of Consumer Affairs; 2007.

43. Knight JR, Sanchez LT, Sherritt L, et al. Outcomes of a monitoring program for physicians with mental and behavioral health problems. *Journal of Psychiatric Practice.* 2007;13(1):25–32.

44. Grant D, Alfred KC. Sanctions and recidivism: an evaluation of physician discipline by state medical boards. *Journal of Health Politics, Policy, and Law.* 2007;32(5):867–885.

45. Anders G. A top physician earns a fortune repairing knees in Vail, Colo. *Wall Street Journal.* April 8, 1993:1.

46. Francis T. HCA chief enjoying the private life. *Wall Street Journal.* January 7, 2008.

47. CEO Compensation. Forbes.com. 2006. http://www.forbes.com/lists/2006/12/AKWH.html. Accessed September 30, 2008.

CHAPTER SEVEN

1. National Center for Health Statistics. *Health, United States, 2007, with Chartbook on Trends in the Health of Americans.* Table 121. Hyattsville, MD: National Center for Health Statistics; 2007.

2. National Center for Health Statistics. *Health, United States, 2007, with Chartbook on Trends in the Health of Americans.* Table 120. Hyattsville, MD: National Center for Health Statistics; 2007.

3. National Center for Health Statistics. *Health, United States, 2007, with Chartbook on Trends in the Health of Americans.* Table 125. Hyattsville, MD: National Center for Health Statistics; 2007.

4. National Center for Health Statistics. *Health, United States, 2007, with Chartbook on Trends in the Health of Americans.* Data table for Figure 6. Hyattsville, MD: National Center for Health Statistics; 2007.

5. Alemayehu B, Warner WE. The lifetime distribution of health care costs. *Health Services Research.* 2004;39(3):627–642.

6. Hogan C, Lunney J, Gable J, et al. Medicare beneficiaries' costs of care in the last year of life. *Health Affairs.* 2001;20(4):188–195.

7. Skinner J, Wennberg JE. Exceptionalism or extravagance? What's different about health care in South Florida? *Health Affairs* (Suppl web exclusives). 2003;W3-372-5.

8. Bodenheimer T. High and rising health care costs—part 1: seeking an explanation. *Annals of Internal Medicine.* 2005;142:842–947.

9. Bodenheimer T. High and rising health care costs—part 2: technologic innovation. *Annals of Internal Medicine.* 2005;142: 932–937.

10. National Center for Health Statistics. *Health, United States, 2007, with Chartbook on Trends in the Health of Americans.* Table 123. Hyattsville, MD: National Center for Health Statistics; 2007.

11. McMahon JA, Drake DF. Inflation and the hospital. In: Zubkoff M, ed. *Health: A Victim or Cause of Inflation?* New York: Milbank Memorial Fund; 1976:130–148.

12. Ham C. Priority setting in health care: learning from international experience. *Health Policy.* 1997;42: 49–66.

13. Carroll RJ, Horn SD, Soderfeldt B, et al. International comparison of waiting times for selected cardiovascular procedures. *Journal of the American College of Cardiology.* 1995;25:557–563.

14. Sobolev BF, Fradet G, Hayden R, et al. Delay in admission for elective coronary-artery bypass grafting is associated with increased in hospital mortality. *BCM Health Services Research.* 2008;(8):185–191.

15. Riley GF. Trends in out-of-pocket healthcare costs among older community dwelling Medicare beneficiaries. *American Journal of Managed Care.* 2008;14(10):692–696.

16. Furman J. Health reform through tax reform: a primer. *Health Affairs.* 2008;27(3):622–632.

17. Wise PH. The transformation of child health in the United States. *Health Affairs.* 2004;23:9–25.

18. Reinhardt UE. Does the aging of the population really drive the demand for health care? *Health Affairs.* 2003;22(6): 27–39.

19. Goldman DP, Smith JP, Sood N. Immigrants and the cost of medical care. *Health Affairs.* 2006;25(6): 1700–1711.

20. Woolhandler S, Campbell T, Himmelstein DU. Costs of health care and administration in the United States and Canada. *New England Journal of Medicine.* 2003;349:768–775.

21. Aaron HJ. The costs of health care administration in the United States and Canada: questionable answers to a questionable question. *New England Journal of Medicine.* 2003;349(8):801–803.

22. Mehr RL, Commack E. *Principles of Insurance.* Homewood, IL: R.D. Irwin; 1980.

23. Fowles JB, Weiner JP, Knutson D, et al. Taking health status into account when setting capitation rates. *Journal of the American Medical Association.* 1996;276:1316–1321.

24. Pauly MV, Blavin FE. Moral hazard in insurance, value-based cost-sharing, and the benefits of blissful ignorance. *Journal of Health Economics.* 2008;27(6):1407–1417.

25. Chase M. Cancer tab: pricey drugs put squeeze on doctors. *Wall Street Journal.* July 8, 2008:A1.

26. Smith PC, Witter SN. *Risk Pooling in Health Care Financing: The Implications for Health System Performance.* Washington, DC: The World Bank; 2004. http://siteresources.worldbank.org/HEALTHNUTRI TIONANDPOPULATION/Resources/281627–1095698140167/Chap9SmithWitterRiskPoolingFinal.pdf. Accessed October 25, 2008.

27. Anderson OW. *Blue Cross since 1929: Accountability and the Public Trust.* Cambridge: Ballinger, 1975.

28. Kaiser Family Foundation and Health Research and Educational Trust. Employer health benefits 2006 annual survey. 2006. http://www.kff.org/insurance/7527/upload/7527.pdf. Accessed October 27, 2008.

29. Rundle RL. Kaiser to offer savings accounts for lower cost health coverage. *Wall Street Journal.* November 15, 2004:B6.

30. Zhang J. To your health: the easy part is opening an HAS account—the hard part is doing it right. *Wall Street Journal.* July 14, 2008:R5.

31. Hall MA, Conover CJ. For-profit conversion of Blue Cross plans: public benefit or public harm? *Annual Review of Public Health.* 2006;27:443–463.

32. Ginzberg E. Improving health care for the poor: lessons from the 1980s. *Journal of the American Medical Association.* 1994;271:464–467.

33. Mathews AW. Medicare battle looms as costs keep climbing. *Wall Street Journal.* October 30, 2008.

34. Actuarial Standards Board. Actuarial Standard of Practice No. 32: Social Insurance. Washington, DC: American Academy of Actuaries; 1998.

35. Riley GF, Warren JL, Potosky AL, et al. Comparison of cancer diagnosis and treatment in Medicare fee-for-service and managed care plans. *Medical Care.* 2008;46(10):1108–1115.

36. Haberer JE, Garrett B, Baker LC. Does Medicaid managed care affect access to care for the uninsured? *Health Affairs.* 2005;24(4):1095–1105.

37. Landon BE, Schneider EC, Normand SL, et al. Quality of care in Medicaid managed care and commercial health plans. *Journal of the American Medical Association.* 2007;298(14):1674–1681.

38. Goldman DP, Joyce GF. Medicare Part D: a successful start with room for improvement. *Journal of the American Medical Association.* 2008;299(16):1954–1955.

39. Social Security Administration. Medicare part B premiums: new rules for beneficiaries with higher incomes. SSA Publication No. 05–10161. 2007. www.socialsecurity.gov/mediinfo.htm. Accessed October 30, 2008.

40. Browne A. Chinese doctors tell patients to pay upfront, or no treatment. *Wall Street Journal.* Dec. 5, 2005:1.

41. National Center for Health Statistics. *Health, United States, 2007, with Chartbook on Trends in the Health of Americans.* Tables 28, 29. Hyattsville, MD: National Center for Health Statistics; 2007.

42. Steinhauer J. No medical insurance means tough and creative choices. *New York Times.* March 2, 1999:1.

43. Soltis C. Uninsured grads risk finances, future coverage. *Wall Street Journal.* August 7, 2007:B6.

44. Anderson GF. From "soak the rich" to "soak the poor": recent trends in hospital pricing. *Health Affairs.* 2007:26(3):780–789.

45. Fuchs VR. National health insurance revisited. *Health Affairs.* 1991;10(4):7–17.

46. Employee Benefit Research Institute. Estimates of the Current Population Survey. March 2002, 2003, and 2004 supplements.

47. Greenwald HP, O'Keefe S, DiCamillo M. Why employed Latinos lack health insurance: a study in California. *Hispanic Journal of Behavioral Sciences.* 2005;27:517–532.

48. Martinez B. Cash before chemo: hospitals get tough. *Wall Street Journal.* April 28, 2008:A1.

49. Martinez B. Healthy funding at M.D. Anderson. *Wall Street Journal.* April 28, 2008:A15.

CHAPTER EIGHT

1. Pasteur L et al. Summary report of the experiments conducted at Pouilly-le-Fort, near Melun, on the anthrax vaccination. *Yale Journal of Biology and Medicine.* 2002;75:59–62. (Originally published in *Comptes Rendus de l'Academie des Science.* 1881;92:1378–1383.)

2. Lewis S. *Arrowsmith.* New York: Grosset & Dunlap; 1925.

3. Rickels K, Zaninelli R, McCaffery J, et al. Paroxetine treatment of generalized anxiety disorder: a double-blind, placebo controlled study. *American Journal of Psychiatry.* 2003;160:749–756.

4. Sulheim S, Holme I, Ekeland A, Bahr R. Helmet use and risk of head injury in Alpine skiers and snowboarders. *Journal of the American Medical Association.* 2006;295:919–924.

5. Cutler DM. Declining disability among the elderly. *Health Affairs.* 2001;20(6):11–27.

6. Yin RK. *Case Study Research.* Thousand Oaks, CA: Sage; 2003.

7. Davis BT, Pasternack MD. Case 19-2007: a 19-year-old college student with fever and joint pain. *New England Journal of Medicine.* 2007;356:2631–2637.

8. U.S. Department of Health and Human Services. Congressionally mandated evaluation of the state children's health insurance program: final report to Congress. Contract no. HHS-100-01-0002; MPR Reference no. 8782-130. 2005. http://www.urban.org/UploadedPDF/411249_SCHIP.pdf. Accessed December 3, 2007.

9. Patrick DL, Grembowski D, Durham M, et al. Cost and outcomes of Medicare reimbursement for HMO preventive services. *Health Care Finance Review.* 1999;20(4):25–43.

10. Greenwald HP, Beery WL, Pearson D, et al. Polling and policy analysis as resources for advocacy. *Journal of Public Administration Research and Theory.* 2003;13:117–191.

11. Campbell DT, Stanley JC. *Experimental and Quasi-Experimental Designs for Research.* Boston: Houghton Mifflin; 1963:2.

12. Feldman AC, Smith DH, Perrin N, et al. Reducing warfarin medication interactions: an interrupted time series evaluation. *Archives of Internal Medicine.* 2006;166:1009–1015.

13. Fetterman DM, Wandersman A (eds.). *Empowerment Evaluation Principles in Practice.* New York: Guilford Press; 2005.

14. Garrison LP, Lubeck D, Lalla D, et al. Cost-effectiveness analysis of trastuzumab in the adjuvant setting for treatment of HER2-positive breast cancer. *Cancer.* 2007;110(3):489–498.

15. Konski A, Speier W, Hanlon A, et al. Is proton beam therapy cost-effective in the treatment of adenocarcinoma of the prostate? *Journal of Clinical Oncology.* 2007;25(24):3603–3608.

16. Stanford University Office of Research Administration. http://ora.stanford.edu/notes/default.asp. Accessed December 7, 2007.

17. Moses H, Dorsey, Matheson, Thier SO. Financial anatomy of biomedical research. *Journal of the American Medical Association.* 2005;294(11):1333–1342.

18. Moertel CG, Fleming TR, Creagan ET, et al. High-dose vitamin C versus placebo in the treatment of patients with advanced cancer who have had no prior chemotherapy: A randomized double-blind comparison. *New England Journal of Medicine.* 1985;312:137–141.

19. Moertel CG, Fleming TR, Rubin J. A clinical trial of amygdalin (Laetrile) in the treatment of human cancer. *New England Journal of Medicine.* 1982;306:201–206.

20. Brown S. The history of breast cancer advocacy. *The Breast Journal.* 2003;9(Suppl. 2):S101–S103.

21. Deyo RA, Psaty BM, Simon G, et al. The messenger under attack: intimidation of researchers by special-interest groups. *New England Journal of Medicine.* 1997;336(16):1176–1180.

22. The a-Tocopherol, h Carotene Cancer Prevention Study Group. The effect of vitamin E and h carotene on the incidence of lung cancer and other cancers in male smokers. *New England Journal of Medicine.* 1994;330:1029–1035.

23. Gray J, Mao JT, Szabo E, et al. Lung cancer chemoprevention. *Chest.* 2007;132:56S–68S.

24. Peterson AV, Kealey KA, Mann S, et al. Hutchinson smoking prevention project: long-term randomized trial in school-based tobacco use prevention—results on smoking. *Journal of the National Cancer Institute.* 2000;92:1979–1991.

25. Ioannidis JPA. Why most published research findings are false. *PLoS Medicine.* 2(8):696–701.

26. Ioannidis JPA. 2005. Contradicted and initially stronger effects in highly cited clinical research. *Journal of the American Medical Association.* 2005;294:218–228.

27. King RT. Biotechnology: the tale of a dream, a drug and data dredging. *Wall Street Journal* (Eastern edition). Feb 7, 1995:B1.

28. Joyce FS. Medical school undergoing inquiry on false data. *New York Times.* May 27, 1983:12.

CHAPTER NINE

1. Montori VM, Guyatt GH. Progress in evidence-based medicine. *Journal of the American Medical Association.* 2008;300(15):1814–1816.

2. Shaman H. What you need to know about pay for performance. *Healthcare Financial Management.* October 2008:92–96.

3. Centers for Medicare and Medicaid Services. Hospital quality initiative overview. 2008. www.cms.hhs.gov/hospitalqualityinits. Accessed December 30, 2008.

4. Felt-Lisk S, Barrett A, Nyman R. Public reporting of quality information on Medicaid health plans. *Health Care Financing Review.* 2007;28(2): 5–16.

5. Chernew ME, Rosen AB, Fendrick AM. Value-based insurance design. *Health Affairs.* 2007;26(2): W195–W203.

6. Donabedian A. Evaluating the quality of medical care. *Milbank Quarterly.* 1966;44(3), Part 2:166–203.

7. Neuhauser D. Ernest Amory Codman, MD. *Quality and Safety in Health Care.* 2002;11:104–105.

8. Newhouse JP, Manning WG, Morris CN, et al. Some interim results from a controlled trial of cost sharing in health insurance. *New England Journal of Medicine.* 1981;305(25):1501–1507.

9. Bindman AB, Grumbach K, Osmond D, et al. Preventable hospitalizations and access to health care. *Journal of the American Medical Association.* 1995;274(4): 305–311.

10. Brook RH, Caren JK, Lohr KN, et al. Quality of ambulatory care: epidemiology and comparison by insurance status and income. *Medical Care.* 1990;28(5):329–433.

11. Wells KB, Manning WG Jr, Duan N, et al. Cost-sharing and the use of general medical physicians for outpatient mental health care. *Health Services Research.* 1987;22(1):1–17.

12. Zwanziger J, Melnick GA, Bamezai A. The effect of selective contractive contracting on hospital costs and revenues. *Health Services Research.* 2000;35(4):849–867.

13. Mukamel DB, Zwanziger J, Bamezai A. Hospital competition, resource allocation, and quality of care. *BMC Health Services Research.* 2002;2(1):10–19.

14. Trinh HQ, Begun JW, Luke RD. Hospital service duplication: evidence on the medical arms race. *Health Care Management Review.* 2008;33(3):192–202.

15. Konetzka RT, Sochalski J, Volpp KG. Managed care and hospital cost containment. *Inquiry.* 2008;54(1): 98–111.

16. Newhouse JP. *Free for All: Lessons from the Rand Health Insurance Experiment.* Cambridge: Harvard; 1993.

17. Dixon A, Greene J, Hibbard J. Do consumer-directed health plans drive change in enrollees' health care behavior? *Health Affairs.* 2008;27(4):1120–1131.

18. Rowe JW, Brown-Stevenson T, Downey RL, et al. The effect of consumer-directed health plans on the use of preventive and chronic illness services. *Health Affairs.* 2008;27(1):113–120.

19. Brook RH, Ware JE Jr, Rogers WH, et al. Does free care improve adults' health? Results from a randomized controlled trial. *New England Journal of Medicine.* 1983;309(23):1426–1434.

20. Greenwald HP. HMO membership, copayment, and initiation of care for cancer: a study of working adults. *American Journal of Public Health.* 1987;77:461–466.

21. Hsu J, Price M, Huang J, et al. Unintended consequences of caps on Medicare drug benefits. *New England Journal of Medicine.* 2006;354(22):2385–2386.

22. Trivedi AN, Rakowski W, Ayanian JZ. Effect of cost sharing on screening mammography in Medicare health plans. *New England Journal of Medicine.* 2008;358(4):375–383.

23. Chandra A, Gruber J, McKnight R. *Patient Cost-Sharing, Hospitalization Offsets, and the Design of Optimal Health Insurance for the Elderly.* Working paper W12972. Cambridge, MA: National Bureau of Economic Research; 2007.

24. Manning WG, Leibowitz A, Goldberg GA, et al. A controlled trial of a prepaid group practice on use of services. *New England Journal of Medicine.* 1984;310(23):1505–1510.

25. Feldman R, Dowd B, Gifford G. The effect of HMOs on premiums in employment-based health plans. *Health Services Research.* 1993;27(6):779–811.

26. Sullivan K. On the "efficiency" of managed care plans. *Health Affairs.* 2000;19(4):139–148.

27. Ware JE, Brook RH, Rogers WH, et al. Comparison of health outcomes at a health maintenance organization with those of fee-for-service care. *Lancet.* 1986;1(8488):1017–1022.

28. Baker LC, Afendulis C. Medicaid managed care and health care for children. *Health Services Research.* 2005;40:1466–1488.

29. Greenwald HP, Henke CJ. HMO membership, treatment, and mortality risk among prostatic cancer patients. *American Journal of Public Health.* 1992;82(8):1099–1104.

30. Guadagnoli E, Landrum MB, Peterson EA, et al. Appropriateness of coronary angiography after myocardial infarction among Medicare beneficiaries. *New England Journal of Medicine.* 2000;343:1460–1466.

31. Ferris TG, Blumenthal D, Woodruff PG, et al. Insurance and quality of care for asthma. *Journal of General Internal Medicine.* 2002;17:905–913.

32. Baker LC, Afendulis C. Medicaid managed care and health care for children. *Health Services Research.* 2005;40:1466–1488.

33. Greenwald HP, Henke CJ. HMO membership, treatment, and mortality risk among prostatic cancer patients. *American Journal of Public Health.* 1992;82(8):1099–1104.

34. Guadagnoli E, Landrum MB, Peterson EA, et al. Appropriateness of coronary angiography after myocardial infarction among Medicare beneficiaries. *New England Journal of Medicine.* 2000;343:1460–1466.

35. Ferris TG, Blumenthal D, Woodruff PG, et al. Insurance and quality of care for asthma. *Journal of General Internal Medicine.* 2002;17:905 913.

36. Feldman PH, Murtaugh CM, Pezzin LE, et al. Just-in-time evidenced-based e-mail "reminders" in home health care: impact on patient outcomes. *Health Services Research.* 2005;40(3):865–885.

37. Fischer MA, Avorn J. Economic implications of evidence-based prescribing for hypertension: can better care cost less? *Journal of the American Medical Association.* 2004;291(15):1850–1856.

38. Glickman SW, Ou FS, DeLong EB, et al. Pay for performance, quality of care, and outcomes in acute myocardial infarction. *Journal of the American Medical Association.* 2008;297:2373–2380.

39. Shaman H. What you need to know about pay for performance. *Healthcare Financial Management.* October 2008:92–96.

40. Vonnegut M. Is quality improvement improving quality? A view from the doctor's office. *New England Journal of Medicine.* 2007;357:2652–2653.

41. Landro L. What's new (or improved) in health sites. *Wall Street Journal.* January 7, 2009:D1.

42. Ferris TG, Blumenthal D, Woodruff PG, et al. Insurance and quality of care for asthma. *Journal of General Internal Medicine.* 2002;17:905–913.

43. Pronovost PJ, Miller M, Wachter RM. The GAAP in quality measurement and reporting. *Journal of the American Medical Association.* 2007;298(15):1800–1802.

44. Farber M, Bosch M, Wollersheim H, et al. Public reporting in health care: how do consumers use quality-of-care information? A systematic review. *Medical Care.* 2009;47(1):1–8.

45. Goldman DP, Leibowitz AA, Robalino DA. Employee responses to health insurance premium increases. *American Journal of Managed Care.* 2004;10(1):41–47.

46. Hibbard JH, Slovic P, Peters E, et al. Is the informed choice policy approach appropriate for Medicare beneficiaries? *Health Affairs.* 2001;20:199–203.

47. McWilliams JM, Zaslavsky AM, Meara E, Ayanian JZ. Health insurance coverage and mortality among the near-elderly. *Health Affairs.* 2004;23:223–232.

CHAPTER TEN

1. Thucydides. *The History of the Peloponnesian War.* New York: Dutton; 1950.

2. Marcus MB. Ginkgo doesn't block Alzheimer's. *USA Today.* November 19, 2008:1.

3. Cilliers L, Retief FP. Medical practice in Graeco-roman antiquity. *Curationis.* 2006;(2):34–40.

4. Brody SN. *The Disease of the Soul: Leprosy in Medieval Literature.* Ithaca: Cornell University Press; 1974.

5. Horton R. Infection: the global threat. *New York Review of Books.* 1995:42(6).

6. Schafer D. Aging, longevity, and diet: historical remarks on calorie intake reduction. *Gerontology.* 2005;51(2):126–130.

7. Selikoff IJ, Churg J, and Hammond EC. Asbestos exposure and neoplasia. *Journal of the American Medical Association.* 1964;188:142–146.

8. McCain JA. Making access to quality and affordable health care a reality for every American. *Journal of the American Medical Association.* 2008;300(16):1925–1926.

9. Obama B. Affordable health care for all Americans: the Obama-Biden plan. *Journal of the American Medical Association.* 2008;300(16):1927–1928.

10. Woolf SH. The power of prevention and what it requires. *Journal of the American Medical Association.* 2008;299(20):2437–2439.

11. McGinnis JM, Foege WH. Actual causes of death in the United States. *Journal of the American Medical Association.* 1993;270(18):2207–2212.

12. Bryce J, Daelmans B, Dwivedi A, et al. Countdown to 2015 for maternal, newborn, and child survival: the 2008 report on tracking coverage of interventions. *Lancet.* 2008;371(9620):1247–1258.

13. Child vaccinations reach goal. *Wall Street Journal.* July 27, 2005:D5.

14. Broder KR, Cortese MM, Iskander JK, et al. Preventing tetanus, diphtheria, and pertussis among adolescents. *Morbidity and Mortality Weekly Review.* 2006;55(RR03):1–34.

15. Voordouw AC, Sturkenboom MC, Dieleman JP, et al. Annual revaccination against influenza and mortality risk in community-dwelling elderly persons. *Journal of the American Medical Association.* 2004;292(17):2089–2095.

16. Pignone M, Rich M, Teutsch SM, et al. Screening for colorectal cancer in adults at average risk: a summary of the evidence for the US preventive services task force. *Annals of Internal Medicine.* 2002;137:132–141.

17. Mandel JS, Bond JH, Church TR, et al. Reducing mortality from colorectal cancer by screening for fetal occult blood. *New England Journal of Medicine.* 1993;328:1365–1371.

18. Rollins G. Developments in cervical and ovarian cancer screening: implications for current practice. *Annals of Internal Medicine.* 2000;133(12):1021–1024.

19. U.S. Preventive Services Task Force. *The Guide to Clinical Preventive Services 2008: Recommendations of the U.S. Preventive Services Task Force.* Washington, DC: Agency for Healthcare Research and Quality; 2008.

20. Whiteman DC, Green AC. Melanoma and sun exposure: where are we now? *International Journal of Dermatology.* 1999;38:481–489.

21. Beyrer C. HIV epidemiology update and transmission factors: risks and risk contexts—16th International AIDS Conference Epidemiology Plenary. *Clinical Infectious Diseases.* 2007;44:981–987.

22. Kannel WB. Some lessons in cardiovascular epidemiology from Framingham. *American Journal of Cardiology.* 1976;37(2):269–282.

23. Wilson WF, D'Agostino RB, Levy D, et al. Prediction of coronary heart disease using risk factor categories. *Circulation.* 1998;97:1837–1847.

24. Kannel WB. Some lessons in cardiovascular epidemiology from Framingham. *American Journal of Cardiology.* 1976;37(2):269–282.

25. Paffenbarger RS Jr, Hyde RT, Wing AL, et al. The association of changes in physical-activity level and other lifestyle characteristics with mortality among men. *New England Journal of Medicine.* 1993;328:538–545.

26. Lee IM, Sesso HD, Oguma Y, Paffenbarger RS Jr. The "weekend warrior" and risk of mortality. *American Journal of Epidemiology.* 2004;160(7):636–641.

27. Stampfer MJ, Hu FB, Manson, et al. Primary prevention of coronary heart disease in women through diet and lifestyle. *New England Journal of Medicine.* 2000;43:16–22.

28. Mozaffarian D, Katan MB, Ascherio A, Stampfer MJ, Willett WC. Trans fatty acids and cardiovascular disease. *New England Journal of Medicine.* 2006;354(15):1601–1613.

29. Hu FB, Willett WC. Optimal diets for prevention of coronary heart disease. *Journal of the American Medical Association.* 2002;288(20):2569–2578.

30. Miyagi S, Iwama N, Kawabata T, et al. Longevity and diet in Okinawa, Japan: the past, present, and future. *Asia Pacific Journal of Public Health.* 2003;15(Suppl.):S3–S9.

31. Kris-Etherton PM, Harris WS, Appel LJ, et al. Fish consumption, fish oil, omega-3 fatty acids, and cardio-vascular disease. *Circulation.* 2002;106:2747–2757.

32. Wingard DL, Berkman LF, Brand RJ. A multivariate analysis of health-related practices. *American Journal of Epidemiology.* 1982;116(5):765–775.

33. Berkman LF, Syme SL. Social networks, host resistance and mortality: A nine-year follow-up study of Alameda County residents. *American Journal of Epidemiology.* 1979;109:186–204.

34. Haan M, Kaplan GA, Camacho T. Poverty and health: prospective evidence from the Alameda County Study. *American Journal of Epidemiology.* 1987;125:989–998.

35. Yen IH, Kaplan GA. Poverty area residence and changes in physical activity level: evidence from the Alameda County Study. *American Journal of Public Health.* 1998;88(11):1709–1712.

36. Doll R, Peto R. The causes of cancer: quantitative estimates of avoidable risks of cancer in the United States today. *Journal of the National Cancer Institute.* 1981;66(6):1196–1308.

37. Prentice RI, Caan B, Chlebowski RT, et al. Low-fat dietary pattern and risk of invasive breast cancer: the Women's Health Initiative Randomized Controlled Dietary Modification Trial. *Journal of the American Medical Association.* 2006;295(6):629–642.

38. Koushik A, Hunter DJ, Spiegelman D, et al. Fruits, vegetables, and colon cancer risk in a pooled analysis of 14 cohort studies. *Journal of the National Cancer Institute.* 2007;99(19):1471–1483.

39. Maruti SS, Willett WC, Feskanich D, et al. A prospective study of age-specific physical activity and pre-menopausal breast cancer. *Journal of the National Cancer Institute.* 2008;100(10):728–737.

40. Bodenheimer T, Wagner EH, Grumbach K. Improving primary care for patients with chronic illness. *Journal of the American Medical Association.* 2002;288(14):1775–1779.

41. The Meth Project. What is the Meth Project? 2008. http://www.methproject.org/About_Us/index.php. Accessed November 25, 2008.

42. Evans RI, Rozelle RM, Mittelmark M, et al. Deterring the onset of smoking among children: knowledge of immediate psychological effects and coping with peer pressure, media pressure, and parents modeling. *Journal of Applied Social Psychology.* 1978;8:126–135.

43. Schinke SP, Gilchrist LD. Preventing substance abuse with children and adolescents. *American Journal of Public Health.* 1985;75:665–667.

44. McAfee TA. Quitlines: a tool for research and dissemination of evidence-based cessation practices. *American Journal of Preventive Medicine.* 2007;33(6Suppl.).S357–S367.

45. Greenwald HP, Beery WL. *Health for All: Making Community Collaboration Work.* Chicago: Health Administration Press; 2002.

46. Frieden TR, Bassett MT, Thorpe LE, Farley TA. Public health in New York City, 2002–2007: confronting epidemics of the modern era. *International Journal of Epidemiology.* 2008;37(5):966–977.

47. Foundation for a Healthy Kentucky. General Support for Health Advocacy Grantees. 2007. http://www.healthyky.org. Accessed November 27, 2008.

48. Greenwald HP, Beery WL, Pearson D, et al. Polling and policy analysis as resources for advocacy. *Journal of Public Administration Research and Theory.* 2003;13:117–191.

49. Alpha-Tocopherol Beta Carotene Cancer Prevention Study Group. The effect of vitamin E and beta carotene on the incidence of lung cancer and other cancers in male smokers. *New England Journal of Medicine.* 1994;330:1029–1035.

50. Peterson AV, Kealey KA, Mann SL, et al. Hutchinson smoking prevention project: Long-term randomized trial in school-based tobacco use prevention—results on smoking. *Journal of the National Cancer Institute.* 2000;92:1979–1991.

51. Farquhar JW, Fortmann SP, Flora JA, et al. Effects of communitywide education on cardiovascular disease risk factors: the Stanford Five City Project. *Journal of the American Medical Association.* 1990;264: 359–365.

52. Puska P, Nissinen A, Toumilehto J, et al. The community-based strategy to prevent coronary heart disease: conclusions from the ten years of the North Karelia Project. *Preventive Medicine.* 1986;15:176–191.

53. Wagner EE, Koepsell TD, Anderman C, et al. The evaluation of the Henry J. Kaiser Family Foundation's Community Health Promotion Grant Program: design. *Journal of Clinical Epidemiology.* 1990;44(7): 685–699.

54. Wagner EH, Wickizer TM, Cheadle A, et al. The Henry J. Kaiser Family Foundation's health promotion grant program: findings from an outcome evaluation. *Health Services Research.* 2002;35(3):561–589.

55. Park Y, Hunter DJ, Spiegelman D, et al. Dietary fiber intake and risk of colorectal cancer. *Journal of the American Medical Association.* 2005;294:2849–2857.

56. Koushik A, Hunter DJ, Spiegelman D, et al. Fruits, vegetables, and colon cancer risk in a pooled analysis of 14 cohort studies. *Journal of the National Cancer Institute.* 2007;99(19):1471–1483.

57. Gotzsche PC, Olsen O. Is screening for breast cancer with mammography justifiable? *Lancet.* 2005;355: 129–134.

58. Gotzsche PC, Nielson M. Screening for breast cancer with mammography. *Cochrane Database Systematic Reviews.* 2006;4:CD001877.

59. Prentice R, Anderson GL. The Women's Health Initiative: lessons learned. *Annual Review of Public Health.* 2007;29:131–150.

60. Gillman MW, Cupples LA, Millen BE, et al. Inverse association of dietary fat with development of ischemic stroke in men. *Journal of the American Medical Association.* 1997;278:2145–2150.

61. Dorgan JF, Brown C, Barrett M, et al. Physical activity and risk of breast cancer in the Framingham Heart Study. *American Journal of Epidemiology.* 1994;139:662–669.

62. Patrick, DL, Grembowski D, Durham M, et al. Cost and outcomes of Medicare reimbursement for HMO preventive services. *Health Care Financing Review.* 1999;20(4):25–43.

63. Charlier M. In the name of fitness many Americans grow addicted to exercise. *Wall Street Journal.* October 1, 1987:1.

64. Zinser L, Schmidt MS. Ready to race, reminded of risks. *New York Times.* November 4, 2007:1.

65. Schlesinger JM. Second-hand smoke study ruled invalid. *Wall Street Journal.* July 20, 1998.

66. Marantz PR, Bird ED, Alderman MH. A call for higher standards of evidence for dietary guidelines. *American Journal of Preventive Medicine.* 2008;34(3):234–240.

67. Koushik A, Hunter DJ, Spiegelman D, et al. Fruits, vegetables, and colon cancer risk in a pooled analysis of 14 cohort studies. *Journal of the National Cancer Institute.* 2007;99(19):1471–1483.

68. Pignone MP, Ammerman A, Fernandez L, et al. Counseling to promote a healthy diet in adults: a summary of evidence for the U.S. Preventive Services Task Force. *American Journal of Preventive Medicine.* 2003;24(1):75–92.

69. Orleans TC, Schoenbach VJ, Wagner EH, et al. Self-help quit smoking interventions: effects of self-help materials, social support instructions, and telephone counseling. *Journal of Consulting and Clinical Psychology.* 1991;59(3):439–448.

70. Pierce JP, Gilpin EA, Emery SL, et al. Has the California tobacco control program reduced smoking? *Journal of the American Medical Association.* 1998;280:893–899.

71. Fernandes MM. The effect of soft drink availability in elementary schools on consumption. *Journal of the American Dietetic Association.* 2008;108(9):1445–1452.

72. Freedman AM. Amid ghetto hunger, many more suffer eating wrong foods. *Wall Street Journal.* December 18, 1990:A1.

73. Greenwald HP. Getting the most out of health promotion. *Business and Health.* 1987;4(11):40–42.

74. Taira DA, Safran DG, Seto TB, et al. The relationship between patient's income and physician discussion of health risk behaviors. *Journal of the American Medical Association.* 1997;278(17):1412–1417.

75. Relman AS. Encouraging the practice of preventive medicine and health promotion. *Public Health Reports.* 1982;97(3):216–219.

76. Russell LB. *Is Prevention Better Than Cure?* Washington, DC: Brookings; 1986.

77. Casey CG, Iskander JK, Roper MH, et al. Adverse events associated with smallpox vaccination in the United States. *Journal of the American Medical Association.* 2005;294(21):2734–2743.

78. Mandelblatt JS, Lawrence WF, Womack SM, et al. Benefits and costs of using HPV testing to screen for cervical cancer. *Journal of the American Medical Association.* 2002;287(18):2372–2381.

79. Mansnerus L. Making a case for death. *New York Times.* May 5, 1996.

80. Rosenthal E. When healthier isn't cheaper. *New York Times.* March 16, 1997:4.

CHAPTER ELEVEN

1. Fuchs V. *Who Shall Live? Health, Economics, and Social Choice.* New York: Basic Books; 1974.

2. Guttmacher Institute. State funding of abortion under Medicaid. 2008. http://www.guttmacher.org/statecenter/spibs/spib_SFAM.pdf. Accessed March 24, 2008.

3. Borger C, Smith S, Truffer, et al. Health spending projections through 2015: changes on the horizon. *Health Affairs.* 2005;25:w61–w73.

4. McKnight R. Medicare balance billing restrictions: impacts on physicians and beneficiaries. *Journal of Health Economics.* 2007;26(2):326–341.

5. Begun JW, Crowe EW, Feldman R. Occupational regulation in the states: a causal model. *Journal of Health Politics, Policy, and Law.* 1981;6(2):229–254.

6. Weinstock R, Vari G, Leong BG, Silva JA. Back to the past in California: a temporary retreat to a Tarasoff duty to warn. *Journal of the American Academy of Psychiatry and the Law.* 2006;34:523–528.

7. U.S. Department of Health and Human Services. Centers for Medicare & Medicaid Services 42 CFR Part 483 [CMS–3121–F] RIN 0938–AM55 Medicare and Medicaid Programs; Requirements for Long Term Care Facilities; Nursing Services; Posting of Nurse Staffing Information Federal Register Vol. 70, No. 208. October 28, 2005: 62065–62073.

8. George Bugbee: a first-person profile (Part 2). *Health Services Research.* 1981;16(4):459–466.

9. Butler P. ERISA implications for state "pay or play" employer-based coverage. Supplement D to the report— challenges and alternatives for employer pay-or-play program design: an implementation and alternative scenario analysis of California's "Health Insurance Act of 2003" (SB 2). Washington, DC: Institute for Health Policy Solutions; 2005.

10. Drinkard J. In Congress, "we simply have too much power." *USA Today.* January 9, 2006.

11. Beery WL, Greenwald HP, Marzotto T. *The Designation of Rural Areas in California.* Los Angeles: The California Endowment; 2006.

12. Braun S. The history of breast cancer advocacy. *The Breast Journal.* 2003;9(Suppl. 2):S101–S103.

13. Carpenter DP. The political economy of FDA drug review: processing, politics, and lessons for policy. *Health Affairs.* 2004;27:52–63.

14. Brown LD. *Politics and Health Care Organization: HMOs as Federal Policy.* Washington, DC: Brookings; 1983.

15. Bergthold L. Crabs in a bucket: the politics of health care reform in California. *Journal of Health Politics, Policy, and Law.* 1984;9(2):203–222.

16. Johnson H, Broder D. *The System: The American Way of Politics at the Breaking Point.* Boston: Back Bay; 1997.

17. Ludlam JE. *Health Policy—the Hard Way: An Anecdotal Personal History by One of the California Players.* Pasadena, CA: Hope; 1998.

18. Kolko G. *The Triumph of Conservatism.* New York: Free Press; 1977.

CHAPTER TWELVE

1. Rich S. 1989. Hill decisions due on Medicare surtax: "catastrophic" health plan faces major benefit cuts, possible repeal. *Washington Post.* October 1, pg. A20.

2. Balz D. 1989. A display of "gray power" in politics: elderly vocal, active in opposition to catastrophic care bill. *Washington Post.* September 17, pg. A8.

3. Sidel VW. Feldshers and "feldsherism": the role and training of the feldsher in the USSR. *New England Journal of Medicine.* 1968;278:934–940, 981–992.

4. Horn JS. *Away with All Pests: An English Surgeon in People's China: 1954–1969.* New York: Monthly Review Press; 1969.

5. Glaser WA. How expenditure caps and expenditure targets really work. *Milbank Quarterly.* 1993; 71(1):97–127.

6. Hanratty B, Zhang T, Whitehead M. How close have universal health systems come to achieving equity in use of curative services? A systematic review. *International Journal of Health Services.* 2007; 37(1):89–109.

7. Pilote L, Saynina O, Lavoie F, et al. Cardiac procedure use and outcomes in elderly patients with acute myocardial infarction in the United States and Quebec, Canada, 1988 to 1994. *Medical Care.* 2003;41(7):813–822.

8. Gatta G, Capocaccia R, Coleman MP, et al. Toward a comparison of survival in American and European cancer patients. *Cancer.* 2000;89(4):893–900.

9. Black D. *Inequalities in Health: The Black Report.* Harmondsworth, Eng.: Penguin; 1982.

10. Esmail N. Imagine: a universal health system without waiting lists. *National Post.* Oct. 17, 2007:A18.

11. O'Neill JE, O'Neill DM. Health status, health care, and inequality: Canada vs. the US. *Forum for Health Economics and Policy.* 2008;10(1): Article 3.

12. Steinbrook R. Private health care in Canada. *New England Journal of Medicine.* 2006;354(16):1661–1664.

13. Wallace J. Our ailing medical system: 69% of voters believe health care has not improved under McGuinty government. *Toronto Sun.* September 17, 2007:5.

14. Iglehart JK. Health care reform: the states. *New England Journal of Medicine.* 1994;330:75–79.

15. Long SK, Masi PB. Access and affordability: an update on health reform in Massachusetts, fall 2008. *Health Affairs.* 2009;28(4):W578-W587.

16. Medicare Early Access Act of 2005, HR 2072, 109th Cong, 1st Sess (2005). http://frwebgate.access.gpo.gov/cgi-bin/getdoc.cgi?dbname=109_cong_bills&docid=f:h2072ih.txt.pdf. Accessed October 19, 2007.

17 McWilliams M, Meara E, Zaslavsky AM et al. 2007. Health of previously uninsured adults after acquiring medicare coverage. *Journal of the American Medical Association;* 298(24):2886–2894. J. Michael McWilliams; Ellen Meara; Alan M. Zaslavsky; et al.

18. Knowlton B, Sack K, Pear R. 2009. Obama making push on health as GOP steps up criticism. *New York Times.* July 21.

19. *New York Times.* 2009. A public health plan. June 21, Sec. 4, pg. 7.

20. Adamy J, Mackler L. 2009. Small business faces bug bite: House health bill penalizes all but tiniest employers for not providing insurance. *Wall Street Journal.* July 15.

21. Connolly C. 2009. Like car insurance, health coverage may be mandated. a proposed requirement that all Americans have policies has broad support among reformers. *Washington Post.* July 22.

22. Sessions SY, Lee PR. 2008. Using tax reform to drive health care reform. *Journal of the American Medical Association.* 300 (16): 1929–1931.

23. Groopman J, Hartzband P. 2009. Why "quality" care is dangerous. *Wall Street Journal.* April 8, pg. 13.

24. Dluhy RG, MvMahon GT. 2008. Intensive glycemic control in the ACCORD and ADVANCE trials. *New England Journal of Medicine.* 358(24):2630–3.

25. Glickman SW, Ou FS, DeLong ER, et al. 2007. Pay for performance, quality of care, and outcomes in acute myocardial infarction. *Journal of the American Medical Association.* 297 (21): 2373–80.

INDEX

Page references followed by *fig* indicate an illustrated figure; followed by *t* indicate a table, followed by *p* indicates a photograph.